COMMUNICATION
from the INSIDE OUT
STRATEGIES FOR THE ENGAGED PROFESSIONAL

D1410846

COMMUNICATION
from the INSIDE OUT
STRATEGIES FOR THE ENGAGED PROFESSIONAL

Karen Mueller, PT, PhD

Professor
Program in Physical Therapy
Northern Arizona University
Flagstaff, AZ

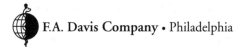 F.A. Davis Company • Philadelphia

F. A. Davis Company
1915 Arch Street
Philadelphia, PA 19103
www.fadavis.com

Printed in the United States of America

Last digit indicates print number: 10 9 8 7 6 5 4 3 2 1

Publisher: Margaret M. Biblis
Acquisitions Editor: Melissa A. Duffield
Manager of Content Development: George W. Lang
Developmental Editor: Jill Rembetski
Art and Design Manager: Carolyn O'Brien

As new scientific information becomes available through basic and clinical research, recommended treatments and drug therapies undergo changes. The author(s) and publisher have done everything possible to make this book accurate, up to date, and in accord with accepted standards at the time of publication. The author(s), editors, and publisher are not responsible for errors or omissions or for consequences from application of the book, and make no warranty, expressed or implied, in regard to the contents of the book. Any practice described in this book should be applied by the reader in accordance with professional standards of care used in regard to the unique circumstances that may apply in each situation. The reader is advised always to check product information (package inserts) for changes and new information regarding dose and contraindications before administering any drug. Caution is especially urged when using new or infrequently ordered drugs.

Library of Congress Cataloging-in-Publication Data

Mueller, Karen (Mary Karen)
  Communication from the inside out : strategies for the engaged professional/Karen Mueller.
      p. ; cm.
  Includes bibliographical references and index.
  ISBN 978-0-8036-1877-0
  1. Physical therapist and patient. 2. Communication in medicine. I. Title.
  [DNLM: 1. Physical Therapy (Specialty) 2. Professional-Patient Relations. 3. Communication. 4. Interprofessional Relations. WB 460 M597c 2010]
  RM705.M84 2010
  615.8'2--dc22

2009043005

To David,
whose unwavering love and
encouragement sustains me from the inside out.

Preface

As a future physical therapist, you will soon be joining a profession dedicated to the improvement of quality of life, which is broadly defined as the degree to which one derives life satisfaction. Obviously this definition suggests that quality of life is a multidimensional construct that includes elements related to physical, emotional, and psychological well-being.

As you know, entrance into the physical therapy profession requires an intensive course of rigorous academic training to assure your competence in the evaluation, diagnosis, and treatment of the spectrum of diseases and conditions that limit movement and function. The theoretical basis of this training derives from a growing number of scientific disciplines including anatomy, physiology, and biomechanics. Accordingly, the unique application of these skills in the context of patient management has often been considered as the science of physical therapy. Furthermore, the validity and clinical efficacy of these skills can be supported through scientific inquiry and *evidence,* the consummate "holy grail" by which the value of our professional interventions is measured.

Proficiency in our scientific body of knowledge, while inarguably crucial to professional success, is of little value unless it is embedded in the context of a respectful, supportive, and empowering therapeutic partnership. In order for this partnership to succeed, another set of skills is also critical, and many of these involve effective communication. In the practice of physical therapy, we are called to communicate numerous virtues to those we serve and with whom we work. These include empathy, compassion, encouragement, and optimism. In order to exude these qualities with any level of authenticity within the broader context of health-care delivery, (e.g., in our workplace, profession, and society at large), we must finesse our communication on many distinct but overlapping levels. Furthermore, in order to maintain the passion needed to empower our patients, we must continually stoke the fires of engagement. This too involves proficiency in our interactional skills.

Because these virtues cannot be objectified in the typical language of scientific research, they have become known as the *art* of our profession. This distinction should not be misconstrued to imply a lesser level of importance, but without a substantial body of evidence (or even an idea of which disciplines to examine in order to find it), we have perhaps conveyed this impression by default, leaving our future practitioners to develop these skills on their own. This is an unfortunate predicament and my central reason for writing this book.

This text addresses communication from a comprehensive theoretical perspective involving three levels of communication (internal, external, and instrumental), which evolve from the inside out. Wherever possible, evidence is provided to support this perspective. In many cases, the work in this text is the author's attempt to present and integrate existing or emerging concepts in a unique and hopefully useful way.

In presenting this theoretical model, the first step was to explore communication from the standpoint of other disciplines who also view it as an important element in quality of life. To that end, much of the research in this text is from the realm of psychology, where quality of life is measured by levels of resilience, optimism, and self-efficacy. Evidence from this discipline supports the text's central premise that these attributes are shaped and conveyed in our communication. In addition, the professions of nursing, education, and organizational behavior have also yielded a rich harvest of information that can serve to enrich our understanding of the complexities of communication.

As our marvelous physical therapy profession continually expands its body of knowledge, it is my sincere hope that the contributions of these disciplines will be better understood and appreciated. Our mission to enhance quality of life in all areas of our scope of influence (namely, personal, professional, and social) stands to benefit enormously.

In the hope of perhaps assisting this process, I am honored to present this text.

KAREN MUELLER PT, PhD

Professor
Northern Arizona University, Program in Physical Therapy
Flagstaff, AZ

Reviewers

REVIEWERS

Charles J. Gulas, PT, PhD, GCS
Dean, School of Health Professions
Maryville University
St. Louis, MO

Susan Hallenborg Ventura, PT, MEd, PhD
Director of Clinical Education and Associate
Clinical Professor
Physical Therapy
Northeastern University
Boston, MA

Rhonda K. Stanley, PT, PhD
Associate Professor
Physical Therapy
University of Texas at El Paso
El Paso, TX

Valerie Strunk, MS, PT
Director of Clinical Education, Lecturer
Physical Therapy
Indiana University
Indianapolis, IN

Melinda J. Suto, PhD (Education), MA (OT), BS (OT), OTR
Senior Instructor
The University of British Columbia
School of Rehabilitation Sciences, Division
of Occupational Therapy
Vancouver, British Columbia, Canada

Kris Vacek, OTD, OTR/L
Chair and Associate Professor
Occupational Therapy
Rockhurst University
Kansas City, MO

Denise Wise, PT, PhD
Chair, Associate Professor
Physical Therapy
The College of St. Scholastica
Duluth, MN

STUDENT REVIEWERS

Jessica Lee Lassiter, ATC
DPT student (3rd year)
Physical Therapy
Indiana University—Purdue University
Indianapolis
Indianapolis, IN

Lynn Taylor, SPT
Physical Therapy
Indiana University—Purdue University
Indianapolis
Indianapolis, IN

Contents

The Foundations of Engaged Professionalism and Effective Communication

Part 1 introduces the building blocks of effective communication and professionalism, which are explored in subsequent chapters. A primary purpose of Chapter 1 is to provide evidence suggesting that continuous social change demands the ongoing development of communication skills. In addition, active learning strategies that will be used throughout the text are presented and described. In Chapter 2, the concept of *engagement* is presented as the application of effective communication skills to professionalism and work satisfaction. Chapter 3 explores specific elements associated with the choice of an optimal line of work, presenting a spectrum of three domains (job, career, and mission) that direct attitudes and values.

CHAPTER 1

Communication Revisited

"In the beginner's mind, there are many possibilities,
but in the expert's there are few."

Shunryu Suzuki,
Zen Mind, Beginner's Mind

Chapter Overview

This chapter begins with the exploration of two common assumptions that may contribute to the belief that communication skill training is unnecessary in doctoral-level physical therapy (PT) education. These two assumptions are countered with evidence suggesting that today's physical therapist must confront unique communication challenges that require ongoing skill development. Of particular significance is the increasing number of technologically based communication options at our disposal. Each of these options affords specific benefits and liabilities that must be considered in order to optimize communication in all contexts. In order to facilitate this consideration, a theoretical Communication Pyramid is introduced as a reflective model to guide the selection of optimal modes of interaction.

A major theme of this text is that happy, authentic, and successful individuals view personal and professional interaction as a seamless continuum involving three levels of communication. These are defined as internal, external, and instrumental communication. This chapter provides a theoretical framework linking these three communication levels to *engaged professionalism.* Engaged professionals possess the virtues of commitment, empowerment, and a sense of mission. Most important, engaged professionals use the three levels of communication to promote effective change in self, profession, and society.

Finally, the chapter presents key experiential learning activities that will be used throughout the text to facilitate the development of skill at each of the three levels of communication.

Key Terms

Affective domain

American Physical Therapy Association

Federation of State Boards of Physical Therapy

National Physical Therapy Examination

The Value of Communication: Patients Will Not Care How Much You Know Until They Know How Much You Care

The value of effective communication skills in the practice of health-care delivery, including PT, is inarguable. Communication has been called "the most important element of practice that health professionals must master."[1] Effective communication is associated with greater patient adherence, improved patient outcomes, and patient satisfaction. Thus, as health-care delivery has become more competitive, every related discipline has recently directed increasing attention to the development of this skill. Professions serving as points of entry into the health-care system—such as medicine, nursing, and physical therapy—have a critical responsibility in this regard.

Accordingly, communication skills training has become a top priority in U.S. medical schools in the past 10 years. Prior to this, studies of physician–patient interactions revealed patterns of communication that were less than successful. One study showed that physicians interrupted their patients within the first 18 seconds of an initial interview, with only 23% of patients completing their sentences.[2] In 1999, the American Association of Colleges of Medicine Medical School Objectives Project issued a report stating the need to ensure that future physicians "aren't just skilled in the art of diagnosing and treating disease, but are also skilled in managing and communicating with their patients."[3] The report went on to outline several communication-based outcomes to be achieved by all medical students, one of which is to communicate effectively with patients, their families, colleagues, and others with whom they must interact in the execution of their duties.

Effective communication skills have also been shown to be a critical prerequisite at all levels of PT practice. In a recent study of 343 physical therapists in supervisory roles, the perceived importance of 75 different managerial skills was examined. Effective communication skills were ranked first.[4] The development of expert clinical practice is also grounded in the development of communication skills involving patient interaction, collaborating with and teaching patients and families, and the ability to discuss a patient's plan of care.[5]

BOX 1-1: Opening Exercise: Some Communication Challenges in Physical Therapy Practice

Consider each of the communication challenges below, then identify one goal for your own communication skills development. Make notes as you identify each goal.
Suggestion: After reading each statement, begin with: "The most important challenge for me in this situation would be . . ."

1. Establishing rapport with a new patient who is fearful that PT will be painful
2. Communicating your findings (which indicate a poor prognosis for benefit from physical therapy) to the patient and family
3. Presenting and defending your plan of care to a physician who disagrees with it
4. Discussing a denial of your insurance claim for patient treatment with a claims manager

Readying the Path for Your Journey

"What more can I possibly learn about communication?" As a teacher of communication skills in a PT program for more than 20 years, I probably hear this question from my students more often than any other. Thus, it is obviously an important question, and one worthy of a thoughtful reply.

In a word, the answer is "YES." But in order to make an intellectually compelling case for this response, we will explore two assumptions that may contribute to the belief that there is nothing more to learn about communication, or that it is not a worthwhile topic in doctoral PT education (Box 1-2).

BOX 1-2:   Two Less-Than-Helpful Assumptions About Communication

ASSUMPTION #1:

Either you are born with good communication abilities or you are not, and nothing will change this.

ASSUMPTION #2:

Quantity equals quality (doing something a lot means it will naturally be done well).

Let us explore each of the assumptions in turn. This should be below as it is not an assumption.

Assumption #1: Either you are born with good communication abilities or you are not, and nothing will change this.

Reality #1: Communication must be practiced to remain effective.

Like any other form of expertise, communication is a *learned skill* that you must practice in order to excel. As with any skill, the pursuit of excellence in communication requires the willful decision to direct our energies toward its realization. And as with any area of expertise, the pursuit of communication excellence requires a commitment to continue *its ongoing development throughout our lives.* Accordingly, we would probably consider it ludicrous to ask Olympic athletes or virtuoso musicians whether they "practice" their craft, because it is understood that there are always new dimensions of expertise to be realized as new demands emerge within a body of knowledge.

Reality #2: New communication challenges are always emerging. These require the development of new communication skills.

As the level of complexity increases in society as a result of technological advancement and the increasing demands of a global economy, new challenges emerge that require an increasingly sophisticated level of communication skill.

For example, consider how the Internet has affected communication. On the positive side, without leaving our homes, we can instantaneously communicate with countless persons across the world at any time of day. We can obtain volumes of information on any imaginable subject in a matter of seconds. We can shop, pay bills, and even find a date. We can also represent ourselves in any manner we choose or say whatever we want from the presumed safety of our computer station.

These are all intoxicating possibilities, but they are not without risk. The Internet creates an illusion of anonymity that engenders new and unprecedented challenges to trust, honesty, and integrity. For example, confidential or sensitive information that was once shared discreetly in a face-to-face conversation between two individuals can now be made available to millions of persons with a single keystroke. Consider the following true examples.

1. A public health worker walked away with a computer disk containing the names of 4,000 people who tested positive for HIV. The disks were sent to two newspapers.[6]
2. A physical therapist was terminated from a small-town private practice after a patient discovered offensive material on the therapist's MySpace blog.
3. A university president suddenly resigned after a local newspaper leaked a series of e-mails containing sexually harassing comments made to a university staff member.[7]

On an even larger scale, the widespread availability of anonymously generated confidential information can create unprecedented challenges to longstanding legal and ethical mores. Consider the real-life example contained in **Box 1-3**.

BOX 1-3: What Defines Cheating?

Almost every student has had an experience where a classmate who stood to gain from the information has asked, "So, how was the test?" Do you think that providing any form of information to your classmate (such as, "You better be sure you know all muscles in the forearm") could be considered cheating?

If you are like most students today, you have probably had this experience so often that you do not consider such a response to have ethical implications. This begs the question of the parameters by which we define *cheating*. Taking this a step further, would you be enabling your classmate to cheat if your answer were more specific (e.g., "There were three questions on the brachial plexus")? What if you wrote down every question you remembered and gave it to your classmate? What if you posted these questions on the Internet?

If your answers are inconsistent, it is interesting to consider the grounds on which you would justify your position. Like so many ethical dilemmas, there are often no black-and-white boundaries by which we can determine the "rightness" or "wrongness" of a given situation. Often it takes an extreme case to force examination of a gray-zone issue. The following situation is an example.

Successful completion of the **National Physical Therapy Examination** (NPTE) is required in order to obtain licensure for the legal practice of physical therapy in the United States. The NPTE is written, administered, and scored on behalf of all state licensure boards in the United States by the **Federation of State Boards of Physical Therapy** (FSBPT). In recent years, the examination has evolved from a pen-and-paper format to one that is administered by computer.

In 2002, it was discovered that questions from the NPTE had been posted on the Internet with the obvious potential for widespread cheating on the examination. Virtually overnight, the FSBPT faced a massive threat to the security of the NPTE. Of equal concern was the threat to public safety at the hands of physical therapists who cheated on the very examination intended to assure their competence.

The insinuation of technology into the NPTE thus created a new and pressing ethical legal dilemma that required an immediate response from the FSBPT. Of foremost importance was the construction of an inarguable definition of *cheating*, along with an equally inviolable means to prevent it. Accordingly, the FSBPT developed an examination security policy that strictly prohibits the sharing or solicitation of any information in any format about the NPTE. This policy is posted clearly on the "examination information" page of the FSBPT Web site[8] and also includes a statement that persons who violate this policy may be denied a license to practice PT.

Assumption #2: Quantity equals quality (doing something a lot means that it will naturally be done well).

Reality #1: We are spending less time in face-to-face communication.

Humans are social beings with the ability to develop deeply personal, authentic bonds with others. Obviously, such bonds are not likely to result from an overreliance on impersonal and anonymous forms of communication. We can spend our energies on only a finite number of tasks in a given day, so that time devoted to one activity will be spent at the expense of another. According to a study at Stanford University,[9] persons who spend more than 10 hours a week on the Internet also report a 15% decrease in social activities and a 25% decrease in time talking on the phone with friends and family. The 2008 Pew Internet & American Life Project reported that 67% of Americans working 41 to 50 hours a week use the Internet "constantly" or "several times a day" to communicate with colleagues.[10] While these workers report that this activity increases their productivity, they note that it also cuts into their time away from work and contributes to the feeling of being "always on." These findings raise interesting questions about the relationship between reliance on technological forms of communication and decreased opportunities to practice the art of face-to-face social interaction. What do your own experiences indicate?

The increasing reliance on electronic forms of communication can make the challenges of face-to-face communication even more difficult. Over the years, I have seen significant increases in the numbers of students who identify the ability to initiate and sustain a personal conversation as their biggest communication concern. These students astutely acknowledge that there is a huge "disconnect" between their comfort and abilities in electronic versus real-life interaction, and they are concerned about their ability to establish rapport with patients in a clinical setting.

This concern is further underscored by social science researchers who have studied the decline in face-to-face communication resulting from the widespread use of technological approaches. According to Michael Bugeja, Director of the Greenlee School of Journalism at Iowa State University[11]:

> Friendships are very difficult. They require investment in time and energy. When you can add or delete a friend with the click of a key, you are really avoiding the interpersonal practice that's going to shape your character as you grow older.
> The more we use technology, the less time we have to nurture our primary relationships. Many of us, including students, are depressed because of stress or addiction and seek self-help using the same digital gadgets that are the source of our problems, visiting Web sites or social networks instead of resolving issues interpersonally, face-to-face.

Reality #2: Quality communication involves the conscious choice to connect with the speaker.

Even though most of us have been communicating since the day we were born, we can all readily distinguish between those who do it well and those who do not, regardless of the format. The difference between the two relates to *connecting*, which involves a purposeful choice. To that end, each of us can probably easily recall face-to-face situations where we failed to connect with a person who spoke to us, whether it was ignoring a parent asking us to take out the garbage or tuning out a roommate's complaints about a disastrous date. Perhaps we have allowed days (or even weeks) to go by without responding to letters, phone messages, or e-mails, leaving their authors to assume that we don't care about them. In each of these situations, on some level, we *chose* (either consciously or unconsciously) *not* to connect. When we withhold our connections from others, we may contribute to misunderstandings and injured relationships. A major element of communication then, is first, the conscious decision to actively listen, which means that *we choose to devote our full attention to a person speaking to us.*

As you will discover further on in the text, active listening is not easy, especially in a culture that values multitasking and efficiency. As you will also learn, both in your classes on neuroscience and further on in this book, the human brain cannot attend to two different tasks *simultaneously.* Rather, it rapidly alternates focus between two such demands, so that the quality of attention to both is decreased.

Assuming that we choose to actively listen, our ability to connect will also hinge on whether we can respond in the empathic manner that invites validation and builds trust.

Reality #3: Abuses of technology can challenge effective communication.

As we have discussed thus far, technological forms of communication such as the Internet and cellular phone can be tremendously useful by enabling us to communicate with anyone, anywhere. However, communication challenges arise when we use poor judgment in the use of these technologies.

For example, let's say that you are having difficulties with a classmate with whom you are working on a class project. This person has taken credit for your ideas and has even suggested that you are not contributing to the group effort. As these transgressions mount, you find your anger slowly building. Then, after a particularly frustrating interaction, you go home and compose a flamingly vulgar and insulting e-mail about this classmate. Although your intention is simply to send it solely to one sympathetic classmate, you mistakenly select the wrong recipient address. With a single keystroke, off goes this blistering invective to your entire PT class list serve.

The problem of "e-mail regret" is yet another example of the many emerging communication challenges that have arisen from the abuse of technological communication. In this case, there are no reliable methods to retract an offensive e-mail once the "send" button has been activated.

To forestall this problem, Gmail, the free e-mail service provided by Google, initiated a unique new feature titled "Mail Goggles" in 2008.[12] Modeled after automobile devices, which require a person to prove their sobriety by performing a specific task (such as entering numbers on a keypad on the door) to gain vehicle entry, Mail Goggles requires successful completion of math problems as a prerequisite to sending late-night e-mails.

As the need for Mail Goggles suggests, the anonymity of e-mail provides a sense of insulation that can disinhibit our sense of appropriate social boundaries for communication. For example, we have all perhaps been party to e-mail disclosures at a level of intimacy that we would never employ in a face-to-face situation. In addition, this boundary distortion may even goad us toward expressions of hostility and aggression that we wouldn't dream of inflicting on others in real time. Terms such as *cyberbullying* and *cyberstalking* underscore the prevalence and severity of these distorted forms of communication. For example, a 2007 report by the nonprofit Pew Internet & American Life Project reported that one-third of all teenage Internet users reported that they had been bullied online.[13] Another study reported that increased levels of personal disclosure online by teenagers were associated with higher rates of depression.[14] The severity of this problem came to light in 2007, when a 13-year-old girl committed suicide after a MySpace relationship with a boy named "Josh" suddenly turned mean. Sadly, it was later discovered that "Josh" never existed. Furthermore, he was created by the overzealous mother of one of the victim's friends in retaliation for a recent falling out with her daughter.[15]

Inappropriate use of technological communication can be dangerous in other ways. Several studies have documented the dangers of driving a car while using a cellular phone. These studies have suggested that the impairments associated with cell phone use on the road were equivalent to those associated with driving while intoxicated[16] and that cell phone use while driving resulted in a fourfold increase in the risk of a motor vehicle accident.[17] In 2002, cell phone use while driving accounted for 2,600 fatalities.[18] In the summer of 2007, five teenagers were killed in a motor vehicle accident that occurred while the driver of the car was sending a text message from her cell phone.[19]

The Ultimate Reality: Skilled Communicators Effectively Use All Forms of Communication

Now that we have explored two common misperceptions about communication, you are hopefully intrigued and excited about the many challenges and opportunities that await you in the quest of further developing your skills. As the previous discussion has suggested, these challenges and opportunities have never been greater.

Perhaps one of the most important challenges for the engaged professional is to effectively harness the power of all forms of communication. Beginning in the following section and continuing throughout the text, a new model is presented to help you meet this challenge.

The Communication Pyramid

With so many forms of communication available to us, we are constantly selecting among numerous options. What considerations might drive our choices? In our time-pressed society, many of us may base our selection on a desire for efficiency. Thus, given our societal "need for speed," it is no surprise that electronic methods of communication are increasingly becoming a first choice for many persons. As suggested previously, many U.S. workers believe that electronic communication has enhanced their productivity and opportunities for networking.

At an unconscious level, however, we may also select electronic approaches because they allow us to avoid an uncomfortable face-to-face dialogue. If we are completely honest with ourselves, we can probably all recall a time that we avoided such an interaction through use of an e-mail or text message.

In many cases, the use of electronic communication methods over personal interaction can be both *efficient* (communicating quickly) and *effective* (making the true meaning of our message clear), thus saving us time and energy for other valuable activities. However, there are other times when these more impersonal electronic methods can contribute to misunderstandings, thus damaging our relationships. In such an instance, our communication may have been efficient but not effective. This often occurs when electronic communication is used for emotionally charged situations such as the delivering of unpleasant news. For example, a physical therapist who had provided vacation coverage in a hospital for more than 20 years was devastated to learn of the termination of his employment through an e-mail message from the director of the PT department.

Although the purpose of communication might be described simplistically as the "exchange of information" between individuals, it is, in fact, a complex interaction that is highly dependent on sensory input. In reality, we communicate with our entire beings, using the sensory modalities of vision, hearing, and tactile sensation to add emotion and meaning to our words. Because these sensory modalities of communication are nonverbal, they are collectively known as *paralanguage*, or perhaps more commonly, *body language*. Much study has been devoted to the understanding of these nonverbal elements of communication, and it is generally understood that they are instrumental in conveying the true meaning of our words.

The communication pyramid integrates these nonverbal, sensory elements into three levels as shown in **Figure 1-1**. The purpose of the pyramid is to provide guidelines that promote effectiveness rather than efficiency as the *primary consideration* in our communication method choice. Because paralanguage is a critical element in effective communication, it is a fundamental element in this model.

Beginning from the bottom, three levels are shown in **Figure 1-1**. These levels represent the most common forms of communication delivery, beginning with face-to-face interactions and moving toward electronic methods. These levels are also delineated by decreasing levels of paralanguage components, which are noted at the right of the pyramid. The benefits and drawbacks inherent in the various types of communication are illustrated on the left of the pyramid.

It is important to understand that the pyramid is not intended to convey any judgment about the value of the communication approaches in each of the three levels. Rather, the purpose of the pyramid is to provide guidelines for appropriate usage of these various methods in effective communication. As we move into our discussion on external communication further on in the text, you will encounter several examples that highlight the importance of appropriate communication at each level.

At this point in the text, it is appropriate to provide an overview of the levels as they relate to the availability of the components of paralanguage. From there, we can then explore the application of these levels to your communication as a physical therapist.

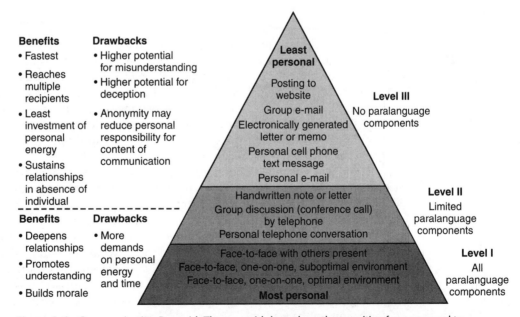

Benefits
- Fastest
- Reaches multiple recipients
- Least investment of personal energy
- Sustains relationships in absence of individual

Drawbacks
- Higher potential for misunderstanding
- Higher potential for deception
- Anonymity may reduce personal responsibility for content of communication

Benefits
- Deepens relationships
- Promotes understanding
- Builds morale

Drawbacks
- More demands on personal energy and time

Least personal
Posting to website
Group e-mail
Electronically generated letter or memo
Personal cell phone text message
Personal e-mail

Level III
No paralanguage components

Handwritten note or letter
Group discussion (conference call) by telephone
Personal telephone conversation

Level II
Limited paralanguage components

Face-to-face with others present
Face-to-face, one-on-one, suboptimal environment
Face-to-face, one-on-one, optimal environment
Most personal

Level I
All paralanguage components

Figure 1–1. Communication Pyramid: The pyramid shows how the transition from personal to electronic forms of communication decreases the availability of the sensory components of paralanguage (sensory, auditory, visual, kinesthetic), which are used to convey emotional content and meaning. This transition is depicted by three levels, shown on the right. The benefits and drawbacks of the three levels of communication are shown on the left.

Level I

Level I involves face-to-face interactions in which all components of paralanguage are available for communication. Visual input allows us to see the facial expressions, body language, and gestures of the speaker, providing valuable information about his or her emotional state. The presence of visual input thus allows us to interpret the spoken and unspoken meanings of the speaker's words more accurately.

Other forms of sensory input are valuable as well. Auditory sensory input—including volume, pacing, and inflection of the speaker's voice—also provides important information about the speaker's state of mind and intended meaning. Kinesthetic input, including the speaker's movement and the distance from which we are being addressed, further illuminates the meaning of the words, as does tactile input (e.g., if the speaker puts a hand on your shoulder while speaking).

In addition, as noted within the pyramid, face-to-face communication involves the choice of physical setting, which may be an important consideration depending on the purpose, emotional intensity, and desired effect of the exchange. For example, consider the impact of the physical setting in providing emotional support to an elderly woman who is distraught over her husband's recent stroke. Accordingly, optimal settings would be those that are consistent with the purpose of the interaction and that provide the fewest possible distractions.

Obviously, it is not always possible to control the setting for communication, and it is important to note that suboptimal settings may pose additional challenges to the communication interaction. Such might be the case if you were confronted by an angry patient in a busy PT gymnasium in which other patients were present. Given the distractions of such an environment, it might be difficult to create the quiet atmosphere needed to promote emotional de-escalation.

Level II

When communication is exchanged via the telephone, the type of sensory input is purely auditory; this is a potent modality that conveys significant information through the voice qualities described previously. Nevertheless, the absence of visual and kinesthetic input can provide challenges in the interpretation of emotional cues afforded by facial expression and body language. Accordingly, in making the important decision of whom to hire in a PT practice, few employers would use the telephone as their preferred interview method. Consider what can be learned from a job applicant through his or her facial expressions, eye contact, and gestures.

When we deliberately choose to write a note or letter by hand, the act of putting pen to paper to reflect our thoughts takes more concentration than typing on a keyboard (assuming a level of proficiency in the latter). Because there is no automatic "delete" or "spell check" in handwritten communication, we must be more attentive to the words we choose. Thus, handwritten notes or letters convey a level of thoughtful attentiveness. Accordingly, they are still commonly used in expressions of sympathy and gratitude (sympathy cards and thank-you notes, respectively). Finally, unlike few other forms of communication, handwritten notes leave a personal legacy that can have a lasting impact. Consider for example, how the written diaries of Anne Frank or Helen Keller have continued to speak to generations of readers.

Finally, there is an enduring personal element in a page on which a person has inscribed words in his or her own hand. Most serious art collectors will only consider original paintings or sculptures as worthy of their collections. As handwriting is replaced increasingly by electronic text, how will the concept of "original" be defined in the future?

Level III

Electronic forms of communication, such as text messages and e-mail, remove all components of paralanguage, leaving us to interpret information entirely from the decoding of alphabetical symbols. In the absence of other additional sensory inputs, the potential for misinterpretation of the messages increases, as does its anonymity. Thus, it is not surprising that electronic forms of communication may be considered impersonal, especially if they convey emotional content. Interestingly, as we become more reliant on electronic communication formats such as text messaging and e-mail, face-based symbols, known as emoticons (e.g.,☺), are now being used to provide cues about emotional content. Thus, it could be said that these emoticons are an attempt to provide an electronic substitute for the information conveyed in the paralanguage of facial expression.

BOX 1-4: Traveling the Communication Pyramid

Below is a list of common communication interactions. Using the communication pyramid (see **Figure 1-1**), select the level you would prefer to <u>deliver</u> the interaction.

1. Informing a friend that you will be 1 hour late for an engagement
2. Giving positive feedback to a coworker
3. Asking to borrow money from a family member
4. Apologizing for hurting a friend's feelings
5. Ending a dating relationship
6. Inviting a large group of friends to a party at your house
7. Sending holiday greetings to friends
8. Resigning from a job
9. Informing a professor that you will not be in class for several days
10. Informing a classmate about the unexpected death of a close mutual friend

DISCUSS THE FOLLOWING:

1. The rationale for your choices. Under which circumstances might the communication level you selected change?
2. Go down the list again, this time, considering the level you would prefer for *receiving* the information. Are there any differences from the first list?

▌Navigating the Pyramid as a Physical Therapist

Upholding Our Legacy

The PT profession has a long history of combining the science of healing with the art of caring. This art is carried out largely through physical contact with our patients. Thus, the bottom line is that despite the ongoing and explosive advances in medical care (including telemedicine), most PT services are provided at the face-to-face level. Thus, it is critical to be skilled in the area of interpersonal communication, which is the supporting base from which all subsequent levels of interaction are built. In other words, expertise at the face-to-face level of communication will provide a solid base for other forms.

You Must Consciously Connect With Your Patients

As a physical therapist, you will personally interact with countless individuals who have a vast array of significant concerns to share. They will include patients, family members, colleagues, supervisors, and case managers. In a given work day, where you will likely be consumed with many important tasks, you will need to decide whether to connect with each of these individuals in a meaningful and authentic manner. This will be a choice for you every day and one that will need to be mindfully repeated throughout your life and career.

As you will discover in this text, the decision to connect with others is only the first step in the development of engaged communication, but it is the most important one. You will also need strong interpersonal skills to gain your patients' trust so that they can share important concerns with you. You will need to display keen sensitivity and awareness of socially and professionally communication-appropriate boundaries. These communication requirements will necessitate strong skills in the area of *emotional intelligence (EQ)*. The elements of EQ and how they relate to your internal and external communication skills are examined in the next section, and you will be given several exercises to facilitate your development of these skills.

Exciting Interpersonal Communication Challenges Await You

As a physical therapist, you will be faced with the challenge of effectively communicating in situations that may be new to you, as with persons who are in severe pain, very frightened, or facing significant life changes. These new and unique situations will require you to deepen your communication skills related to compassion, empathy, negotiation, and problem solving. For example, how do you respond to the patient with a C7 spinal cord injury whose main concerns are whether she will be able to parent her teenage children and return to work? How do you negotiate with a case manager for 1 additional week's stay at a rehabilitation center on behalf of a patient with stroke, because the family needs more time for education so that he may be able to return home safely?

The challenges presented by our patients affect all members of the health-care team, who must be specifically trained to respond appropriately. A 2004 article in *Academic Medicine*, the journal of the Association of American Medical Colleges, states that "persistent evidence indicates that the communication skills of practicing physicians do not achieve the goals of patient satisfaction, strengthening health outcomes and decreasing malpractice litigation." This statement was made to support the need for integrating communication training into the family medicine clerkships of medical students.[20]

When It Comes to Communication Skills Training, Attitude Is Everything

Although you may not particularly feel the need for a course (or a textbook) devoted entirely to communication, recent studies of physicians, nurses, and allied health practitioners show that communication training improves several dimensions of patient care, including evaluation skills, functional outcomes, and patient satisfaction.[21,22] Despite these benefits, you are not likely to work toward building a skill that you don't view as important or in which you already feel highly confident. In either case, the "beginner's mind" quote at the start of this chapter may be helpful as a reminder to you to keep an open mind.

In the course of my faculty experiences, I have sometimes observed that the students who are most resistant to communication skills training are often the same ones who face interpersonal difficulties during their internships. Ironically, many of these students also see themselves as excellent communicators. These observations were validated in a study of medical students demonstrating a relationship between perceptions of good communication skills and lack of receptivity toward communication training. Furthermore, many of these students stated that they felt communication skills training was too "soft" (i.e., nonscientific) a topic for inclusion in a medical school curriculum. However, many of these same students rated their communication skills significantly *lower* after such training. The authors of this study suggested that perhaps one impact of communication skills training is to reduce overconfidence to a more realistic level. Because humility is likely to be interpreted more favorably than arrogance when it comes to communication, this finding may bode well for optimal patient care in the long run.[23]

Technological Forms of Communication Will Become Increasingly Important in Physical Therapy Practice

In addition to the many face-to-face demands of PT practice, electronic forms of communication are playing an increasingly important role. Thus you will also need to be skilled in the use of electronic forms of communication for documentation, billing, and interdisciplinary care. As more persons turn to the Internet for medical information, you are likely to have patients inquire about information they obtained online. These requests will call on your ability to obtain evidence for the validity of this information, and the Internet can provide you with an efficient means of obtaining this. For example, the **American Physical Therapy Association** (APTA) provides members-only access to *Hooked on Evidence*, an online repository of evidence from peer-reviewed journals pertaining to numerous PT interventions and examination procedures.[24] On a larger scale, you will also need to be familiar with the provisions of the Healthcare Information Portability and Accountability Act of 1996 (HIPAA). HIPAA involves several policies regarding the appropriate use and disclosure of "protected information" pertaining to a person's health care. HIPAA was enacted in part to protect patient confidentiality after widespread violations occurred as a result of Internet abuse. Thus, adherence to HIPAA policy is critical for ethical and legal PT practice.

Guiding Assumptions for This Text

Communication Skills Affect All Areas of Your Life

Although this text explores communication from the perspective of professionalism and its relationship to effective PT practice, the reality is that good communication skills cannot be practiced within the isolation of a single life context. In other words, you are a person first and then a citizen of society with many roles, one of which will hopefully be as a physical therapist. The skills, attitudes, and behaviors in one context will naturally overlap to some degree with those of the others in which you function. This text is grounded in an evidence-based, interactive model that links communication with self and others to professional engagement and work satisfaction (**Figure 1-2**).

The major premise of the model is that communication is the vital link between self and others. Thus, communication is the critical prerequisite for our ability to achieve professional engagement in our work. In turn, engaged professionalism empowers us to become agents of change. As we widen our scope of influence, we can affect both our

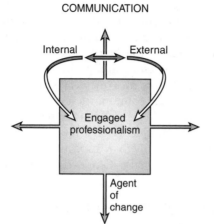

Figure 1–2. Interactive model linking communication and professional engagement to becoming an agent of change for the benefit of ones profession and his/her society.

profession and society. Physical therapists have long recognized the importance of such a scope of influence, as noted by the APTA's 2020 Vision Statement,[25] which states:

By 2020, physical therapy will be provided by physical therapists who are doctors of physical therapy, recognized by consumers and other health care professionals as the practitioners of choice to whom consumers have direct access for the diagnosis of, interventions for, and prevention of impairments, functional limitations, and disabilities related to movement, function, and health.

Communication Starts From the Inside Out

The communication skills needed to affect change at the professional and societal levels begin from within. Communication begins with self-awareness, which is expressed in our internal communication—the messages we give ourselves. Our internal communication creates a personal outlook, which is then expressed in our external communication—our interactions with others. In other words, our work satisfaction and our ability to make positive changes in our profession and the society it serves depend to a great extent on how effectively we communicate. Finally, we use both internal and external communication as the instrument by which we drive positive change in society, empowering and transforming those with whom we interact. This is the essence of instrumental communication.

At this point in your life, as you contemplate the investment of considerable effort and resources toward the goal of becoming a physical therapist, you are probably hoping that these efforts will lead you to enjoyable and satisfying work that makes a difference in the lives of others. This text will assist you in the development of the communication skills you will need to flourish as an engaged professional.

Here are the other guiding assumptions that are systematically explored in the upcoming chapters of this text.

1. Our communication is a reflection of how we see ourselves; self-assessment can help us develop and maintain a healthy point of view.
2. Communication is first *internal*; consisting of our self-talk, our outlook, and the emotional intelligence factors of self-awareness, self-control, and the ability to read emotions in others.
3. Internal communication sets the stage for the quality of our interactions and our ability to effectively direct our lives.
4. Internal communication can be consciously changed to promote confidence, optimism, and self-motivation.
5. Internal communication directs our *external communication*—our dialogues with others. The skills for external communication include emotional and social intelligence. These skills help us manage ourselves and our relationships in positive, growth-enhancing ways.

6. Instrumental communication is the use of both internal and external communication to effect change. Inherent in this skill is the ability to negotiate, manage conflict, and provide information in way that promotes self-efficacy.

Engagement is the work satisfaction that results when challenges are interesting and within our present or emerging level of competence. Work satisfaction is also enhanced when we have the ability to control our work to some degree and, most important, when we are committed to the outcome involved. Another important factor related to engaged professionalism (and work satisfaction) includes involvement in a professional support network. Persons who are engaged in their work are more likely to practice safely and ethically than those who are not. Communication, professional engagement, and work satisfaction are interrelated, and the area over which we have the most control is communication.

Provisions for Your Journey: Learning Approaches for the Affective Domain

Domains of Learning

Throughout your educational process, in each of your courses, you will find yourself presented with a myriad of diverse information pertaining to three domains of learning.[26] These include *knowledge* (information to commit to memory), *psychomotor skills* (tasks to perform), and *attitudes* (values to internalize and demonstrate in your work).

As you know from your considerable educational experiences thus far, you are more likely to learn and remember information (regardless of which domain it is in) when it is made personally relevant in some way. The manner in which this happens will depend on the type of information. For example, the need to learn anatomy becomes readily obvious when you are examining a patient with a knee injury, as would be the need to know how to perform a manual muscle test when your examination of this patient requires an assessment of knee strength. As you prepare for direct patient care in the course of your PT education, you will first demonstrate your command of this knowledge through written and practical examinations that are meant to provide an objective measure of your learning. In most PT curriculums, you will need to demonstrate a certain level of competence on these objective measures before beginning the full-time clinical education portion of your coursework.

The area of communication falls into what is known as the **affective domain** of learning.[20] This domain pertains to the development of attitudes and values. As you know from your own life experience, attitudes and values are deeply personal and are instilled through a variety of sources such as your parents, teachers, culture, and religion. Given the personal element of the affective domain, it is difficult to measure learning through an objective examination. Valuable methods for affective domain learning include group discussion, case studies, and personal reflection.

In order to engage you in the learning process involving the affective domain, this text employs several approaches to place the content in the context of real-life situations and scenarios. These examples will all be real, accrued from my own direct experiences as well as those of my colleagues and, most important, my students. The following section introduces you to each unique feature of this text.

Champ and Blockhead

Perhaps when you were younger, you read a children's magazine called *Highlights*. A regular feature of this publication (which began in 1948 and continues today) was a pair of young boys named Goofus and Gallant. Each month, the boys demonstrated examples of both rude and polite behavior (i.e., "Goofus bosses his friends around. Gallant asks, 'What would you like to do?'"). Throughout the 60-year history of *Highlights*, Goofus and Gallant have demonstrated the mores of social behavior to several generations of readers.

The discussion of appropriate communication behaviors lends itself well to a "Goofus and Gallant" approach, albeit with more of a tongue-in-cheek attitude given the adult audience of this text. Accordingly, examples of both ineffective and effective communication will be demonstrated by two characters: Champ (Communication Hero And Master Professional) and Blockhead (Big Lack Of Communication Knowledge Has Everyone Avoiding Dialogue).

The conceptualization of these characters was based on the human form, but in the interest of gender equality, they are androgynous. Furthermore, creative license has been used to illustrate communication-related "anatomic" features that represent assets (in the case of Champ) or deficits (in the case of Blockhead).

The anatomies of Blockhead and Champ are depicted in **Figures 1-3** and **1-4.**

Again, for the sake of gender equity, Champ and Blockhead alternate between male and female. In each chapter, they find themselves facing a communication challenge pertaining to the topic at hand, with Champ demonstrating a desirable response and Blockhead fumbling.

The purpose of the Champ and Blockhead features is to give you an opportunity to discuss and explore the approaches to a specific communication challenge in professional practice. Although Champ and Blockhead's responses to their ongoing communication challenges may seem extreme (i.e., too good or too bad to be true), this is again a purposeful attempt to widen the range of possibilities. Accordingly, in your

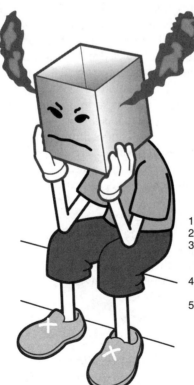

Biggest **L**oser **of C**ommunication
Know-**H**ow **E**xtinguishes
Authentic **D**ialogue

1. Empty head: Doesn't think before talking.
2. No ears: Doesn't listen to others.
3. Sour expression reflects ineffective internal communication resulting in pessimistic outlook.
4. Smoke from head reflects constant frustration from poor communication.
5. Posture reflects lack of engagement.

Figure 1–3. Anatomy of Blockhead.

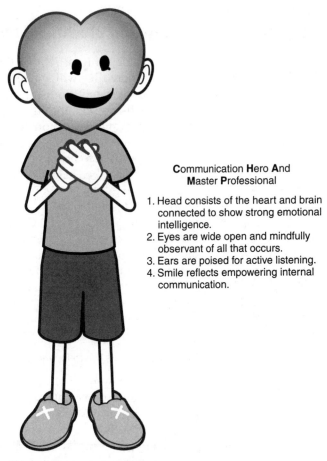

**Communication Hero And
Master Professional**

1. Head consists of the heart and brain connected to show strong emotional intelligence.
2. Eyes are wide open and mindfully observant of all that occurs.
3. Ears are poised for active listening.
4. Smile reflects empowering internal communication.

Figure 1–4. Anatomy of Champ.

discussions, you will be asked to consider appropriate communication strategies that fall somewhere in between their behaviors. As Champ and Blockhead's experiences are presented throughout the book, you will also be asked to analyze these in terms of the consequences that relate to either their lack or abundance of communication skills.

There may be times when you can relate more to the responses of either Champ or Blockhead, and this too is no accident. None of us communicate with perfect skill all the time, but we can learn from the times when we fall short. Thus, most of us are probably Champs most of the time and Blockheads occasionally. With this in mind, I hope that Champ and Blockhead will help you assess and develop the level of your communication skills in a manner that is nonthreatening, enlightening, and at times, light-hearted. Here is an example to get you started.

Field Notes

Field notes are records of observations made during engagement with an area of knowledge or interest. For the purposes of this text, the field under observation is communication, and the observations that you will make will pertain to the behaviors, attitudes, and feelings that arise within yourself as you interact with the material.

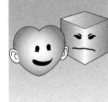

Champ and Blockhead Meet Their PT School Classmates

It is the first day of PT school for Champ and Blockhead. As they drive to the PT program building where they will spend the next 2 years with 40 other persons, they are both nervous and excited. Both want to make a good impression on their classmates and become well-accepted into their new learning community. Thus, their minds are filled with thoughts and ideas about how they will engage with their classmates when they meet for the first time. However, despite their similar hopeful intentions, each will have a rather different approach to how they present themselves. Their approaches are reflected in their self–talk, as described below.

Blockhead thinks, "I'm going to meet a group of really smart, accomplished people. I'm really nervous, but I want everyone to know that I have earned my place in this class. I'll just tell people about my 4.0 GPA, my manager's position at ALLFIT Health Club, and the fact that my dad owns a professional football team. By the end of the day, I'll have slipped these tidbits into my conversations. I hope that will help me make a great impression."

Champ thinks, "I'm going to meet a group of really interesting people who have probably done some amazing things. Like, I wonder who has traveled to Europe, I wonder who plays in a band, or if anyone has run a marathon. I can't wait to ask everyone what they're looking forward to about being in PT school. I wonder if they are as nervous as I am. By the end of the day, I hope I know something interesting about everyone in the group."

Questions: Discuss the following in a small group or with a partner.

1. Meeting a new group of people who will play an important role in your life is certainly a communication challenge. What sort of thoughts, fears, and emotions went through your head on your first day of PT school? How did these drive your conversational approach?
2. What impact is Blockhead likely to convey given his or her thought process? How might this process affect his or her conversational approach?
3. What impact is Champ likely to convey given his or her thought process? How might this thought process affect his or her conversational approach?
4. Is it appropriate to talk about personal accomplishments in a setting like the first day of school? Can this be done in a humble manner?
5. Are there any drawbacks to a conversational approach that involves mostly asking questions? How can this be done in a way that is not intrusive?

Field notes are used widely in the social and behavioral sciences and are valuable records of the learning process; they are most useful as a record of progress for the student. In many ways, they can be considered a part of class notes for the course utilizing this textbook.

Throughout this text, you are invited to record your observations and reflections related to the topic at hand. The field notes assignments in the text include specific questions and exercises to which you can respond in one or two paragraphs. The first field notes exercise appears in Chapter 2.

There is also a journaling aspect of the field notes in which you will be invited to monitor the strengthening of a specific communication skill of your choosing. In Chapter 2, you will be invited to complete a communication self-assessment and to identify an area of communication to develop for the duration of an academic term. My students have done this in our communication class for the past several years and have found it to be very valuable.

It is suggested that you keep your field notes separate from other course notes so that their continuity will not be interrupted. You might want to use a notebook or special computer file for this purpose.

Many of you may already be recording your insights in a journal or diary. Since the age of 8, I have been recording my observations and reflections about the events of my personal and professional life. I will share examples of these entries at the end of Chapters 1 and 3, in the hope that you might find them encouraging (and perhaps even entertaining).

Talking Points

Learning is task-specific, which means that the best way to learn a specific skill is to practice that skill directly. Thus, in the area of communication, the best way to develop your skills is to communicate!

Throughout the text, questions, or *talking points,* are provided for you to discuss. You can discuss these talking points with other classmates in a small or large group either in or out of class. Talking about an issue is a very helpful way of exploring and developing your thoughts and ideas. Many of my students have also enjoyed recording their reflections about these discussions in their field notes. Accordingly, talking point and field note questions are combined throughout the text.

Clinical Scenarios

A major goal of this text is to help you develop your communication skills in the context of your future clinical practice. Thus, throughout the text, you will find short examples of how the content at hand might present itself in a clinical setting. You will then be able to process this information through talking points, field notes, or other activities. All of these clinical scenarios are taken from my own experiences as well as those of my colleagues.

Take Home Menu

At the end of each chapter, you will find suggestions for activities that can be done either in or out of class that will provide further opportunities to explore the material presented. The Take Home Menu section can be used as desired (hence, the term "menu"), and can be used to provide insights for use in your field notes or to share with classmates as a talking point.

Making the Most of Your Communication Journey

Every journey worth taking has its challenges, and in the area of communication, this may involve talking about things that make us uncomfortable. Although this is certainly not the intent of this text, you may find that some of the content or resultant discussions may lead you to such a place. Should this occur, the first thing to keep in mind is to take care of yourself and keep your balance. *The most important way to do this is to share at your comfort level.* Trust yourself to know what this level is. If you would like an approach to help you monitor this, Chapter 3 will include a section on a self-monitoring scale known as *Subjective Units of Discomfort.*

So enjoy your process, as this will help you to learn this material most effectively and to do what your own wisdom tells you is the best for your growth. Finally, your instructors can be a tremendous source of support in this process. If they are like the vast majority of PT faculty I have had the privilege to know, they will be there for you if you need them.

This text was written with great hope and confidence that you, the reader, have many marvelous gifts that can one day lead you to become an engaged professional in the discipline of PT. Simply put, this means that you will use your profession for your own good as well as that of your patients, your profession, and the society in which you live. As an individual who has been in this profession for over 30 years, I can assure you that the journey to develop your communication skills to realize this outcome can be among the most rewarding of your life. Over the years, my students (many of whom have become wonderful friends and colleagues) have underscored this conviction.

Implications for PT Practice

1. Despite the increasing use of technological forms of communication, PT care is delivered primarily in a face-to-face context. Thus, physical therapists must possess strong interpersonal communication skills.
2. As more health-care consumers turn to the Internet for medical information, physical therapists will need to skillfully use this technology to acquire evidence supporting their interventions.
3. Physical therapists are being called by their professional organization, the APTA, to become the recognized providers of care in the areas of movement and function. The realization of this goal will involve the use of effective communication skills by physical therapists in all areas of practice.

Chapter Summary

1. No matter what your current communication skill level might be, societal changes, particularly those involving the use of technology as a means of communication, pose continued challenges to this skill. Ongoing skill development in the area of communication is critical to meet these societal changes.
2. Effective communication skills are the first step to being professionally engaged. In turn, professional engagement empowers us to make important contributions to our profession and to society at large.

References

1. Roberts L, Bucksey SJ. Communicating with patients: what happens in practice? *Phys Ther.* 2007;87(5): 586-593.
2. Beckman HB, Frankel RM. The effect of physician behavior in the collection of data. *Ann Intern Med.* 1984; 101:692-696.
3. Association of American Medical Colleges, Medical School Objectives Project. *Report III: Contemporary Issues in Medicine: Communication in Medicine.* Washington DC: Association of American Medical Colleges; 1999.
4. Schafer DS. Three perspectives on physical therapy managerial work. *Phys Ther.* 2002;82(3):228-236.
5. Jensen GM, Gwyer J, Sheperd K, Hack L. Expert practice in physical therapy. *Phys Ther.* 2000;80(1):28-52.
6. Bacon J. AIDS confidentiality. *USA Today*, October 10, 1996:A1.
7. Ex-NAU President Sent Suggestive E Mails to University. *UA News*, November 15, 2001. http://wc.arizona.edu/papers/ 95/62/01_5.html. Accessed November 14, 2008.
8. Federation of State Boards of Physical Therapy. Exam information. http://www.fsbpt.org/exams/index.asp. Accessed June 26, 2007.
9. Stanford University. The Internet study: more detail. http://www.stanford.edu/group/siqss/Press_Release/press_detail.html. Accessed November 13, 2008.
10. Pew & Internet American Life Project. Networked workers, September 24, 2008. http://www.pewinternet.org/PPF/r/264/report_display.asp. Accessed November 13, 2008.
11. Bugeja M. *Interpersonal Divide: The Search for Community in the Technological Age.* London: Oxford University Press; 2005.
12. Cheng J. Mail Goggles: A breathalyzer test for your Gmail. *Ars Technica*, October 7, 2008. http://arstechnica.com/news.ars/post/20081007-mail-goggles-a-breathlyzer-test-for-your-gmail.html. Accessed November 14, 2008.

13. Pew Internet & American Life Project. Parents and teens survey, October–November, 2006. http://www.pewinternet.org/pdfs/PIP%20Cyberbullying%20Memo.pdf. Accessed July 5, 2007.

14. Ybarra ML, Alexander C, Mitchell KJ. Depressive symptomatology, youth internet use and online interactions: a national survey. *J Adolesc Health.* 2005;36(1):9-18.

15. FOXNews.com. MySpace mom linked to Missouri teen's suicide being cyber-bullied herself. December 6, 2007. http://www.foxnews.com/story/0,2933,315684,00.html. Accessed November 14, 2008.

16. Strayer DL, Drews FA, Crouch DJ. A comparison of the cell phone driver and the drunk driver. *Hum Factors.* 2006;48(2):381-391.

17. McCartt AT, Hellinga LA, Bratiman KA. Cell phones and driving: review of research. *Traffic Inj Prev.* 2006;7(2):89-106.

18. Clayton M, Helms B, Simpson C. Active prompting to decrease cell phone use and increase seat belt use while driving. *J Appl Behav Anal.* 2006;39(3):341.

19. Mahoney J. Text message ban for drivers mulled. *Daily News Albany,* July 17, 2007. http://www.nydailynews.com/news/2007/07/17/2007-07-17_textmessage_ban_for_drivers_mulled.html. Accessed August 27, 2007.

20. Egnew TR, Mauksch LB, Greer T, Farber S. Integrating communication training into a required family medicine clerkship. *Academic Med.* 2004;79(8):737-743.

21. Parry R. Are interventions to enhance communication performance in allied health professionals effective, and how should they be delivered? Direct and indirect evidence. *Patient Educ Counseling.* 2008;73:186-195.

22. Ammentorp J, Sabroe S, Kofoed PE, Mainz J. The effect of training in communication skills on medical doctors' and nurses' self-efficacy: a randomized controlled trial. *Patient Educ Counseling.* 2007;66:270-277.

23. Rees C, Sheard C. The relationship between medical students' attitudes towards communication skills learning and their demographic and education related characteristics. *Med Educ.* 2002;36(11):1017-1027.

24. American Physical Therapy Association. Hooked on evidence. http://www.hookedonevidence.com. Accessed July 5, 2008.

25. American Physical Therapy Association. 2020 Vision Statement. http://www.apta.org/AM/Template.cfm?Section=Vision_20201&Template=/TaggedPage/TaggedPageDisplay.cfm&TPLID=285&ContentID=32061. Accessed July 5, 2007.

26. Bloom BS. *Taxonomy of Educational Objectives, Handbook I: The Cognitive Domain.* New York: David McKay Co Inc; 1956.

Take Home Menu: Activities for Paired or Small Group Discussion

1. Experimenting With the Communication Pyramid (see Figure 1-1)

For the next week, be mindful of your choices with respect to your levels of communication. What drives your choices the most (e.g., efficiency, ability to reach more persons, convenience)?

At least once in the next week, consciously move your communication with a friend or family member toward a more personal mode on the pyramid. For example, if you usually talk with a given friend through e-mail, give him or her a phone call. If it is possible to arrange a face-to-face visit, do so.

Questions:

   A. How was the quality of your communication affected by the use of a more personal approach?

   B. Is it possible to truly deepen a relationship without personal contact every now and then? Which factors guide your decision to move toward more personal contacts?

   C. Is it ever appropriate to move up the pyramid to limit communication? Why or why not?

   D. On a given day, what percentage of your communication is at level 1, level 2, and level 3 on the pyramid? Why do you think this is so? What changes would you make if this were an option?

2. Get to Know the APTA Website

Log onto http://www.apta.org to explore the website of your professional organization. Pretend that you are a consumer trying to learn about PT. What can you learn from this website? In what ways does the APTA website help inform the public about the PT profession in a manner consistent with the 2020 vision statement?

CHAPTER 2

Engaged Professionalism: The Benchmark of Effective Communication

"The first is vision, for without vision there can be no forward movement. The second is faith in the purpose...
keen, alive, kindled with enthusiasm. The third is courage to overcome all odds and difficulties."

The response of Mary McMillan, First APTA president, to the question, "What does it take to be a successful innovator?"

"I don't know what your destiny will be, but one thing I do know: the only ones among you who will be really happy are those who will have sought and found how to serve."

Albert Schweitzer, MD,
Nobel Laureate

Chapter Overview

Have you ever wondered what it takes to remain passionate and invested throughout the course of a career? The above quotations highlight two interconnected attributes, both of which are supported by effective communication. The first is *engagement,* the focused alignment of personal resources with a meaningful purpose outside of oneself. The second is *engaged professionalism,* the application of values and knowledge in the service of work that benefits society. This chapter explores the concepts of engagement and engaged professionalism from a life-work perspective while emphasizing communication skills, which enhance interactions in both realms.

Key Terms

Job satisfaction	Engagement	Engaged professionalism
Positive psychology	Core values	

Take This Job and Love It: The Essence of Engaged Professionalism

As you consider your future career as a physical therapist (PT), what excites you the most? What do you hope to accomplish? What contributions do you hope to make? Although these questions may be difficult to address while you are in the thick of your physical therapy studies, you are likely to find that they can be easily answered by physical therapists who continue to find meaning in their work. Most likely, these therapists are making positive contributions at many levels, which affect their patients, their coworkers, and their professional colleagues. These therapists embody a quality called *engaged professionalism*. Like you, they may have entered the profession with the worthy goal of helping others. In addition, as their professional skills developed, they probably found new opportunities to apply these in exciting and creative ways. Such therapists are likely to tell you that even after decades of practice, that they have never stopped learning. Luckily for us, many of these therapists are actively practicing in our midst. The following section describes such an individual.

A Compelling Example of Engaged Professionalism

Each year, the APTA Student Assembly names a physical therapist "living legend" who is invited to speak at the National Student Conclave. These individuals (who include Florence Kendall and Shirley Sahrmann) have all made professional contributions that have shaped our profession in groundbreaking ways. The living legends series is an inspiring opportunity for future physical therapists to interact with some of the most brilliant innovators of our profession.

In 2008, the honoree was Stanley Paris, PT, PhD, FAPTA, the founder of the APTA Orthopedic Section and its first president. The list of Paris's professional accomplishments alone is staggering and includes authorship of numerous books and articles on the topic of manual PT. He has received our profession's top honors, including the Mary McMillan Lectureship (2006) and designation as an APTA Catherine Worthingham Fellow. This award gives the honoree the distinguished title of "Fellow of the American Physical Therapy Association" (which is noted by the letters FAPTA).

Paris's personal life is equally underscored by numerous accomplishments. He has twice swum the English Channel, sailed around the world, and completed the World Championship Ironman Triathlon. In 2008, at the age of 70, Paris attempted to become the oldest person to swim the English Channel. In an extraordinary gesture of professional self-sacrifice and goodwill, Paris took on this mission as a way to raise money for the APTA Foundation for Physical Therapy (which provides grants for professional research). Paris explained his reasoning behind this generous gesture in his online weblog[1]: "My life's passion is taking on challenges and succeeding by planning well and by displaying tenacity. I have done it all my life in sports and have applied it to my professional and business careers."

Unfortunately Paris was unsuccessful in his swimming attempt. Nevertheless, he was instrumental in raising considerable support for research. Foundation President Richard Shields, PT, PhD, FAPTA, lauded Paris for his efforts in securing funds that will "create possibilities for physical therapist researchers to push the boundaries of science while, most importantly, improving the quality of life and well-being of the patients we serve every day."[2]

Paris's actions are a compelling demonstration of *engaged professionalism*, in which a cohesive set of values allows the seamless integration of life and work for the benefit of others. When our ideals overlap in this way, it becomes easier to prioritize the demands of our lives as well the resources they require. As you will discover in the coming sections, a significant aspect of maintaining our engagement is the effective management of our personal, emotional, and physical resources.[3] When all elements of our lives are guided by consistent values, it becomes easier to determine the best use of our resources, as the example of Stanley Paris illustrates.

The word *engagement* is probably familiar to us in its most conventional form, that being a public announcement by two individuals of their intent to marry. Embedded in this intent, of course, is a commitment. In a broader sense, the term *engagement* thus is a synonym for a commitment between persons and the people or organizations with whom they interact. In 2000, the PT profession articulated its commitment to society in its 2020 Vision Statement. This commitment includes doctoral-level preparation, the integration of scientific evidence into clinical decision making, and the demonstration of the highest level of professionalism.[4]

As you may already realize, engagement in life and engaged professionalism are interrelated attributes. In order to become agents of change for the good of our profession and society, we must first tend the homes fires of our personal health, energy, and focus. If we view our work as a vital expression of our best selves, then our attitudes, behaviors, and relationships will tend to synchronize in a consistent, self-renewing manner. In contrast, a rigid separation between one's work and personal life has been shown to contribute to dissatisfaction in each.[5] Research suggests that those who can move flexibly and spontaneously between their roles in life and work have a greater sense of balance and satisfaction in both. Workplace initiatives that promote integration between employees' professional and personal lives can be helpful and are becoming more common. These include provision of on-site child care, flexible hours, and opportunities to work from home. In 2004, the Center for Work-Life Policy was established as a means of "designing, promoting and implementing policies that enhance productivity and enhance personal/family wellbeing."[6] **Figure 2–1** shows the flow of engagement between life and work.

Talking Points/Field Notes

My Best Attributes for Life Engagement and Engaged Professionalism

Reflect on three of your best personal qualities. Consider traits that have been acknowledged by your friends, family members, or coworkers or traits that you are proud of. Address the following questions either through a small group discussion and/or through reflection in your field notes.

1. Describe these qualities. How well have they served you in both your personal and work life (or student role) thus far?

2. How have you adapted these traits for appropriate use in each situation?

3. How have you developed these traits in each situation?

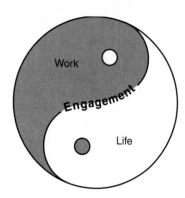

Figure 2–1. The flow of engagement between work and life promotes satisfaction in both realms.

Engagement and Engaged Professionalism Are Driven by Values

Values are sets of attitudes that guide our interactions in all contexts of our lives. Consequently the nature of our values also guides our behaviors and their consequences. Thus if we are driven by greed, we may accumulate material wealth at the expense of our relationships. If we are driven by compassion, we may seek a life of service to others.

Two classes of values have been identified.[7] *Terminal values* pertain to desired life outcomes (such as accumulation of wealth or social recognition) and *instrumental values* relate to everyday modes of behavior (such as kindness), which presumably lead to the desired end. If our instrumental values are not line with our terminal ones, it is unlikely that our daily actions will lead us toward the life we desire. An example of this might be a person whose long-term desire for optimal health is undermined by the immediate gratification of a fast-food diet. **Boxes** 2-1 and 2-2 illustrate examples of these values.

BOX 2-1:   Values for Life and Work

1. A meaningful career
2. Financial success
3. Prestige and recognition
4. Use of talents and abilities
5. A supportive work environment (supervisors, colleagues)
6. Freedom to make decisions and direct work
7. Opportunities for promotion and advancement
8. Opportunities for new learning
9. Security and stability
10. Interesting challenges
11. Flexible work hours
12. Vibrant physical health and fitness
13. A strong social network
14. Pleasurable hobbies and interests
15. A comfortable home
16. A strong sense of spirituality
17. A loving family
18. Physical attractiveness
19. A pleasant city or community in which to live
20. Opportunities for travel
21. A safe and peaceful world
22. OTHER (add as desired)

BOX 2-2:   Personal Values for Everyday Interactions

1. Loyalty
2. Honesty
3. Trustworthiness
4. Dependability
5. Compassion
6. Assertiveness
7. Enthusiasm
8. Commitment
9. Tenacity
10. Affection
11. Humor
12. Equanimity
13. Confidence
14. Competence
15. Optimism
16. Joyfulness
17. Pleasure
18. Humility
19. Wisdom
20. Open-mindedness
21. Fairness
22. Popularity
23. Creativity
24. Courageousness
25. Freedom
26. OTHER (add as desired)

The link between values and actions is so compelling that many professions, including medicine[8] and nursing,[9] have adopted their own sets of guiding *core values*. In the context of our discussion, it can be said that core values are a set of guiding ideals that support engaged professionalism in a specific discipline.

In 2003, the APTA board of directors adopted a consensus-based document including seven professional core values describing "what the graduate of a physical therapist program and the individual practitioner ought to be demonstrating in their daily practice that would reflect professionalism."[10] **Table 2-1** lists the seven core values of the American Physical Therapy Association.

The APTA Core Values document includes a self-assessment that helps physical therapists determine how they are integrating the related behaviors in the context of their work. In the following exercise, you will have the opportunity to identify the core values of your own life-work situation.

Talking Points/Field Notes

My Core Values for Engagement

Review the values listed in **Tables 2-1** and **2-2**. Rank your top 10 values in each table. Then consider your ideal life 5 years from now as you answer the following questions. Do this individually at first (you can write these in your field notes). Then, if you are comfortable sharing your ideas, discuss them in a small group.

1. Where are you working? Consider the setting (acute care, orthopedics, etc.).

2. What are your primary responsibilities?

3. What are you most proud of in your work?

4. What are you most excited about in your work?

5. What do you enjoy most about your work?

6. What are your work goals?

7. Where are you living?

8. Who are you with?

9. What are the other valuable elements of your life (hobbies, interests, new experiences, etc.)?

10. What is the most important thing in your life?

As you answer these questions, consider the role of your prioritized values. How might they guide you for optimal work-life success? How might they challenge you (e.g., if you ranked honesty as a top value, how might you respond in a work setting where your supervisor asked you to bill patients in a fraudulent manner?). Consider how your values might inform your choices with respect to working and living in general. Finally, consider the happiest persons you know. What examples does he or she provide about the role of values in optimal life-work engagement?

Table 2–1.	**The Seven Core Values of the American Physical Therapy Association**
Accountability	Active acceptance of the responsibility for the diverse roles, obligations, and actions of the physical therapist including self-regulation and other behaviors that positively influence patient/client outcomes, the profession, and the health needs of society.
Altruism	Primary regard for or devotion to the interest of patients/clients, thus assuming the fiduciary responsibility of placing the needs of the patient/client ahead of the physical therapists' self-interest.
Compassion and caring	Compassion is the desire to identify with or sense something of another's experience; a precursor of caring. Caring is the concern, empathy, and consideration for the needs and values of others.
Excellence	PT practice that consistently uses current knowledge and theory while understanding personal limits, integrates judgment and the patient/client perspective, challenges mediocrity, and works toward the development of new knowledge.
Integrity	The possession of and steadfast adherence to high ethical principles or professional standards.
Professional duty	The commitment to meeting one's obligations to provide effective physical therapy services to individual patients/clients, to serve the profession, and to positively influence the health of society.
Social responsibility	The promotion of mutual trust between the profession and the larger public, which necessitates responding to societal needs for health and wellness.

Used with permission of the American Physical Therapy Association.

Communication Is the Medium of Engaged Professionalism

Effective communication is the vehicle by which we convey the elements of engaged professionalism in our dialogues with self and others. Consider the various levels of dialogue that must be addressed in order to maintain an empowering outlook through which we feel capable of making positive contributions in our various life roles. This empowerment originates from within and pertains to our *internal communication*. Internal communication consists of our mental dialogue with self, through which we view our lives as vibrant with optimism at best or darkly pessimistic at worst. Not surprisingly, engaged individuals have learned to harness their self-talk toward a more optimistic orientation, which promotes self-efficacy and goal attainment. Because few goals are met solely through our own efforts, we must also be effective in our *external communication*, through which we gain support for our vision in the context of interpersonal dialogue. For example, although Stanley Paris's goal to swim the English Channel was born from his internal passion and sense of possibility, he required the support of many individuals to help him attempt this. Thus, in order to gain such support, effective external communication skills are essential. Finally, the ability to educate others and negotiate needs (in Paris's case, financial support from his colleagues at St. Augustine University) are elements of *instrumental communication,* in which internal and external dialogues become the instruments of positive change. As you move through this text, you will find each of these levels explored in detail, and you will be guided to continue developing them in service of a life and a career that you love. Keeping in mind that the profession of PT is grounded in evidence, it is important to recognize that the concept of engagement is gaining considerable validation through a body of scientific knowledge known as *positive psychology*.

Table 2–2. Classification of 6 Virtues and 24 Character Strengths

Virtue/Strength	Description
Wisdom and knowledge	**Cognitive strengths that facilitate learning and use of knowledge**
Creativity	Thinking of novel and productive ways to do things
Curiosity	Taking an interest in all ongoing experiences
Love of learning	Mastering new skills and bodies of knowledge
Perspective	Being able to provide wise counsel to others
Courage	**Emotional strengths involving the exercise of will to accomplish goals in the face of opposition**
Authenticity	Speaking the truth and presenting oneself in a genuine way
Bravery	NOT shrinking from threat, challenge, difficulty, or pain
Persistence	Finishing what one starts
Zest	Approaching life with excitement and energy
Humanity	**Interpersonal strengths that involve "tending and befriending" others**
Kindness	Doing favors and good deeds for others
Love	Valuing close relationships with others
Social intelligence	Being aware of the motives and feelings of self and others
Justice	**Civic strengths that underlie healthy community life**
Fairness	Treating all people the same according to the notions of fairness and justice
Leadership	Organizing group activities and seeing that they happen
Teamwork	Working well as a member of a group or team
Temperance	**Strengths that protect against excess**
Forgiveness	Forgiving those that have done wrong
Modesty	Letting ones accomplishments speak for themselves
Prudence	Care of ones choices, not saying or doing anything that might later be regretted
Self-regulation	Regulating what one does and feels
Transcendence	**Strengths that forge connections to the larger universe and provide meaning**
Appreciation of beauty	Noticing and appreciating beauty, excellence, and/or skilled performance in all domains of life
Gratitude	Being aware and thankful for good things that occur
Hope	Expecting the best and hoping to achieve it
Humor	Liking to laugh and tease, bring smiles to others
Religiousness	Beliefs about the higher purpose and meaning of Life

From Seligman MEP, Steen TA , Park N, Peterson C. Positive psychology progress: Empirical validation of interventions. *Am Psychol.* 60(5):410, 2005. Courtesy of the American Psychological Association.

Elements of Engaged Professionalism

Optimal Psychological Health: The Study of Positive Psychology

In recent years, the health and social sciences have broadened their areas of study to include not only the examination of dysfunction and illness but also the elements that constitute the highest levels of human function. A solid understanding of the limits of human performance (or what we can strive for) is particularly important in determining the effectiveness of therapeutic interventions. Accordingly, the science of PT involves the delivery of therapeutic interventions that maximize quality of life through the achievement of optimal physical function. In the area discipline of psychology, this includes the study of what constitutes optimal emotional health and mental functioning. Thus, the area of *positive psychology* is devoted to the scientific exploration of attitudes and behaviors that contribute to life satisfaction, happiness, and enjoyment in all life roles (i.e., hobbies, family, work, community).

Until the advent of this positive emphasis, the field of psychology was largely invested in the study of mental illness and dysfunction. In the years after World War II, this emphasis was further validated by preferential grant funding from newly formed government agencies such as the Veterans Administration (1946) and the National Institute for Mental Health (1947).[11] In the 1950s and '60s, a few psychologists attempted to promote happiness through the field of "popular psychology" (also known as "pop psych"), but sadly, many of the related theories and treatments were disseminated to the public in the form of "self-help" books, with little evidence for their support.

In 1998, Martin Seligman became the president of the American Psychological Association and dedicated his tenure in this role to the study of optimal mental health. Since that time, he has published over 200 articles and 20 books in this area. These scientific publications provide compelling evidence for the support of positive psychology theory and intervention. Of particular interest is the study of factors related to engagement and work-life satisfaction. This knowledge can thus promote the facilitation of these virtues in the workplace.

Positive psychology also employs an individual focus, having recently identified six virtues and 24 character strengths related to optimal psychological function (see **Table 2-2**).

Seligman and colleagues have also developed and validated methods by which each of us can develop these optimal virtues and attitudes for happiness and life-role satisfaction. In a 2005 randomized clinical trial of 577 subjects, they explored the impact of five specific interventions and one control exercise on self-ratings of happiness and depression.[12] Three of the exercises were found to have a significant impact on increasing happiness and decreasing depressive symptoms for up to 6 months. One of these interventions (which they called the *gratitude visit*) involved writing and personally delivering a letter of gratitude to a person whose kindness had not ever been acknowledged. Another exercise involved writing down three good things that had occurred each day for a week.

Seligman also founded the Positive Psychology Center at the University of Pennsylvania, where he and his colleagues continue to develop and explore interventions for optimal happiness and well-being. Any interested persons can take any one of the several measures of optimal functioning and even participate in ongoing research by registering on Seligman's University of Pennsylvania website.[13] The most exciting evidence from positive psychology suggests that to a considerable degree, *we can consciously change our attitudes and outlook in a positive direction.*[14] As you will discover, this finding is of major importance for our study of communication, because *our attitudes and outlook are largely a result of our internal communication.*

Because most adults spend a significant number of their waking hours engaged in some form of work, a growing area of focus in positive psychology is the exploration of factors related to job satisfaction. The following discussion describes many of these factors.

Intrinsic and Extrinsic Factors Related to Engagement

In the increasingly competitive and demanding arena of health care, concerns about productivity have become increasingly important. Because growing evidence supports engagement as a major contributing factor to productivity, managers have increasingly directed attention toward the development of workplace environments that promote employee satisfaction.

Environmental elements are generally considered external or "extrinsic" factors and relate to things such as salary, job security, company policies, and working conditions. Thus, engagement can be increased to a considerable degree by pleasant surroundings, a good income, and options for flexible work hours. In addition, recognition in the form of awards and public acknowledgment can also help to maintain workplace morale and engagement. For example, one supervisor colleague instituted a "Blue Hippo" award in her PT department as a humorous but sincere effort to recognize individual staff efforts. The award became a beloved tradition within the department as staff members looked forward to finding the blue rubber creature on a different desk each month.

In addition to extrinsic elements in the workplace, a significant proportion of engagement and motivation arises from within. These internal elements are known as "intrinsic factors" and relate, first, to perceptions of the potential for psychological growth and a sense of accomplishment and, second, to a sense of empowerment to achieve such potential. Also included in the realm of intrinsic motivators are the needs for autonomy (to self-direct the scheduling of work and determination of appropriate work methods), competence (the skills to effectively address work-related challenges), and meaning (a sense that the work has a positive effect on others).[15] Research on the relative importance of extrinsic versus intrinsic factors indicates that intrinsic factors are the most important for engagement and work satisfaction. However, this research also indicates that extrinsic factors must also be present at a certain level in order to prevent workers from being frustrated in their efforts to grow professionally.[16,17] For example, a person's intrinsic need for professional development opportunities may be greatly enhanced by a work culture that provides financial support for continuing education. Achieving a balance between extrinsic and intrinsic motivators can be a significant challenge for managers, especially in difficult economic times.

Hardiness: Control, Challenge, and Commitment

In 1984, a model of workplace "hardiness" was developed around three behaviors related to job satisfaction, physical health, and emotional well-being.[18] These are control, challenge, and commitment. In the workplace, these behaviors affect both individuals and the organizations they serve. In addition, the greater spheres of ones profession and society at large can also be affected.

Control

Control pertains to self-efficacy, the perception that one has the ability to "make things happen." With respect to PTs, beginning at the *individual level*, this would involve the behaviors related to managing stress, maintaining healthy personal relationships, and the continuing development of professional competence. At the *organizational level*, this could involve the ability to plan the schedule of patients for the day and to structure the time spent with each one according to his or her needs. It can also include a level of professional autonomy—that is, the ability to make decisions related to each patient's plan of care. At the *professional level*, this could involve membership and support of APTA, for example, serving on a state task force to determine fair reimbursement for PT services by insurance companies. At the *societal level*, this could include community involvement, such as providing scoliosis screening in the elementary schools of your city.

Each of us knows the sense of satisfaction that results when we are able to make a positive change within our scope of influence. This satisfaction is a large component of engagement. Accordingly, most physical therapists will tell you that their greatest source of professional satisfaction is the ability to make a difference in lives of their patients.

Challenge

Challenge can be defined as striving (being engaged) toward a novel task that is viewed as being slightly beyond one's current capability. Obviously, if the task is totally familiar or easily accomplished, the sense of striving is lost, and thus also the sense of challenge. An example of a reasonable challenge might be the decision by a healthy but sedentary person to take up jogging for exercise, with the goal of completing a 1-mile run within 2 weeks. On the other hand, if this same person decided to complete a 26-mile marathon within 2 weeks, the likely result would be stress, a sense of being overwhelmed, and finally disengagement from the goal. Jobs with the lowest levels of satisfaction often involve continuous repetition of work that is not challenging. Thus the obvious result is boredom, frustration, and disengagement.

Commitment

Commitment is the sustained dedication of one's attention and efforts toward a person or endeavor. One of the most important ways we demonstrate commitment is through communication. In the workplace, the commitment of those in leadership toward those they serve must be considered genuine and actively demonstrated in valuable ways. At the individual level, most physical therapists commit to maintaining the highest possible level of competence. At the organizational and professional levels, physical therapists commit to providing their patients with positive regard and competent care. At a societal level, APTA has made the commitment to be the provider of choice for disorders affecting movement, function, and quality of life.

Energy Resources

As you will quickly learn in your work as a physical therapist, your patients' most valuable resource for the accomplishment of functional tasks (which will vary tremendously in terms of each individual's goals) will be their ability to apply physical, emotional, cognitive, and spiritual *energy* toward their rehabilitation effort. If you have ever attempted to attend class with a bad cold or other illness (a behavior that your professors and classmates will likely discourage), you can surely understand how the resultant lack of energy affects your learning.

The concept of energy as the major currency of engagement is receiving increasing attention in the United States, where employees have the longest work week in the industrialized world.[19] When coupled with our relentless emphasis on productivity and top performance, it is easy to see how many workers are simply unable to muster the energy to sustain their efforts. The result can be fatigue, burnout, and disengagement.

Thus an important approach to maintaining full engagement is to take care of ourselves in order to optimize our energy resources.[3] This "resource management" approach involves the integration of the same health-supporting behaviors that you will soon be promoting in your patients: adequate rest, stress management, good nutrition, exercise, and the cultivation of a healthy belief system that supports a sense of meaning. As you well know if you practice any of these behaviors, they produce results that are well worth the effort.

In managing our resources, we often benefit from the encouragement of others. Thus effective communication also has a key place in enabling us to direct our energies toward desired outcomes in all areas of our lives. The same is true for our patients.

Field Notes/Talking Points

My Energy Resource Management Program

1. What activities do you engage in to cultivate your energy in the following areas?

   a. Physical energy: all aspects physical well-being

   b. Emotional: an outlook that promotes freedom from undue stress and cultivates peace, happiness, and optimism

   c. Mental: focus, attention, memory for learning

   d. Spiritual: beliefs that give meaning and purpose to your life

2. In what ways do these activities enhance the quality of your life?

3. What goals might you have to sustain your energy resources during the course of your PT education? Describe these and consider a realistic plan for their achievement.

Clinical Scenario

Exploring Resources in the Context of the Patient Interview

Rachel is a 32-year-old mother of three children between the ages of 2 and 7. She is not currently employed outside the home. Rachel arrives at your outpatient PT clinic for a fitness assessment and training program. The results of your assessment indicate that she is healthy, with no risk factors or conditions that would prevent her from full participation in an exercise program. Rachel is motivated to begin an exercise program but mentions that she is often to too tired and busy to do so.

Discuss the following with a partner:

1. What questions from you might help Rachel explore realistic options for exercise?

2. What energy resources are important for Rachel to maintain in order to meet the demands of her day? How might you explore this with her?

3. How do you explore exercise options with Rachel?

4. Describe a way in which Rachel might fit some level of exercise into her busy life.

As this discussion has demonstrated, many studies have explored the construct of engagement, and each has contributed important insights suggesting that engagement is the interaction of several contributing elements. These are summarized in **Table 2-3**.

Having examined these characteristics, let us now direct our attention to how these might play out in the PT workplace.

Table 2–3. Factors Contributing to Engagement in the Workplace

Individual Factors	Work Resources	Work Features
Interest in work	Social support from colleagues and supervisors	Autonomy/control
Joy in one's work	Coaching and mentorship	Interesting variety of tasks
Conscientiousness (ability to be thorough, organized, goal-directed)	Feedback on performance	Ability to identify work tasks and complete to one's satisfaction
Commitment to mission of organization	Availability of challenges, opportunities for growth	Perceived task importance
Skills and competence	Time	
Desire for growth	Tools/equipment	
Virtues and character strengths		
Physical resources to meet work requirements (energy endurance, strength)		

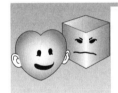

Champ and Blockhead Go to Work

The 6:30 alarm goes off in two separate apartments inhabited by two different PTs. Each of them has been out of PT school for 2 years.

Champ eagerly bounds out of bed, ready to begin his day working as a staff physical therapist in the burn unit of his city's major teaching hospital. He chose physical therapy after working as a PT tech and seeing the impact the staff therapists had on their patients' lives. After graduating from PT school, he carefully sought employment in a setting where he would be able to continue learning, receive mentorship, and find professional opportunities for advancement. This morning, he will provide an in-service presentation to the student interns in the PT department and then treat patients for the rest of the day. After work, he plans to join some colleagues for a 45-minute jog and some dinner before spending the evening at his local APTA district meeting, where he is leading a journal club. Champ is exploring new interventions for burn care and would like to do an interdisciplinary project on functional outcome measures in burn rehabilitation. He loves his work as a PT and enjoys sharing his ideas with colleagues, students, and fellow team members. He feels appreciated for his contributions and that he has regular opportunities to make a positive impact on his patients. He enjoys mentoring the many PT students who come through the department and plans to become an APTA credentialed clinical instructor within the next year. He is grateful to be a physical therapist and sees himself as staying in the profession for many years ahead.

Continued

Blockhead is not so eager to begin his day. He entered the PT profession because he was told that he could do very well financially and work without anyone telling him what to do. He didn't bother to learn about the profession before applying to PT school, but being naturally very intelligent, he had good grades that easily gained him acceptance into a program. Right out of PT school, he looked for a job that would give him the highest salary and the ability to be his own boss. Without too much difficulty, Blockhead found a high-paying job as the sole therapist in a small community hospital outpatient clinic. Unfortunately, in his eagerness to accept this position, he failed to ask about its requirements. Now, much to his dismay, he is required to see at least 30 patients a day per the productivity standards of the corporation that hired him. With no one to mentor him, Blockhead makes patient-care decisions based on what he remembers from his academic program. Because he is saving money to buy an expensive car, he does not belong to APTA (he thinks the dues are too high) and has not been to a continuing education course since graduation. Blockhead finds himself increasingly overwhelmed and disinterested in his work. He has recently begun to experience problems sleeping and has found that he is usually too tired to eat well or to exercise. He is also starting to regret his decision to become a physical therapist.

Consider:

1. Which factors in each job would enhance your motivation and engagement?
2. Which factors in each job would decrease your motivation and engagement?
3. What justification might you have for taking either job?
4. What suggestions might you have for Blockhead in order to increase his engagement?

Perhaps, while you were reading this discussion on engagement, you thought of persons in your own life who exemplify the best and worst of this attribute. As a future physical therapist and member of the workforce, you might also wonder what to expect in terms of the overall engagement levels of its members, both within and without our profession. The following discussion explores these questions and provides some encouraging insights.

Engagement in the U.S. Workforce

In 2001, the Gallup Organization published a study examining engagement in the U.S. workforce, using a measure called the "Gallup Q12 Employee Engagement Survey."[20]

The Q12 is a copyrighted assessment and training tool consisting of 12 questions that highlight various elements related to engagement in the workplace. Thise tool can be used to assess the level of employee engagement or to help managers develop this attribute in the persons they supervise. Examination of the Q12 indicates that the constructs of control, challenge, and commitment are addressed within the 12 questions. For example, control is explored in terms of whether the employee knows what is expected; commitment is measured by the perceived presence of committed colleagues; and challenge is related to the availability of opportunities for learning. Using this tool, the Gallup study identified three levels of engagement and the number of U.S. workers in each:

1. **Engaged employees:** These individuals feel a connection to their workplace. They feel supported and encouraged to be innovative and to move their workplace forward. According to the Gallup study, *28% of the U.S. workforce fell into this category in 2001.*

2. **Unengaged employees:** These individuals are "checked out" and are merely putting in their time without an investment of energy toward improving their workplace situation. According to the Gallup study, *54% of the U.S. workforce fell into this category in 2001.*

3. **Actively disengaged employees:** These individuals are visibly unhappy in their workplace. They spread their discontent and undermine the efforts of their colleagues. According to the Gallup study, *17% of the U.S. workforce fell into this category in 2001.*

The study went on to say that actively disengaged employees were absent from work 3.5 more days a year than other workers, for a total 86.5 million days. Furthermore, the study suggested that "actively disengaged" employees who are fundamentally disconnected from their jobs cost the U.S. economy between $292 and $355 billion a year.

Engagement in the Physical Therapy Profession

What are the implications of this study for PT? It should be obvious that disengagement could have serious consequences in terms of the quality of patient care. Accordingly, data on physical therapists who have been reported to their state boards for licensure infractions suggests that physical therapists who work alone, who do not belong to APTA, and who do not regularly attend continuing education are more likely to have complaints lodged against them (which can result in legal sanctions, including the loss of licensure).

On a more positive side, physical therapists as a whole demonstrate that they are engaged in their work. In one study,[21] 88% of 164 PT graduates from one program indicated that if they had to choose their careers all over again, they would choose PT.

On a broader scale, in a 2007 study by the National Opinion Research Center (NORC) at the University of Chicago, *physical therapists ranked second of all professions in the level of their job satisfaction,* with more than 75% reporting that they were "very satisfied."[22] This finding was based on data from over 27,500 randomly selected individuals who had been surveyed since 1988. An excerpt of the study findings is shown in **Table 2-4.**

The director of this survey, which was supported by the National Science Foundation, was quoted as saying, "the most satisfying jobs are . . . those involving caring for, teaching, or protecting others." Perhaps one of the most telling findings of the survey was the revelation that persons who are highly satisfied with their work view their careers as "callings"; they have a sense that a part of their life purpose is to do such work. To this end, a physical therapist with 23 years of experience was quoted as saying, "I believe that I was probably

Table 2–4.   Job Satisfaction Rankings From the National Opinion Research Center Study of 27,500 Americans

Rank	Highest Job Satisfaction	Lowest Job Satisfaction
1	Clergy	Roofers
2	Physical therapists	Waiters, Servers
3	Firefighters	Laborers (not construction)
4	Education administrators	Bartenders
5	Painters and sculptors	Hand packers and packagers

From Rose B. Money really can't buy happiness, study finds. *Chicago Tribune,* April 17, 2007.

put on this earth to make someone's life a little easier, that's what I get out of my job. I get rewarded every day." The opportunities for involvement in this marvelous profession look very promising. The *Tribune* article also reported that PT is now considered one of the top six best jobs for college graduates because of the increasing demand for services from aging baby boomers (the 80 million persons born between 1946 and 1964).

Engagement "Insurance": Membership in the American Physical Therapy Association

Our discussion about the elements of engagement has examined several features including feedback, mentorship, and networking with colleagues. While supportive relationships with colleagues in our own workplace can be tremendously valuable, it is easy to develop a sense of professional tunnel vision if that is the sole arena of interaction. Especially in times of significant change or challenge, membership in the national professional organization can provide an invaluable source of information and support. One of the most valuable ways to network with colleagues is by being a member of our national professional organization, APTA. As you will hopefully discover in your future, membership in APTA has countless benefits; a recent study suggested that one of these includes the enhancement of job satisfaction.

In the past several years, one of the most significant sources of professional upheaval was the Balanced Budget Act of 1997, which included a legislative initiative to produce a $40 billion reduction in Medicare payments to health-care providers. These initiatives resulted in widespread closures of skilled nursing facilities, which negatively affected PTs through job layoffs, mandatory salary cuts, and a decrease in employee benefits.

In 2000, APTA published the results of its annual member employment survey, which provides important information about the demographics and work patterns of the profession. The 2000 report examined these variables during the tumultuous and demoralizing period immediately following the Balanced Budget Act. Nevertheless, one of the most provocative findings of this report was the discovery of significantly higher levels of job satisfaction among APTA members compared with nonmembers. In addition, APTA members experienced less "job turbulence" than nonmembers, indicating that membership in the organization, along with the inherent opportunities for networking and peer support, provided a stabilizing influence that helped to maintain engagement.[23]

Implications for You as a Physical Therapy Student

You are entering a marvelous profession that has a demonstrated legacy of engaged practitioners. As the body of knowledge increases and the demands for our services escalate, you will be called to direct your engagement at three levels—individual, professional, and societal (see Figure 2–1). Communication will be the most important tool helping you to succeed in this endeavor.

In the next chapter, using the elements of engagement described previously, we begin our exploration of communication from the internal assessment of our strengths and resources. From there, we go on to explore how to develop these and share them with others. Again, and always, *this is a process embedded in our communication.*

Implications for PT Practice

1. As PTs, we can enhance our engagement first by appropriate self-care and then by continuously seeking opportunities to learn and grow. We can also support our

professional engagement by involvement in APTA, participation in continuing education, and seeking work settings in line with our interests and values.

2. Effective communication is the vehicle whereby we can demonstrate and enhance our engagement as well as that of our patients.

Chapter Summary

1. Engagement is the ability to direct personal virtues and energy resources toward efforts that challenge and empower us.
2. The study of positive psychology can help us to cultivate attitudes and virtues that support engagement.
3. The concepts of control, commitment, and challenge describe attributes that promote engagement in our endeavors.
4. Being fully engaged in our work allows us to be positive agents of change for the good of ourselves, our profession, and society at large.

Take-Home Menu

1. Engagement Interview

A. With a classmate, interview a person (a physical therapist if possible) who enjoys his or her work. Using the information presented in this chapter, inquire about the following:
   – The features of the workplace that promote engagement
   – The challenges he or she is enjoying
   – How much freedom this person has to direct his or her efforts
   – This person's attitudes about the value of the work
   – How he or she manages energy for the best

B. After the interview, reflect on the results by discussing your findings with a group of classmates. What similarities emerged? What can you learn from these engaged persons?

2. Further Learning Opportunities in Positive Psychology

If you are interested in learning more about positive psychology, Dr. Martin Seligman has two related websites that can provide further information. They are:

A. http://www.authentichappiness.sas.upenn.edu/ This website provides information on web-based educational programs for increasing personal happiness, resilience, and engagement. You can also participate in Dr. Seligman's research related to positive psychology.

B. http://www.ppc.sas.upenn.edu/ppquestionnaires.htm. This website provides a list of assessments pertaining to various elements of positive psychology. Many of these are available to take online.

3. Professional Engagement Exercise: Get Involved in the APTA

A. Attend the next meeting of your state or local chapter of the APTA with some (or all!) of your classmates. This is a marvelous opportunity to begin learning about the issues, challenges, and opportunities that await you in your profession. Make it a point to talk to at least one therapist that you don't know, and learn more about the value of APTA membership.

B. Learn more about opportunities for student involvement in the APTA. The APTA website— http://www.apta.org—has a specific link to student information. Share this with classmates and discuss ways in which you can become involved in these activities (including the Student Assembly and the Student Conclave).

References

1. Paris on La Manche: Stanley Paris's attempt at becoming the oldest person to swim the English Channel ("La Manche"), made to benefit physical therapy. February 6, 2008. http://stanleyparis.blogspot.com/2008_02_01_archive.html. Accessed January 25 2009.

2. PT makes record English Channel swim attempt. July 28, 2008. http://www.apta.org/AM/Template.cfm?Section=Home&CONTENTID=50671&TEMPLATE=/CM/ContentDisplay.cfm. Accessed January 25 2009.

3. Loehr J, Schwartz T. *The Power of Full Engagement.* New York: Free Press; 2003.

4. American Physical Therapy Association: Vision 2020: http://www.apta.org/AM/Template.cfm?Section=Vision_20201&Template=/TaggedPage/TaggedPageDisplay.cfm&TPLID=285&ContentID=32061. Accessed December 5, 2008.

5. Bulger CA, Matthews RA, Hoffman ME. Work and personal life boundary management: Boundary strength, work/personal life balance, and the segmentation-integration continuum. *J Occup Health Psychol.* 1997;12(4):365-375.

6. Center for Work-Life Policy: Mission Statement: http://www.worklifepolicy.org/index.php/pageID/26. Accessed December 5, 2008.

7. Johnston CS. The Rokeach Value Survey: underlying structure and multidimensional scaling. *J Psychol.* 1995;129:583-598.

8. Howie JGR, Heaney D, and Maxwell M. Quality, core values and the general practice consultation: Issues of definition, measurement and delivery. *Fam Pract.* 2004;21(4):458-468.

9. National League for Nursing. Core Values: http://www.nln.org/aboutnln/corevalues.htm. Accessed December 3, 2008.

10. American Physical Therapy Association. Professionalism in Physical Therapy: Core Values: http://www.apta.org/AM/Template.cfm?Section=Search&section=Leadership&template=/CM/ContentDisplay.cfm&ContentFileID=287. Accessed December 3, 2008.

11. Gable SL, Haidt J. What (and why) is positive psychology? *Rev Gen Psychol.* 2005;9(2):103-110.

12. Seligman MEP, Steen TA, Park N, Peterson C. Positive psychology progress: Empirical validation of interventions. *Am Psychol.* 2005;60(5):410-421.

13. University of Pennsylvania. Positive Psychology Center: http://www.authentichappiness.sas.upenn.edu/register.aspx Accessed December 5, 2008.

14. Seligman MEP, Csikszentmihalyi M. Positive psychology: An introduction. *Am Psychol.* 2000;55(1):5-14.

15. Deci EL, Moller AC. The concept of competence: A starting place for understanding intrinsic motivation and self-determined extrinsic motivation. In: *Handbook of Competence and Motivation.* New York: Guilford; 2005.

16. Herzberg F. *Work and the Nature of Man.* New York: Thomas Y. Crowell; 1966.

17. Carroll E, Dwyer L. The shortage of nurses in NSW: A motivation-hygiene approach to identifying problems and solutions. *Aust Health Rev.* 1998;11(1):4-20.

18. Kobasa S, Maddi S. *The Hardy Executive: Health Under Stress.* Homewood, IL: Dow-Jones Irwin; 1984.

19. CNN. Study: U.S. employees put in the most hours. CNN.Com/Career August 31, 2001. http://archives. cnn.com/2001/CAREER/trends/08/30/ilo.study/. Accessed August 30, 2007.

20. Thackray J. Feedback for Real. *Gallup Management Journal*, March 15, 2001. http://gmj.gallup.com/ content/default.aspx?ci=811. Accessed June 29, 2007.

21. Mueller K. Take this job and love it: Factors related to job satisfaction and career commitment among physical therapists. (Platform presentation, 14th Congress of the World Confederation for Physical Therapy. Barcelona, Spain. June 2003.)

22. Rose B. Money really can't buy happiness, study finds. *Chicago Tribune.* April 17, 2007.

23. American Physical Therapy Association. Survey shows that members are faring better than nonmembers. *PT Bulletin Online.* May 5, 2000;1(17): http://www.apta.org/ AM/Template.cfm?Section=Archives2&Template=/ Customsource/TaggedPage/PTIssue.cfm&Issue=05/05/ 2000#article7979. Accessed July 10, 2007.

CHAPTER 3

YOU on a Mission: Charting Your Course of Engaged Professionalism

The more faithfully you listen to the voice within you,
the better you will hear what is sounding outside.
Only he who listens can speak.

Dag Hammarskjold

Chapter Overview

Most adults spend many of their waking hours engaged in some form of work. How can the quality of this time be optimized so that it is both enjoyable and productive? This chapter begins with an exploration of elements related to the identification of a satisfying line of work, which is the foundation of engaged professionalism.

In the context of work, most adults have jobs, many have careers, and some have a mission. What is the difference? This chapter explores the attitudes and values that differentiate these, providing you with examples and exercises to help you identify and articulate your life-work mission more clearly. Understanding your mission will help you optimize both internal and external communication toward the achievement of your life-work goals.

Key Terms

Holland code	Mission statement
Meyers-Briggs	SWOT analysis

What Is Your Life Calling You to Do?

As you move through the years, you will be confronted with many questions that arise from the convergence of external events in your life and your innermost desires. One of the most important of these will concern the matter of your role and purpose in the provision of service to others. For most of us, this involves the selection of a line of work. As tempting as a life of leisure may sometimes appear, the happiest and most fulfilled individuals are those who have, in the words of the humanitarian physician Dr. Albert Schweitzer, "sought and found a way to serve."[1]

Your decision to pursue a physical therapy (PT) career is likely based on many factors.

Some of us may have discovered our answer early in our lives, perhaps as the result of a life-changing event that led us quite dramatically to our decision. Others may have been attracted to the profession after exploring other less satisfying options.

The stories of how these decisions were made are often revealed during the interview process for PT school. In that context, many applicants speak poignantly of being inspired to choose this profession because of an injury or illness that led them to seek PT intervention. Others talk of being compelled to the same choice after volunteering in a PT department.

Regardless of how these individuals were led to our profession, their inspiring stories suggest that applicants make this career choice *primarily* because of their interactions with engaged physical therapists who passionately demonstrate the rich opportunities our profession offers for making a difference in people's lives. Physical therapists who are so excited about their work that they encourage others to join them are compelling ambassadors of engaged professionalism.

Obviously, not every person who interacts with a physical therapist decides to pursue a career in our profession. In the course of your life thus far, you have undoubtedly interacted with members of numerous professions without aspiring to pursue any of them. Thus, on some level, the opportunities of PT practice resonate with the elements of your personality that seek expression in your work. These elements often come to the fore in the inspired moment where you declare, "I could do that!" This sense of connection with a line of work is no accident and is, in fact, a strong indication that you have found a launching pad for your mission.

As you finish your academic studies and internships, you will further define your place in the PT profession. For example, decisions related to practice setting, specialty area, and your level of professional involvement await you. How will you best direct your interests and energies for a lifetime of engaged professionalism? In other words, how will you serve?

Work as an Expression of Self

Research on career satisfaction indicates that an effective vocational choice involves an optimal "goodness of fit"[2] between the personality of the individual and the demands of a given profession. This concept is the cornerstone of career-choice theory. A significant body of evidence from this area suggests that the closer the match between personal characteristics and job expectations, the greater the likelihood of success, a high level of productivity, and satisfaction.[2]

Psychologist John Holland describes six personality types that seek expression in a choice of work. For each individual, the predominant two or three personality traits of these six (which include realistic, artistic, investigative, social, enterprising, and conventional) constitute their "Holland code." For example, a person with artistic, social, and investigative traits would have a code of "ASI."[3] In turn, this code would direct the individual to the best professions for those traits.

The six personality types, descriptions, and related work areas are listed in **Table 3-1**.

Research on the personality traits of college freshmen aspiring to a career in medicine has demonstrated a prevalence of investigative, social, and artistic personality types.[2] One study of 73 Canadian PT students demonstrated a collective SAI Holland code (social, artistic, intellectual).[4]

Many universities use the Holland Codes as part of their career counseling service program. In several of these programs, students with investigative and social codes are directed towards a career in physical therapy.[5–7]

Table 3–1. Holland's Six Personality Types: Descriptions and Sample Career Choices

Type	Characteristics	Emphasis	Careers
Investigative (thinker)	Intellectual, analytical, curious, independent, scholarly	Working with **ideas** and **things**	Medicine, science, engineering, law, technology, education
Artistic (creator)	Expressive, original, nonconformist, creative, complicated	Working with **ideas** and **people**	Performing arts, graphic design, expressive therapies, author
Social (helper)	Humanistic, collaborative, communicative, helpful, inspiring	Working with **people**	Teaching, health care, counseling, clergy, coaching
Realistic (doer)	Practical, hands-on, physical, mechanically minded, athletic	Working with **things**	Mechanical engineering, law enforcement, information technology, architecture
Enterprising (persuader)	Energetic, sociable, ambitious, risk-taking, persuasive	Working with **data**	Administration, business, investment banking, public relations, retail
Conventional (organizer)	Conscientious, structured, detail-oriented, orderly, precise	Working with **data** and **things**	Accountant, banking, technical writing, clerical, editor

Adapted from Holland J. *Making Vocational Choices: A Theory Of Vocational Personalities and Work Environments.* Lutz, FL: Psychological Assessment Resources, 1997.

Talking Points/Field Notes

Holland Personality Types in Physical Therapy Practice

Consider the following examples of how PTs can apply each of Holland's six personality traits in their work. Rate each of the activities on the following scale:

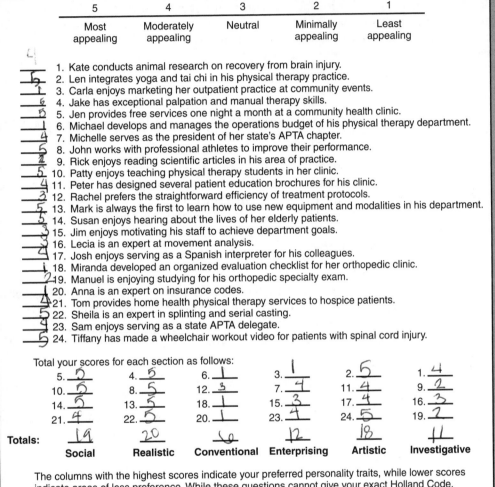

5	4	3	2	1
Most appealing	Moderately appealing	Neutral	Minimally appealing	Least appealing

___ 1. Kate conducts animal research on recovery from brain injury.
_5_ 2. Len integrates yoga and tai chi in his physical therapy practice.
_1_ 3. Carla enjoys marketing her outpatient practice at community events.
_6_ 4. Jake has exceptional palpation and manual therapy skills.
_5_ 5. Jen provides free services one night a month at a community health clinic.
_1_ 6. Michael develops and manages the operations budget of his physical therapy department.
_4_ 7. Michelle serves as the president of her state's APTA chapter.
_5_ 8. John works with professional athletes to improve their performance.
_2_ 9. Rick enjoys reading scientific articles in his area of practice.
_5_ 10. Patty enjoys teaching physical therapy students in her clinic.
_4_ 11. Peter has designed several patient education brochures for his clinic.
_3_ 12. Rachel prefers the straightforward efficiency of treatment protocols.
_5_ 13. Mark is always the first to learn how to use new equipment and modalities in his department.
_5_ 14. Susan enjoys hearing about the lives of her elderly patients.
_3_ 15. Jim enjoys motivating his staff to achieve department goals.
_3_ 16. Lecia is an expert at movement analysis.
_4_ 17. Josh enjoys serving as a Spanish interpreter for his colleagues.
_1_ 18. Miranda developed an organized evaluation checklist for her orthopedic clinic.
_2_ 19. Manuel is enjoying studying for his orthopedic specialty exam.
_1_ 20. Anna is an expert on insurance codes.
_4_ 21. Tom provides home health physical therapy services to hospice patients.
_5_ 22. Sheila is an expert in splinting and serial casting.
_4_ 23. Sam enjoys serving as a state APTA delegate.
_5_ 24. Tiffany has made a wheelchair workout video for patients with spinal cord injury.

Total your scores for each section as follows:

5._2_	4._5_	6._1_	3._1_	2._5_	1._4_
10._5_	8._5_	12._3_	7._4_	11._4_	9._2_
14._5_	13._5_	18._1_	15._3_	17._4_	16._3_
21._4_	22._5_	20._1_	23._4_	24._5_	19._2_

Totals:

_19_	_20_	_6_	_12_	_18_	_11_
Social	**Realistic**	**Conventional**	**Enterprising**	**Artistic**	**Investigative**

The columns with the highest scores indicate your preferred personality traits, while lower scores indicate areas of less preference. While these questions cannot give your exact Holland Code, they can provide insight into the activities you might enjoy in the profession. As you can see, each personality type has useful applications.

After completing this activity, discuss the following questions:

1. How do you hope to use your traits in our profession? What do you hope to accomplish? What do you think are the advantages of these traits?
2. Which areas of less preference do you think are important for professional success? How might you go about strengthening these?
3. How do your scores compare to other members of your class? Are there more similarities or differences?

Continued

Talking Points/Field Notes—cont'd ▬▬▬▬▬▬▬▬▬▬▬▬

The Meyers-Briggs Type Indicator (MBTI)* is another valid and reliable personality assessment tool that is commonly used for career counseling. The MBTI is based on personality types originally developed by psychiatrist Carl Jung. These concepts were further refined by the mother-daughter team of Katharine C. Briggs and Isabel Briggs Meyers, who are credited with developing the MBTI. The MBTI is a self-scored forced-choice inventory through which one rates oneself along four different dimensions.[8] Sixteen different personality types are possible from the combination of these four dimensions. Each of the four dimensions and 16 personality types are equal in value and represent a combination of personal preferences that direct one's attention, decision-making, and lifestyle approach. Descriptions of the four Meyers-Briggs dimensions are shown in **Box 3-1**.

BOX 3-1:   Dimensions of the Meyers Briggs Personality Attributes[8]

INTROVERSION–EXTROVERSION

Introverts tend to focus on the inner world of thoughts, ideas, and perceptions. They may appear quiet in nature. They are thoughtful and reflective and think before speaking. They gain energy from being alone.

Extroverts tend of focus on the outer world of people, places, and events. They are often talkative and outgoing. They may speak before thinking and gain energy from being with others.

SENSING–INTUITION

Sensers prefer information in the form of objective data such as facts, direct observations, and personal experiences. They are present-oriented and think in terms of concrete realities.

Intuitives prefer information in terms of patterns, perceptions, and "gut feelings." They are future-oriented and think in terms of possibilities.

FEELING–THINKING

Feelers prefer to make decisions based on their impact on people, relationships, and emotions.

Thinkers prefer to make decisions based on objective analyses of facts and their impact on tasks and organizations.

PERCEIVING–JUDGING

Perceivers prefer spontaneity, open-endedness, and flexibility in their daily lives.

Judgers prefer schedules, organization, and a planned approach to daily life.

PERSONALITY TYPES: ISTJ, ISFJ, INFJ,INTJ,ISTP, ISFP, INFP,INTP, ESTJ, ESFJ, ENFJ, ENTJ, ESTP, ESFP, ENFP, ENTP

One study of 165 PT students showed an overall ESFJ type, which differed from those of osteopathic, pharmacy, and physician assistant students.[9] Another study of 45 PT students found that those with aspirations to generalist practice had a different MBTI than those who wanted to specialize (ESFJ versus ENFP, respectively).

There are several resources for determining your own Holland code and MBTI preference (see references at the end of the chapter). Regardless what you discover, you will find endless opportunities to express your preference in the PT profession, whether it be in clinical practice, teaching, research, professional leadership, or administration.

Invested for the Long Haul: The Many Opportunities of Our Profession

In addition to the many ways in which you can express the preferred elements of your personality, the PT profession offers virtually countless opportunities for a lifetime of service. Accordingly, the results of the 2006 APTA demographic survey suggest that PTs find plenty of satisfying challenges in their own professional backyards as the years go by. Consequently the average time in the profession for all respondents was 17 years, with the largest group (24%) having been in practice between 21 and 30 years.[10] In June 2007, the APTA demographics survey provided an overview of the distribution of practice settings for 45,406 PTs.[11]

The various areas of PT practice represented by the APTA demographics survey are illustrated in **Figure 3-1**.

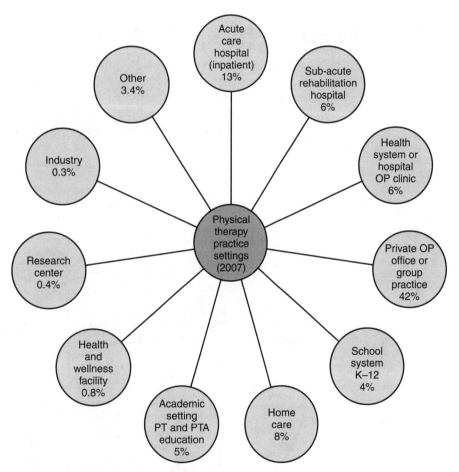

Figure 3–1. Practice Settings of 45,406 physical therapists in 2007. *(Adapted from American Physical Therapy Association. PT Demographics: Practice Settings. Available Online: www.APTA.org.)*

Talking Points/Field Notes

My Professional Aspirations

Reflect on the areas of PT practice shown in Figure 3-1 and answer the following questions, recording your observations in your field notes.

1. Which practice setting interests you the most? Which diagnostic areas would you most enjoy working with?

2. How can you begin to further explore areas of interest in order to prepare for an optimal employment situation after graduation?

3. How might you develop a career within a career in our profession? Which areas might you move toward in future years?

4. In which ways might PT practice be different in the future?

Three Domains of Work: Job, Career, and Mission

As you prepare to work in the PT profession, there are three ways in which you can approach your future involvement. You can define your work as primarily a job, as a career, or as a mission. In those of us who are truly engaged in our work, these three domains form a seamless progression of experiences and opportunities that enrich the lives of all we touch. **Figure** 3-2 describes these three domains.

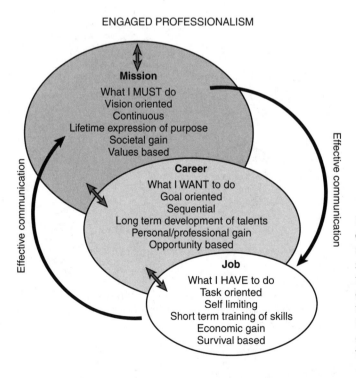

Figure 3–2. Three domains of work: job, career, and mission. The upward arrow suggests that we work from the bottom up as we seek our mission and work from the top down when we find it. In both cases, effective communication is essential for success.

As you will discover in the following pages, the dominant domain from which you approach your work will reflect certain values and attitudes that determine the satisfaction you obtain from your efforts. To begin your consideration of these attitudes and values, consider the case below:

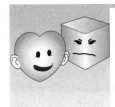

Champ and Blockhead

Champ and Blockhead Receive a Work-Adjustment Opportunity (i.e., Utimatum)

Champ and Blockhead are PTs working in an outpatient facility. Upon arriving for work one Monday, they are called to a staff meeting, where they learn that their facility has been bought out by a nationwide health-care corporation. Under the new corporate owner, the PT staff must meet rigorous productivity requirements. These include performing initial evaluations on at least three patients an hour, with most follow-up treatment done by PT assistants. As a special incentive, the corporation is offering a financial bonus and promotion for the therapist with the most evaluations and the shortest average number of treatments per patient at the end of the year. Therapists who do not wish to accept the new requirements are encouraged to submit their resignations.

Blockhead is excited about the new guidelines, seeing a great opportunity to earn more money and gain recognition. Having recently earned her doctorate in PT, she feels that many aspects of patient care are monotonous. Instead, she would prefer to develop her supervisory skills in order to obtain a more prestigious and powerful administrative position. Thus Blockhead decides to make a little game out of the new guidelines by timing the speed of her evaluations and documentation. She also decides to base her treatments on generic protocols so that she'll be spending less time discussing patient care plans with her three PT assistants. Finally, she agrees to supervise two PT students, promising to "teach them the ropes about time management and efficiency."

Champ loves treating patients and has seen her interventions make a difference in their lives. She also has recently earned a doctorate in PT and feels that her patients require a highly skilled level of care that can be given only by a licensed physical therapist. Because making a positive impact on her patients is more important than money or power, Champ has little interest in following the new guidelines. Nevertheless, because she enjoys new challenges, she decides to arrange a meeting with the new director of rehabilitation to discuss her concerns and to suggest ways of increasing revenue without sacrificing quality of patient care.

Questions:

1. As you look at **Figure** 3-2, describe the differences in Blockhead's and Champ's attitudes about their work.
2. How might their attitudes affect their next move if they are not successful with their approaches to the new guidelines?
3. What are the professional risks and benefits of Blockhead's course of action if she is successful in being the most productive staff member?
4. What alternative strategies could Champ propose in order to remain engaged in her work?
5. Which policies must all physical therapists follow in order to protect themselves and their patients? (Hint: Does your state PT practice act have guidelines regarding the number of support personnel who can be supervised by an individual physical therapist?)

As this example illustrates, the attitudes and beliefs reflected in each domain can have significant implications for our work. Let us now explore each domain in greater detail to provide a further understanding of this impact.

Job: What I Have to Do

A "job" is defined as a regular activity performed in exchange for payment—a specific task or duty that must be carried out.[12] Major elements of defining work as a job are an emphasis on money (working to pay the bills) and seeing work as a means to an end ("working to live").

Although there is nothing wrong with this approach, work satisfaction may drop when remuneration is threatened by budget cutbacks or insurance denials. Indeed, defining work satisfaction by doing whatever pays the best does allow you to reflect on some valuable insights.

Talking Points/Field Notes

Exploring Work as a Job

Discuss the following questions in a small group. Record your observations in your field notes.

1. As a physical therapist, which will be more important to you:

   a. To get reimbursed in order to work?

   b. To work in order to get reimbursed?

   c. How might your work be affected by your answer?

2. Would you rather take a less interesting job for high pay (i.e., a salary that would provide significant discretionary income) or a fascinating job for average pay (which would allow you to live comfortably but modestly)? Explain your choice.

3. Would you rather take a modestly paying job with numerous opportunities for professional development and advancement or a high-paying job without such opportunities? Explain your choice.

4. Would you rather take a modestly paying job in which you could determine your own schedule or a high-paying job with rigid working hours? Explain your choice.

5. What might be the impact on the PT profession if most of us viewed our work as a job?

6. What do your answers tell you about your work values?

Career: What I Want to Do

The term *career* has traditionally been associated with a history of paid employment in a single occupation.[13]

In today's technologically enhanced global economy, the term *career* has evolved to include a continuous process of learning and development that may play out in many different jobs or occupations. In this broader context, a career can encompass all facets and roles of an individual's life.[14]

Activities that contribute to a career can include any life-work opportunity that strengthens an individual's skills, such as volunteer work, travel experiences, community service, or education. In this context, paid employment is but one element of this lifelong skill-development process.

Having decided that the study of PT is in line with your interests and abilities, you will acquire a professional education that will position you to continue your career development in a wide variety of contexts. Building a career in PT means that you will seek opportunities that capture your interests and enhance your talents, where you will be able to meet personal and professional goals through a succession of opportunities for advancement. These typically take the form of promotions, salary increases, and increased responsibilities. However, these opportunities may also involve the advancement of knowledge and skills through clinical residencies, service provision in other countries, or training in technologically based interventions for patient care. Needless to say, as long as your career engages you in this manner, you are likely to be very happy in your work.

Satisfying careers are the result of an optimal match between one's internal resources (interests and talents) and external opportunities (work that engages these resources). Thus, viewing one's work as a career can promote a highly satisfying experience.

Figure 3-3 depicts this balance as a measure of career satisfaction (of course, this balance is promoted, enhanced, and sustained through effective communication).

Like the concept of work as a job, career development relies mostly on external situations and opportunities to guide its trajectory. In the absence of these, loss of direction and resultant frustration can occur. For example, a hospital administrator who decides to pursue a new patient market may be frustrated by staff that resist the initiative owing to lack of interest or expertise.

In contrast, many of those whom we consider contemporary visionaries rely largely on internal guidance to engineer their own innovative opportunities. For example, Steve Jobs, the founder and CEO of Apple Inc., began the company in his garage, building the first mass-produced personal computer (the Apple II). The success of the user-friendly Apple II created a new consumer market that propelled its creator to the helm of a multimillion-dollar company.[15] Jobs summarized his vision in a 2004 interview by saying, "I've always wanted to own and control the technology in everything we do."[16]

In many careers, societal changes may alter the balance between opportunities and interests, resulting in movement among the three work domains. For example, new developments in the area of robotics may eventually result in their integration into clinical practice. Clinicians will thus face a new career opportunity, which will require the development of new skills and knowledge. It is possible (and even likely) that technological advances will affect health-care delivery through the creation of work opportunities in areas that don't yet exist. Depending on our state of mind, we can view emerging trends

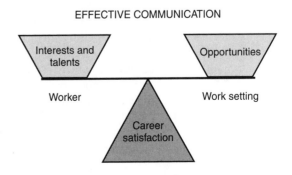

Figure 3–3. Career satisfaction is the result of a balance between the opportunities of the work setting and the interests and talents of the worker. Effective communication can promote, enhance, and sustain this balance.

and opportunities as either threats or invitations. In times of rapid change, a well-defined mission keeps us grounded in our greater life purpose, guiding us toward experiences that facilitate its continued realization.

Talking Points/Field Notes

Reflections on Career

Discuss the following and record these observations in your field notes:

1. What does the term *career* mean to you?

2. Have you ever changed your career direction because it was not in line with your sense of mission?

3. Which of your talents and skills are important for your personal and professional happiness? How do you see the PT profession meeting your needs for their continued development?

4. Which new skills might be required for our profession in the midst of the following societal changes?

   a. Changing racial demographics with rapidly increasing numbers of Hispanic, African American, and Asian citizens?

   b. Robotic-based interventions for motor skills training?

   c. Fully computerized medical records and documentation?

   d. The ability to order diagnostic tests for movement-related disorders?

   e. The ability to prescribe medications to improve functional movement?

   f. The ability to respond to a severe, widespread disaster or war?

Mission: What I MUST Do

A mission can be defined in several ways. Studies of the career decision-making process include concepts with a spiritual emphasis ("What God has put me on Earth to do"),[17] as well as those with a broader societal emphasis ("A transcendent summons to serve the greater good in a meaningful way").[18]

Regardless of how it is defined, the perception of *work as a mission* (which is also called a vocation) is associated with greater self-understanding, enhanced work satisfaction, and higher levels of perceived well-being.[19]

Individuals with a sense of mission also tend to be more highly educated and concerned with social justice.[20] Many seem to have within them a "vibrant life force" (which they perceive as originating from a greater power that permeates their being).[19] This force directs their intentions in a purposeful manner toward the realization of their mission, even compelling them to take personal, financial, and professional risks in the process. Most importantly, persons with a mission are not afraid to work hard in service of their dreams, for great accomplishments require hard work and single-minded dedication.

Throughout the history of humankind, great deeds have been achieved by ordinary people with extraordinary vision. This element of "ordinariness" is a critical aspect of being a person with a mission, because every human being alive has the potential for greatness. This concept is well understood in the realm of positive psychology. Neurolinguistic Programming (NLP) is a theory related to positive psychology. NLP involves the study and application of strategies related to outstanding human success and achievement.[21,22] The concepts of NLP are easy to understand and apply; they begin with these premises:

1. "If one person can do it, any person can do it."
2. "People already have all the resources they need."

Despite the encouragement of these concepts, why don't all of us live up to our greatest dreams? There may be many reasons, and perhaps the biggest is that many of us have yet to articulate our life purpose. If this idea sounds grandiose, consider that it is a common feature of our great leaders and innovators.[21,22] Thus an important starting place is to define our mission. From there, our work can more naturally evolve toward the realization of that purpose. This can be an exhilarating life adventure. A well-directed sense of mission enables us to embrace the future as an empty page on which to inscribe our contributions to society.

We Share and Convey Our Mission Through Communication

Where does communication fit into the scheme of mission? No one achieves a mission in a vacuum. The encouragement and assistance of others is of vital importance. For example, consider the persons behind the scenes of your journey to become a physical therapist. There are likely family members and friends who have provided both tangible and intangible forms of support (money, time, and encouragement). Whether you realize it or not, you have secured this support by your communication, through which you have conveyed your interest and commitment to your career choice of PT. As you enter the profession, you will continue to use communication in the forms of negotiation, motivation, and persuasion in order to secure the support of others—support that will be necessary for the ultimate success of your mission.

Virtually everyone with a mission carries along an inspiring example from history. Appreciation of the trials and triumphs of other ordinary humans is a potent resource for the development and maintenance of mission. The history of PT is full of such examples. The story told in **Box 3-2** is offered to inspire your mission in our profession.

BOX 3-2: How One Woman's Mission Started a Profession: Mary McMillan and the Reconstruction Aides

For a compelling example of a person with a mission and her effectiveness in communicating this to others, we need look no further than the example of Mary McMillan, the founder of the PT profession in the United States and the first president of the American Physical Therapy Association (APTA).[23]

Mary McMillan was born in Massachusetts in 1880. As a young girl, she lost both her mother and sister to tuberculosis. To save her from a similar fate, she was sent to England to be raised by her cousins. Mary was a bright, ambitious young woman; she attended Liverpool University, where her family hoped she would pursue a genteel education in English literature or "domestic science." Instead, fueled by a strong desire to make a difference in the lives of others, she went against her family's wishes and decided to pursue a career in a brand-new area of study: corrective exercise.

Although this might seem like a trivial decision today, the idea of a woman having a career was considered almost brazen during the early 1900s. Nevertheless, Mary's mission forced her to challenge the status quo, compelling her toward a level of education that

---

Continued

BOX 3-2:   How One Woman's Mission Started a Profession: Mary McMillan and the Reconstruction Aides—cont'd

was rare for women of her time (she did graduate work at the Royal College of Surgeons in London).

In 1914, England entered World War I and Mary returned to the United States, where she ran a clinic for the rehabilitation of children with congenital abnormalities. When the United States entered World War I in 1917, the Surgeon General of the U.S. Armed Forces established the first-ever military program for the rehabilitation of injured soldiers. Because the majority of American men were involved in the military, this rehabilitation fell, by default, to women. In a decision that would change health care in this country, Mary McMillan was the first volunteer "reconstruction aide" to offer her services as both a clinician and teacher. In the coming months, she directed the training of several hundred like-minded women who then accompanied her overseas to provide over 3.5 million treatments to 86,000 injured soldiers.[23]

Life as an army reconstruction aide (RA) working on the front lines of battle was far from the comforts of home. The RA living quarters were cold with leaky army barracks with wooden floors that were constantly under water. Undaunted by these conditions, the RAs slept with umbrellas over their beds to keep them dry at night and learned to write their letters home wearing thick gloves to keep their fingers warm. Their working conditions were no better. The first "PT departments" were often the back porches of army barracks or any place where a group of soldiers could be assembled for treatment. To add to their challenges, the RAs were poorly received by the medical staff in the army hospitals to which they were assigned; one nurse made a particularly backhanded prediction when they arrived at their place of work: "You are pioneers. Very few people know what you are for and still fewer want you around. Don't get in the nurses' and doctors' way. Make yourselves scarce....until you have made such a place for yourselves that no ward will be complete without you."[23]Even though the RA program was disbanded at the end of World War I, Mary McMillan and her colleagues sought further opportunities to carry out their mission in the United States. In 1921, she and a group of former RAs met at a New York City restaurant and formed the American Women's Physiotherapeutic Association, the organization now known as the APTA. The goal of their new organization, which has essentially remained unchanged, was to "establish and maintain a professional and scientific standard for those *engaged in the profession.*" Mary McMillan was enthusiastically elected as the first president, and under her leadership a scientific journal was begun (the *P.T. Review,* now known as *Physical Therapy*).

Mary McMillan and her colleagues did not have to wait to find opportunities outside of the military for the application of their skills. As they had predicted, they quickly found themselves immersed in the polio epidemic, where they proved an instrumental force in the rehabilitation of thousands. The rest, as they say, is history.

Engaged Professionals With a Mission Navigate the Three Domains of Work from the Top Down

Engaged professionals use their mission as a sort of internal compass, which directs them toward continuous opportunities for its realization. Therefore the expression of their mission is a consistent attribute of any work they do, and while this work may change and evolve over the course of their lives, it continues to reflect deeply held values that remain constant. This expression was evident in the life of Mary McMillan, whose mission to help others led her to numerous opportunities throughout her career. It is also evident in the life of Steve Jobs and the countless other innovators of our time.

There are many ways in which a person might express his or her mission in the course of life. For example, a person with a mission to educate others might seek a career in academics as an expression of that passion. Contained within that career might be a few less desirable job-like tasks; however, these individuals maintain their engagement because they understand that these tasks are part of a larger picture to which they remain committed.

Career changes can and do happen in the lives of engaged professionals; these usually evolve from the desire to find new forms of expression that are exciting and challenging. Thus, the decision to change careers is made in a top-down manner with respect to the three work domains. Returning to our example of a person with a mission to teach, this individual might leave academics after many years in order to find new ways of educating others. Such options might include writing, mentoring other experienced practitioners, or even teaching in a brand new area of interest.

Until We Find Our Mission, We May Climb Upward Within the Three Work Domains

Many of us do not have a solid sense of our mission fresh out of school. We may therefore seek several different job opportunities before, if we are fortunate, we find one that truly excites us. At that point, we will hopefully be in touch with the values and ideals that are reflected in this work and begin to internalize these as the driving force for future work decisions (which may be independent of salary, benefits, or other external rewards). The internalization of what matters to us, our values, is an important step in selecting work that engages us. If we are successful in uniting our interests and values in the workplace, we will likely find ourselves building a sequence of related jobs and work experiences that many would call a career.

Awareness of our passions, natural gifts, and talents is a crucial prerequisite for finding our mission. In our busy, demanding society, this is not an easy task. It is helpful to examine these entities deliberately in the hope that once identified, they can be aligned through our work.

Exercises to Help You Identify Your Mission

For most of us, the voice of mission begins as a whisper; then, if we listen and acknowledge what we hear, it becomes stronger. In many ways, the voice of our mission is perhaps the most important message to emerge within the scope of our internal communication.

The following exercises can be used now and at any future point to help you identify and develop a guiding mission that will direct your personal and professional goals and keep you engaged throughout the journey.

Talking Points/Field Notes

Defining My Mission

Discuss the following questions in a small group. Please share at your comfort level. You can also record your observations in your field notes.

1. Three Wishes for My Life

If you could be granted three wishes for your life, what would they be? Consider each one in detail, in terms of how it would make you feel, what it would allow you to do, and who it might affect besides you as

Continued

Talking Points/Field Notes—cont'd

an individual. Most importantly, reflect on WHY you chose these, considering perhaps what dreams and desires lie beneath.

2. My Sources of Inspiration

Make a list of the 10 persons who have had the greatest inspiring impact on your life. Next to each name, consider and write:

    a. The main reason they are on your list

    b. Their personal attributes that you most admire

    c. Their accomplishments that you most admire

    d. The most important lesson they have taught you

As you look over your answers, which values and ideals emerge? Write these down and consider their importance in your life.

3. My Life in Review

You are 100 years old and have been asked by one of your grandchildren to write a letter detailing the most important events of your life. The letter should include your personal and professional accomplishments as well as what you most want to be remembered for. What is in your letter?

4. My Personal Verbs

Without censoring yourself, jot down at least 25 action words that pertain to you at this point in your life. For example: running, thinking, reading, creating, learning, loving, talking, laughing, playing the piano, cooking.
As you look over your list, note any similarities. What might these tell you?

5. My Personal Adjectives

Which adjectives describe you? Consider the words you might use to convey the most important elements of who you are and what you stand for. Aim for at least 25 adjectives.

    Examples: enthusiastic, thoughtful, creative, intelligent.

6. How My Best Friends Would Describe Me

Two of your best friends have been asked to describe you by someone who has never met you. What would they be most likely to say?

7. A Theme Song for My Life

What is the theme song for your life? Consider the titles of your favorite songs. What does the title of your theme song say about you?

8. A Special Internship

You have been offered the opportunity to go on an all-expenses-paid trip anywhere in the world to learn a new skill. What would you choose and why?
How might you continue to use this skill in your life once you had learned it?

Writing a Mission Statement

A mission statement is a statement of the purpose, defining principles, and overall intent of a group or individual. In recent years, mission statements have been developed and publicly declared by many businesses and organizations worldwide. Most likely, the university where you are pursuing your PT education has a mission statement that can be accessed on its website. APTA's mission statement is as follows:

> The mission of the American Physical Therapy Association (APTA), the principal membership organization representing and promoting the profession of physical therapy, is to further the profession's role in the prevention, diagnosis, and treatment of movement dysfunctions and the enhancement of the physical health and functional abilities of members of the public.[24]

One of the most powerful ways in which to begin the journey toward the realization of your life goals is to have a clear statement of purpose—in other words, a mission statement. Your mission statement can be short, even as short as a single sentence. It can be written in the context of a life purpose or overall goal. The most important thing is that it be personally meaningful and useful as a guiding statement for the major life decisions that lie ahead.

An Example of a Mission Statement

A few years ago, a new graduate PT wrote the following mission statement: *"My overall life mission is to use my natural enthusiasm for the inspiration of others."*

In the years since then, this therapist has been involved in teaching, writing, and maintaining an active clinical practice. These opportunities continue to provide an outlet for the expression of this person's mission, keeping her engaged and passionate about her work. In times of personal or professional stress, this mission statement has helped this physical therapist to maintain a focus on what matters, providing an attitudinal life jacket for navigating through confusing or difficult times.

Talking Points/Field Notes

My Mission Statement:

1. Write your mission statement. Let it be an honest reflection of who you are and what you hope to do with your life. It can be as long or short as you like to accomplish this. You might consider printing it and putting it in a place where you can see it often.

2. Share your mission statement with one or more classmates. As you listen to each other's statements, note any similarities or differences.

Identifying the Tools of Your Mission: The SWOT Analysis

What Is a SWOT Analysis?

Just as communication is the vehicle through which you will convey your mission to others, your strengths, talents, and skills are the implements with which you will carry it out. Your threats and opportunities are the roads over which you will travel. Thus, another important part of self-assessment is the identification of these elements so that they can be used effectively on your journey through life and work.

SWOT analysis (the acronym SWOT stands for strengths, weaknesses, opportunities, threats) was developed from research conducted at the Stanford Research Institute from 1960 to 1970.[25] This research was funded by Fortune 500 companies to determine effective approaches to long-term planning for business corporations.

SWOT analysis involves the assessment of internal (strengths and weaknesses) and external features (threats and opportunities) of a given work environment in order to assess the capacity for successful growth and change.

Although originally developed as means of assessment for corporate entities, the SWOT analysis model can be readily applied to individuals or groups who are seeking to explore and develop strategies for individual success. The following examples describe applications of the SWOT analysis model at both individual and professional levels.

Application of the SWOT Analysis Model at the Individual Level

Strengths

Strengths consist of two attributes, *talents* and *skills*.[26] Talents are inborn, natural, and generally enjoyable proclivities that come easily to the individual. Skills generally evolve from the directed and repetitive application of talents towards the development of excellence in a specific activity or behavior. For example, the aviator Charles Lindbergh had a natural ability to sense direction, movement, and body position in space. Lindbergh applied these talents to the development of the considerable skills involved in flying an airplane. He then sought opportunities for the application of his skills and talents, being one of the nation's first airmail pilots and even "barnstorming," which involved doing aerial acrobatics at county fairs. His ultimate opportunity presented itself in 1927, when he achieved international fame as the first person to fly nonstop from New York to Paris.[27] As this suggests, successful missions provide an outlet for the expression and development of talents and skills.

Talking Points/Field Notes

Exploring Your Strengths

Reflect on the following questions, then discuss your answers with a classmate. You can also record your observations in your field notes.

Talents

1. Beginning from elementary school, what were your favorite subjects and why did they attract your attention? How have you continued to develop your initial interest in these areas?

2. Which subjects in your PT education come most naturally to you?

3. In what areas did you seem to excel naturally (writing, language skills, art, mathematics)?

4. What were your earliest hobbies and favorite pastimes, and how have these developed over the years?

5. Which activities absorb you so completely that you lose track of time?

6. Which abilities do you most admire in others?

7. Which of your abilities have garnered you consistent praise and recognition throughout your life thus far?

Talking Points/Field Notes—cont'd ■━━━━━━━

Skills

1. In which subjects do you most easily excel in school?
2. Which work assignments are you most likely to volunteer for?
3. What is one accomplishment you would like to achieve in your lifetime?

Relationship of Strengths to Your Mission

1. How do you think your talents and skills can be helpful to you as a physical therapist?
2. How do your talents and skills apply to your mission statement?

Weaknesses: Deficits in Talents or Skill

In contrast to the talents and skills component of strengths, areas of weakness are often those where there is little natural proclivity or interest. When these are lacking, it is unlikely that an individual will seek opportunities for their expression, nor will he or she find such opportunities rewarding. For example, an individual with no talent or skill in math will probably not be well suited to a career such as accounting and financial management. Should she decide to do this for other reasons, she would be likely to find the learning process slower than for areas related to her talent. Obviously, the most satisfied people are those whose work readily allows for the expression of their best attributes.

Nevertheless, it is virtually impossible to completely avoid all activities outside our natural comfort zones of talent and skills. Thus it is important to explore weakness from the perspective of *deficits of talent or skill*. It is important for you to understand that the term *deficit* is meant only to describe and not judge. Talent deficits are best defined as proclivities and abilities that are useful but not critical for success in a given career. An example of a talent deficit could be a lack of artistic ability. This would not likely prevent a physical therapist from being highly successful in their work environment. On the other hand, a physical therapist with such an interest might find unique opportunities to utilize such a talent in the scope of his mission.

Such was the case of Frank Netter, MD, whose outstanding artistic talent led him to create some of the best medical illustrations of the 20th century.[28] In fact, Netter's talent was so extraordinary that he retired from the practice of clinical medicine in order to devote full time to his illustrations. Netter's anatomic drawings were featured in countless textbooks and clinical monographs, where they provided a bird's-eye view of the human body to a generation of health-care practitioners.

A skill deficit is defined as the lack of abilities needed to function in a given environmental context. In the context of PT practice, there are numerous behaviors (skills) that must be developed to a level of competence, regardless of the level of talent or interest. For example, documentation is an important skill for effective PT practice. Yet many PTs dislike documentation because they perceive it as taking valuable time away from patient care—they lack interest in this area relative to their other responsibilities. PTs may also dislike documentation because they are not skilled in efficient and effective strategies—they lack ability in this area. However, documentation is a crucial professional skill required of all therapists and a critical determinant of the ability to maintain a sufficient patient base (i.e., poor documentation may result in the loss of opportunities to treat patients). Thus a physical therapist with a skill deficit in documentation would be well advised to develop efficacy in this professional activity. Fortunately, the increased use of computerized documentation (with its structured format for patient data entry) has streamlined the process by removing the need for time-consuming therapist-generated narratives.

Because skill development involves the repetitive practice of a desired behavior, virtually any skill can be learned in the presence of appropriate motivation and practice (in fact, this is a critical premise of the motor learning principles that you will apply to patient rehabilitation). Therefore it is useful to consider which skills are important for the success of one's current and future career path and develop these accordingly. Thoughtful self-assessment and specific feedback can help an individual to identify these skills and, most importantly, to determine effective strategies for their improvement. The use of written behavioral objectives can be useful in defining the behaviors, conditions, and degree of success in skill development.

Talking Points/Field Notes

Exploring Your Weaknesses

Reflect on the following questions and discuss them with a small group of classmates. You can also record your observations in your field notes.

Talent Deficits

1. Beginning in grade school, which subjects were the least interesting to you? Why do you think this was so?

2. Are there any academic areas in which you struggled because the material didn't come easily to you? What was the outcome?

3. Thus far, which areas in your PT education are the most challenging because they don't come easily to you? How are you addressing these areas to promote your success?

Skill Deficits

1. What skills are involved in the challenging academic areas you identified previously?

2. What specific strategies could you use to improve these skills?

3. Who could you work with to improve these skills?

4. What are your specific desired outcomes for the improvement of these skills?

Opportunities

Opportunities are realized when an invitation for growth is accepted by a well-prepared individual. They can arise from external circumstances indicating a need, such as that created by the numbers of injured soldiers needing rehabilitation during World War I.

Opportunities can also be self-generated, such as the development of a new invention that may help others. Thus, opportunities abound in our lives, but we will not view them as such if they don't involve a chance to grow in a way that we value or if we do not feel prepared to engage in the work involved. Successful and engaged individuals thrive on the acceptance or creation of opportunities in line with their mission, and are consistently on the lookout for such possibilities.

The decision to accept an opportunity is generally based on an assessment of the work involved (i.e., the investment of our talents and skills) relative to the potential for a meaningful outcome. Some opportunities are obvious in their potential to yield success, such as a significant promotion involving new responsibilities. Others may be equally exciting, but with less than certain outcomes, such as developing a new invention without any foreknowledge of its success in the market.

The ability to sustain a healthy life-work balance involves the ability to carefully weigh the benefits and investments of the opportunities that come our way. We also need to be alert to invitations that may appear to be opportunities but which, in reality, are unethical or harmful (for example, accepting a contract with an insurance company that provides financial incentives to providers who restrict services to patients in need). Thus, the decision of whether or not to accept an opportunity requires tremendous self-awareness and personal integrity, which is grounded in honest internal communication.

In identifying opportunities, it might be helpful to consider the needs that arise in life circumstances and then to seek creative ways to meet these through the use of our strengths. When Dr. Netter first began to produce his medical illustrations, it was simply because of his passion for drawing. However, after a period of time, Netter began to develop a reputation for his work and quickly came to realize that there was a special opportunity for him in the marriage of his medical training and his artistic skill. Filling this need led him to produce the expert medical illustrations that are now his legacy.[28]

The legacy of the PT profession is one of ongoing opportunities which arise as members of our profession identify social areas of need which can be addressed through our services. For example, as the 80 million members of the Baby Boomer generation (born between 1946 and 1964) reach retirement, significant opportunities will emerge in our profession that will allow us to address their needs for health, wellness, and continued quality of life.

Talking Points/Field Notes

Exploring Your Opportunities

Reflect on the following and record your observations in your field notes.

1. Consider a time in your life when you were able to meet a need through the use of your talents or skills. What was the outcome?

2. What opportunities do you believe exist in the PT profession today?

3. Which of your talents and skills might these opportunities require?

Threats

While opportunities are external events that allow us to expand the use of our strengths, threats are external events that have the potential to limit these. For example, the closure of your PT educational program would obviously pose a significant threat to the future use of your skills and talents in our profession. Thus, because threats can be an obstacle to our success, it is important to first be aware of them before they affect us in such a manner.

Perhaps the most challenging type of threat is one that is opposes our values system. For example, if we value honesty, it is likely that our relationship with anyone who lies to us would be threatened because of the affront to our values. However, we may also be called to work with those of differing values in the course of PT practice, and must carefully consider whether standing up for our values violates the rights of others. Such is the nature of many ethical dilemmas.

While some threats may pose significant challenges to our values and goals, others may require us to take a fresh approach which results in the creation of an opportunity. Thus, when confronted with what appears to be a threat, it can be helpful to maintain a flexible outlook.

For example, the emphasis on accountability that emerged with managed care appeared at first glance, as a threat to PT practice. As our profession assessed our collective strengths, weaknesses, and opportunities in light of these challenges, many opportunities began to emerge, one of which involved developing and expanding the scientific basis of our profession through a commitment to evidence-based practice. This commitment has enhanced our knowledge base and has allowed us to effectively address the accountability aspect of managed care. It has also given us greater confidence in the value of our interventions. Thus, our profession's willingness to confront our collective strengths and weaknesses has enabled us to transform the threat of accountability to the opportunity of enhancing the efficacy of our practice.

Finally, it is important to note that a great many threats are internally generated, involving exaggerated fears and self-limiting dialogue that prevents us from effectively using our strengths. Many of us grapple with the steady voices of an inner critic or prophet of doom. This is a form of internal communication that can be painful at best and destructive at worst. Again, self-awareness of this tendency can be extremely helpful. In the next chapter on internal communication, we will explore the nature of our inner dialogue or self-talk.

Talking Points/Field Notes

Exploration of Threats

Reflect on the following and discuss with a small group of classmates. You can also record your observations in your field notes.

Affirming Our Values

1. Because most threats come in the form of affronts to our values, it is probably most effective to identify your "nonnegotiables"—that is, ideals that you will attempt to preserve regardless of your circumstances. Thus, consider the following:

   a. What do you value most in life?

   b. What is most important to you for a sense of well-being?

   c. What do you value most in your relationships?

   d. What do you value most in your work?

   e. Complete the following sentence: "In my work as a physical therapist, I will always strive to _____, no matter what the circumstances."

2. What do you think are the greatest threats to the PT profession?

3. Reflect on a time that a threat resulted in an opportunity for you. What was the outcome? What did you learn?

4. Many persons are threatened by change, only because it challenges them to develop new skills. What is your typical reaction to change and why

Clinical Scenario: Take the Promotion or Run?

Richard greatly enjoys his work as the senior PT of the spinal cord unit in a large teaching hospital. His professional colleagues have great respect for his outstanding clinical skills, his friendly and easygoing manner, and his natural leadership skills. One day, he is approached by the director of clinical services, who tells him that because of his recognized expertise, he is being offered a lucrative managerial position that would involve conducting utilization reviews for the PT department. His new responsibilities would include going over clinical documentation and patient records as well as determining budget and staffing needs. Richard is intrigued by the opportunity to learn new managerial skills (and by the substantial increase in salary), but he also recognizes that the activities involved in the new position would take him away from patient care, an activity that he greatly enjoys.

1. How might Richard approach his decision with respect to the three domains of work?
2. How might Richard approach his decision with respect to a personal and professional SWOT analysis?
3. How might Richard make the best use of his existing talents and skills for the good of the new position?

Implications for Physical Therapy Practice

The ongoing demands of providing quality intervention to our patients will be optimally successful if we are engaged in our work. In the coming years, national economic challenges may threaten patient access to health care as well as provider payment for those services. Fortunately, evidence suggests that a sense of mission with respect to our work can fortify us during these challenging times, keeping us mindful of our goals and purpose. With such reinforcement, we can direct our energies to optimally serving our patients, our colleagues, and our society through the consistent exercise of engaged professionalism.

Chapter Summary

This chapter has explored several concepts related to professional engagement and provided suggestions for self-assessment to identify and strengthen these concepts. The major premises explored are these:

1. Each person has a unique combination of personality traits that can be effectively harnessed to allow for their optimal expression in both life and work.
2. As a physical therapist, you can define your work as a job, as a career, or as a mission. Each involves certain beliefs and expectations that can affect work satisfaction.
3. A strong sense of mission will direct your efforts in congruence with your goals and values, leading to engagement and the potential to make significant changes.
4. According to the principles of NLP, in the realm of human potential, nothing is impossible, and humans have the resources they need.
5. An assessment of your strengths, weaknesses, opportunities, and threats will help you to direct your mission appropriately.

Take-Home Menu

1. Engagement Interview

In the next week, talk to at least four other persons who are engaged in their work. Ask them how they chose their profession and how it aligns with their mission statement, interests, and talents.

2. Mission Movie Night

In the next month, with classmates, watch one or two movies about persons whose mission resulted in a significant contribution. Discuss the impact of this mission, as well as the challenges faced by the individual. There are numerous possibilities.

3. Biography Book Club

With classmates, read the biography a person who made a socially significant contribution and get together to discuss the impact of this mission as well as the challenges faced by the individual.

References

1. Albert Schweitzer Quotes: http://www.brainyquote. com/quotes/authors/a/albert_schweitzer.html. Accessed December 26, 2008.
2. Antony JS. Personality-career fit and freshman medical career aspirations: A test of Holland's theory. *Res Higher Ed.* 1998;39(6):679-698.
3. Holland J. *Making Vocational Choices.* 2nd ed. Odessa, FL: Psychological Assessment Resources; 1985.
4. Madill H, Macnab D, Brintell S. Student values and preferences: What do they tell us about program selection? *Can J Occup Ther.* 1989;56(4):171-178.
5. Salisbury University Career Services Office. SU Holland codes, careers and college majors: http://www .hollandcodes.com/support-files/su-careers-majors-and-model.pdf. Accessed December 27, 2008.
6. University of Missouri Career Center. *Guide to Holland Code.*: http://career.missouri.edu/handouts/ Guide%20to%20Holland%20Code%20F2008.pdf. Accessed December 27, 2008.
7. University of Victoria. Occupations by Holland Code: http://careerservices.uvic.ca/resources/Holland_codes_ June_15_05.html. Accessed December 27, 2008.
8. Myers IB, Meyers PB. *Gifts Differing: Understanding Personality Type.* Mountain View, CA: Davies-Black Publishing: 1980, 1995.
9. Hardigan PC, Cohen SR. A comparison of osteopathic, pharmacy, physical therapy, physician assistant and occupational therapy students' personality styles: Implications for education and practice. *J Pharm Teaching.* 1999;7(2):69-79.
10. American Physical Therapy Association: Physical Therapist Demographic Profile, 1999-2006. Available online: http://www.apta.org/AM/Template. cfm?Section=Home&Template=/MembersOnly. cfm&ContentID=46077. Accessed December 18, 2008.
11. American Physical Therapy Association: PT Demographics Practice Settings. Available online: http://www.apta.org/AM/ Template.cfm?Section=Home&TEMPLATE=/CM/ ContentDisplay.cfm&CONTENTID=41549. Accessed December 18, 2008.
12. Job Satisfaction: Strategies to Make Work More Gratifying. Mayo Clinic.Com: http://www.mayoclinic. com/health/job-satisfaction/WL00051. Accessed January 6, 2009.
13. Department of Education and Early Childhood Development, Victoria, Australia. What is a Career?: http://www.education.vic.gov.au/sensecyouth/careertrans/ whatcareer.htm. Accessed January 6, 2009.
14. McMahon M, Tatham P. Career: More than just a job. Dulwich, Australia: Education.aulimited: http://www .myfuture.edu.au/Events/Feature%20Articles/~/media/ Files/Career%20more%20than%20just%20a%20job% 20V2.ashx. Accessed January 15, 2009
15. Viet S. PC-History: http://www.pc-history.org/. Accessed January 16, 2009.
16. BusinessWeek Online. The Seed of Apple's Innovation. October 12, 2004. http://www.businessweek.com/ bwdaily/dnflash/oct2004/nf20041012_4018_PG2_ db083.htm. Accessed January 16, 2009.
17. Dalton JC. Career and calling: Finding a place for spirit in work and community. *New Directions for Student Services.* 2001;95:17-25.
18. Duffy RS. Spirituality, religion and career development: Current status and future directions. *Career Dev Q.* 2006;55:52-63.
19. Wizeniewski A, McCauley C, Rozin P, Schwartz B. Jobs, careers and callings: People's relation to their work. *J Res Personality.* 1997;31:21-33.

20. Duffy RD, Sedlacek WE. The presence and search for a calling: Connections to career development. *J Voc Behav.* 2007;70(3):590-601.
21. The NLP comprehensive training team. Andreas S, Faulkner C (eds). *NLP: The new technology of achievement.* New York: Quill William Morrow, 1994.
22. O'Connor J, Seymour J. *Introducing NLP: Psychological Skills for Understanding and Influencing People.* London: Thorsons; 1990.
23. Murphy A. *Healing the Generations: A History of Physical Therapy and the American Physical Therapy Association.* Lyme, CT: Greenwich Publishing; 1995:56.
24. American Physical Therapy Association, Mission Statement: http://www.apta.org/AM/Template.cfm?Section=Core_Documents1&TEMPLATE=/CM/ContentDisplay.cfm&CONTENTID=32269. Accessed September 11, 2007.
25. BusinessBalls.Com. The Origins of SWOT Analysis: http://www.businessballs.com/swotanalysisfreetemplate.htm. Accessed September 18, 2007.
26. Buckingham M, Clifton D. *Now Discover Your Strengths.* New York: FreePress; 2001.
27. Berg S. *Lindbergh.* New York: Berkley; 1999.
28. *Frank H Netter MD: Artist, Physician, and Influential Master of Human Anatomy:* http://www.graphicwitness.com/netter/bio/netterbio.html. Accessed September 18, 2007.
29. Mueller K. A physical therapy memoir: Finding the path. Arizona Physical Therapy Association, *Arizona Physical Therapy Association Newsletter (APTAN) Update.* January, 1998, p. 4.
30. Mueller K. A physical therapy memoir: Boot camp in Mary McMillan's Army. *Arizona Physical Therapy Association Newsletter (APTAN) Update.* Spring, 1999.

The Author's Perspective on Finding a Mission

Appendix to Chapter 3

If you are the type of person who enjoys learning about the perspective of others, I humbly offer two articles that previously appeared in the *Arizona Physical Therapy Association Newsletter* in the late 1990s. These articles were part of a three part series entitled "A physical therapy memoir" and contain excerpts from my personal journal, written over 30 years ago. These articles are included in the following sections.

A Physical Therapy Memoir: Finding the Path[29]

In the fall of 1976, I was a 19 year old pre-med junior at the University of Missouri. As with many like minded college students of that time, my quality of life was directly proportional to the pinnacles of my social life and grade point average. Both were far from scintillating. My trusted support system had suddenly evaporated in the previous six months. My best friend transferred to another school out of state, others directed their attentions to the lures of romance or sorority life. None of these distractions were forthcoming for me however, as the demands of working and school kept a tight reign on most of my time. But the most troublesome aspect of all was an increasing academic frustration at school, a part of my life that had always provided me with an abiding sense of personal satisfaction and accomplishment.

From the time I dissected my first earthworm in elementary school, I had maintained an interest in the internal workings of the human body. My father, successfully engaged in a career as a physician, also encouraged me, the oldest of his six children, to follow his footsteps. In my family, the call to higher education and a professional career were clear expectations which began when my grandfather sailed to the U.S. from Italy in 1918 with $11.00 in his pocket. Like the majority of immigrants who came to America in search of a better life, my grandfather (who never went beyond elementary school) viewed education as the means to its realization. My father had subsequently internalized this value and now directed it towards myself and my five siblings.

Related to the expectations of my family was also the widely held perception that being a "doctor" (at that time, there was only one kind) was the most prestigious (and thus desirable) career for the sufficiently bright and ambitious. In contrast, health related professions, such as physical therapy, received little consideration by those who destined for medical school, and like most of my ilk, I had no idea as to what practitioners of these disciplines actually did.

Thus indoctrinated as to my future life direction, I had begun my college studies as pre-med psychology major, but found myself struggling to maintain a strong grade point average in a competitive, impersonal, and sometimes hostile educational arena. Most of the premed sciences courses were delivered lecture style in huge auditoriums filled with as many as 300 students. Contact with the course professor was mitigated through an arsenal of grad assistants who kept us at bay. Test averages on most exams were 60% or less. As I accrued scores that were often well below this average, I slogged on despite mounting discouragement.

Feeling desperate, I was finally able to arrange a visit with my organic chemistry professor to discuss an exam on which my performance was utterly dismal. Once in his office, my hopes for any scraps of encouragement went down in flames as he got up from his desk, drew a bell curve on the blackboard and officiously sneered, "The people who don't get into medical school fall into the middle of the curve. Those are folks like you."

With each subsequent pre-med science course, I found myself becoming increasingly disillusioned, not only by my grades, but by the dishonesty of my classmates. I witnessed blatant cheating during exams and for the first time, considered whether I would be able to tolerate these individuals as future colleagues. Fueled by this disillusionment, I began to examine my own goals, interests and hopes for my life.

The long and painful process of internal dialogue that ensued over the next several months slowly led me to the realization that the life balance I wanted above everything was probably not to be easily found in a career as a physician. This self examination allowed me to examine how my interests could be parlayed in to a worthwhile alternative to medical school. Such interests involved physical activity (as part of the new 70's running craze, I had taken up this hobby). They also included a strong interest in acting, wholistic [sic] health, and of course, learning about the human body. As I reflected, I realized that I wanted a career where I could interact with people in a personal way while encouraging them towards meaningful growth related to their health and well being. The nagging little question was, how?

Journal: October 5, 1976

"Keeping in mind that pain is often a prelude to growth, I endure my down days with a hopeful heart. If I could find a suitable alternative path, I could resolve this conflict."

In the words of Dr. Elisabeth Kubler-Ross, there are no accidents in life. Having a vague sense of a major change on the horizon, I kept a receptive outlook, hoping that I would be eventually led to the answer I sought.

My transcendent moment occurred in the lunch line at the student union when I ran into Mark, an old high school classmate, whom strangely, I had never seen on campus until that moment. As we exchanged the usual banter about classes, he mentioned that he was in the process of applying to physical therapy school. This was a profession I had heard about in name only, and I pressed him for details. As he enthusiastically described the possibilities of healing people with injuries and disability, and how he looked forward to interactions in both the physical and psychological realms, I was filled with the sudden conviction that this was a direction I needed to explore. After a short stint volunteering in a physical therapy clinic, I had made my decision. My P.T. school application was in the mail two weeks later, just as the deadline approached.

Journal: January 3, 1977

Tomorrow my fate will be decided: My physical therapy school interview. I spent the day in busy preparation, reading in the medical library. The rest of the week ought to go fast. Time will tell...

I really don't remember much about my physical therapy interview except insipid details like what I wore. I do remember that my interview was a discussion between myself and the entire physical therapy faculty, and that I had to distinguish between handicap and disability (my naively hopeful answer: "a handicap can often be imagined, a disability is usually real").

Journal: January 14, 1977

Well, my life has been saved. Physical therapy it is! I am looking forward to it, because I think that what lies ahead will be good. No matter what happens, it will certainly be interesting.

■ A Physical Therapy Memoir: Boot Camp in Mary McMillan's Army[30]

June 13, 1977: My first day in PT school

At 8:00 a.m. on that memorable first day, I found myself in the PT classroom of Rusk Rehabilitation Center at the University of Missouri clad in a white lab coat and surrounded by the 30 individuals who would be classmates for the next two years. The classroom was pervaded by an expectant tension that was almost palpable. Like me, my comrades were no doubt occupied with the evaluative appraisal of each other, evidence for which we gleaned by furtive sidelong glances across the rows of seats. The flavor of these judgments probably went something like this: "That muscular dude in the tank top and gold chains—his idea of good music is probably the "Village People." Or, "That chick with the long red hair, bangles and flowing gauze—she'll probably want us to sing 'Kumbaya' at class parties."

All of this surreptitious classification was done, of course, while feigning a casual arrogance that no doubt was a careful façade for our various insecurities: (i.e., what if, in this impressive body of intellect, I am merely toenail fungus?) Looking back, I wonder what divinations were made of me that morning, perhaps something like: "Dorothy Hamill" haircut (the short crop that was the rage at the time, so appropriately trendy), faded Levi's jeans and *Mr. Natural* T-shirt (definitely not sorority material).

Our collective reverie was short lived, however, and we were jolted to reality by introductions of the faculty. Here too, first impressions sunk tenacious hooks in our brains. I remember one faculty member in particular, and watching her greet us with her soft spoken enthusiasm, I was instantly overtaken by a sudden, overwhelming conviction: "One day, I am going to teach." That revelation, which so unexpectedly broadsided me that first day, stayed with me; a call I would eventually answer 20 years later.

Faculty introductions complete, we were next oriented to Gross Human Anatomy—in short, our entire waking existence for the next 8 weeks. The regulations were right out of the first day of Kindergarten: Clean up after yourself, take turns, show respect for your teachers (even if they are embalmed). Then, as the objectives of the course were revealed, a somber realization began to sink in: "Say goodbye to your life as you now know it, and to anyone outside these walls: you are now official recruits in Mary McMillan's army. Make her proud! Welcome to PT school!"

Journal: July 2, 1977

Summer school and world of PHYSICAL THERAPY have completely swept me away...All that there is, all thoughts, all actions, revolve around Gross Anatomy. It is the most intense, absorbing, and by far, the most enjoyable educational experience I have ever had. What could be more fascinating than learning all about the marvelously intricate structure of the human body? It is a knowledge that increases my appreciation of life, yet there is an inevitable crassness about the whole thing. Working elbow deep in the muscles and lipids of a dead person hardens you in a way. I could probably now endure seeing the most horrid of wounds or afflictions, except that if they occurred in a living person, then <u>empathy</u> comes into play, and certainly no class will harden me to this.

Part 2

Internal Communication

This section focuses on internal communication, the intrapersonal element of human interaction. Chapter 4 explores the dimensions and impact of self-talk, the internal coaching system that ultimately affects our perceptions of competence, empowerment, and outlook. Mindfulness, the ability to observe ourselves in action without judgment, and to concentrate fully on the present moment, is explored in Chapter 5. Finally, Chapter 6 begins the exploration of the internal aspects of emotional intelligence (EI), or the fundamental building blocks of authentic human interaction.

CHAPTER 4

The Voice Within

"The end comes when we no longer talk with ourselves. It is the end of genuine thinking and the beginning of the final loneliness...The cessation of inner dialogue marks also the end of our concern with the world around us."

Eric Hoffer
American Social Writer

Chapter Overview

Simply put, the way we talk to ourselves directly affects the way we interact with others and hence the way we live in the world. Engaged professionals harness the power of effective internal communication in order to direct their interactions toward positive outcomes. This chapter explores strategies to optimize our self-talk so that we can best shape our communication with others in authentic, meaningful ways.

Key Terms

Explanatory style   Positive psychology

Learned optimism   Subjective units of discomfort

Self-esteem

What Goes Around Comes Around: How We Talk to Ourselves Affects How We Talk to Others

Whether or not we realize it, we are talking to ourselves around the clock, most of the time, without even being aware of doing so. This inner dialogue, known as *self-talk*, is a key element of a reflexive cognitive process known as *automatic thinking*. Like any reflex loop, our moods and overall outlook are direct responses to our internal dialogue. Most of us are not even aware of the nature of this inner conversation; however, recent evidence has demonstrated a direct link between high levels of negative self-talk and depression[1-3] and between high levels of positive automatic thoughts and strong self-esteem.[4]

Just as motor responses can be strengthened through repetitive use, much of our internal dialogue has a habitual tone, which influences our overall outlook. As you will discover, the way we explain the causes, the level of our control, and the events of our lives can dramatically affect both our immediate mood as well as our overall level of optimism or pessimism.

In the course of our daily lives, most of us are unaware of the general tone of our self-talk unless a challenging interpersonal exchange evokes the awareness of a strong emotion (such as anger). Then, as a cascade of angry self-talk raises our level of irritability, we might find ourselves lashing out unexpectedly. Not surprisingly, such behavior may provoke an angry response of similar intensity. This perpetuates a cycle where our self-talk creates an internal mood, which is then conveyed in our interpersonal interactions. Accordingly, the affective responses we receive from others are related to the affect we convey. This cycle is conveyed in **Figure 4-1**.

The following scenario in the lives of Champ and Blockhead is now presented so that you can begin to examine this relationship in the context of a real-life situation.

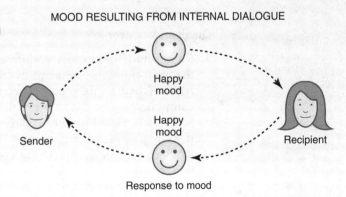

Figure 4–1. The cycle between intrapersonal and interpersonal dialogue.

MOOD RESULTING FROM INTERNAL DIALOGUE

Sender

Happy mood

Happy mood

Response to mood

Recipient

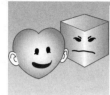

Champ and Blockhead

Champ and Blockhead's Traffic-Jam Self-Talk

Champ and Blockhead both have job interviews for a senior physical therapist position in a brand new rehabilitation facility several miles from each of their homes.

Blockhead sets out in what he considers to be just enough time for a prompt arrival. Three miles into his freeway drive, traffic comes to a standstill because of a major accident that is blocking all lanes. As Blockhead sits tensely in his car, clenching his hands on the steering wheel, the following thoughts circulate in his mind:

Why can't these stupid police just clear the lanes instead of making us all wait? Because of these idiots, I am probably going to be late for this interview. I will probably blow it, and there isn't anything I can do about it! Besides, I am never any good at interviews because the interviewers always try to make me look stupid. This interview will no different, I won't get this job, I will never be able to move forward, and I will never be able to do the things I want. My whole life will just be about getting by.

When Blockhead arrives for his interview, he is anxious, frustrated, and irritable. As his self-talk predicted, the interview does not go well.

Champ sets out early for his interview, hoping to arrive with extra time to walk around the facility beforehand. Upon encountering the same freeway traffic jam, he acknowledges feelings of frustration, then begins to focus on his breathing while beginning this internal dialogue:

This isn't what I hoped for, but it must be far worse for the people in that accident. I will just have to explain the situation if I am late and offer to return if that's the best thing. I am really looking forward to this interview. It is fun to meet new people and learn about new possibilities in this profession. I enjoy the challenge of interesting questions I get on interviews. Even if I don't get this job, it will be a great experience, but I feel really optimistic.

When Champ arrives for his interview, he is alert but generally at ease. His interview is a great success.

Questions for Discussion

1. Champ and Blockhead have different ways of describing the accident ahead. What are the main emotional elements in each of their descriptions?
2. How might the differences between these descriptions and their emotional components affect the ability of these two to manage the stress of the situation?
3. Both Champ and Blockhead realize that they might be late for their interview. How does their self-talk differ in terms of responsibility for the situation?
4. In which ways might Blockhead's self-talk affect his emotional state and his interview performance?
5. In which ways might Champ's self-talk affect his emotional state and his interview performance?

The self-talk elements described in Champ and Blockhead's dilemma represent those of internal communication as a whole. Let us look specifically at these components.

The Functions of Self-Talk

The ongoing dialogue we have with ourselves serves many important purposes, all of which are explored in the next three chapters. Of even more importance to you as a future engaged professional will be the ability to enhance the effectiveness of your internal communication. The field of cognitive psychology has clearly established a relationship between the types of thoughts we have and the quality of our everyday experiences. For example, a preponderance of positive thoughts broadens our sense of personal capability and, in turn, predicts the ability to make desirable behavioral change.[5,6] Positive self-evaluation can enhance self-esteem and build optimism.[7] Moreover, an optimistic outlook improves health outcomes and enhances longevity, even in patients with chronic illnesses such as HIV.[8]

Despite research findings suggesting that our self-talk tends to stabilize as we reach adulthood,[1] there is hope for those of us who tend to view ourselves and our actions through a darker lens. Evidence from positive psychology has demonstrated the efficacy of interventions to promote an optimistic outlook, a happier mood, and a greater sense of personal competence.[9] These approaches are explored further in the following pages.

Let us begin our exploration of internal communication with the same approach you may be taking in your courses in anatomy—with a dissection of sorts. Keep in mind that just as the body systems interact in the service of health, these components interact to produce optimal human interactions. The functions of self-talk are as follows.

Awareness and Accurate Identification of Our Emotions

This is the ability to objectively observe feelings as they arise. The ability to monitor our thoughts, feelings, perceptions, and behaviors is often accomplished through "talking to oneself about oneself."[10] Persons who use self-talk to identify and process their feelings have higher levels of self-awareness and are more skilled at assessing the impact of their actions and behaviors.[11] Self-awareness is thus an important skill in the domain of emotional intelligence, which is the set of skills and behaviors that helps us manage ourselves in our relationships. Emotional intelligence is addressed in Part 3 of this text.

The inability to acknowledge or effectively manage difficult emotions can create physiological manifestations of stress. Thus, self-awareness is an important skill for overall well-being, as is the ability to communicate in ways that effectively support our emotional needs (this communication skill, known as assertiveness, is addressed in Chapter 11).

Finally, the ability to discern our own emotions is a critical prerequisite for *empathy*, the ability to identify feelings in others. As a physical therapist, you will find that empathy is critical for the establishment of a therapeutic partnership with your patients.

Attributions and Explanatory Style: Making Sense of Our Lives

Attributions are explanatory statements about the meaning, implications, and significance of our experiences. For example, one day you go to class, take a test, and receive a grade. Your attributions after this event might include a positive or negative evaluation of the outcome (a *good* grade versus a *bad* one), and a self-statement of who was responsible for it (*your* level of preparation or whether the *professor* wrote a good exam). Furthermore, your attributions would frame this experience in terms of its impact on your life. Accordingly, self-talk around a poor grade might include a far-reaching pervasive statement ("I am a failure, I will never graduate") or a short-term, limited one ("It's just one test. Next time, I'll study harder and do better"). Obviously the nature of your attributions can contribute significantly to your overall mood.

Most adults use a fairly consistent approach to their attributions, so that it can be characterized as an *explanatory style.* The nature of one's explanatory style is related to either an optimistic or pessimistic outlook.[12,13] In addition, a habitually negative or positive explanatory style can affect our level of self-esteem.

An important element of attributions is *self-efficacy*—the perception that our actions can produce the outcomes we desire.[12] The nature of our explanatory style has a direct impact on our sense of self-efficacy. For example, persons whose explanatory style processes life challenges as having a long-term negative impact that is completely out of their control have developed what Seligman calls *learned helplessness.*[13] As physical therapists, we will confront the explanatory styles of our patients. Hopefully, through an effective therapeutic partnership and the use of effective communication, we will be able optimize the self-efficacy of our patients for the good of their functional recovery. First however, it is helpful to develop awareness of our own attributions and how they can be optimized towards empowerment.[13] Because attributions have such an important impact on outlook, their elements are explored in greater detail further on in this chapter.

Development of Self–Esteem

Rosenberg defines self-esteem as a positive or negative orientation toward oneself and thus an overall assessment of one's personal value.[14] Self-esteem has been shown to be related to our perceptions of how effectively we are able to meet our needs for autonomy, competence, and relatedness.[15] Our self-esteem is strongly influenced by early perceptions of support from parents or caregivers; the strength of our academic, artistic, and sports performances; and our success in developing close friendships.[16]

In adulthood, our self-esteem tends to stabilize and has been shown to predict the quality of our social bonds as well as our likelihood of enjoying good health.[17] Fortunately, as in the case of attributions, we can optimize our self-esteem with conscious effort.

The Rosenberg Self-Esteem Scale, shown in **Box 4-1**, is the most widely used measure of its kind in social science research.[18]

In addition to the important psychological functions of self-talk described above, a study of 1,132 college students demonstrated that most of them used self-talk for higher-level cognitive functions such as reasoning and problem solving.[19] Interestingly, a majority of these students were not aware of the extent of their self-talk until they completed a questionnaire exploring this activity. Questions related to the use of self-talk are shown in the **Box 4-2**. How often do you use this important skill?

▌Guiding Assumptions About Internal Communication

Most of us would probably agree that life would be more pleasant and productive if we spoke more kindly to ourselves, and the most promising message in this chapter is that we can learn to do this. The ability to make positive changes in our self-talk is grounded in the following guiding assumptions from Neurolinguistic Programming (NLP), which pertains to the conscious (i.e., neurological) input (i.e., programming) of empowering self-talk (i.e., linguistic) strategies in order to promote life success.[20]

BOX 4-1:   The Rosenberg Self-Esteem Scale

Instructions: Below is a list of statements dealing with your general feelings about yourself. If you strongly agree, circle SA, If you agree with the statement, circle A. If you disagree, circle D. If you strongly disagree, circle SD.

1. On the whole, I am satisfied with myself.	SA	A	D	SD
2. At times, I think I am no good at all.	SA	A	D	SD
3. I feel that I have a number of good qualities.	SA	A	D	SD
4. I am able to do things as well as other people.	SA	A	D	SD
5. I feel that I do not have much to be proud of.	SA	A	D	SD
6. I certainly feel useless at times.	SA	A	D	SD
7. I feel that I'm a person of worth, at least on an equal plane with others.	SA	A	D	SD
8. I wish I could have more respect for myself.	SA	A	D	SD
9. All in all, I'm inclined to think I'm a failure.	SA	A	D	SD
10. I take a positive attitude toward myself.	SA	A	D	SD

Scoring: SA = 3, A = 2, D = 1, SD = 0 for questions 1, 3, 4, 7, and 10. Questions 2, 5, 6, 8, and 9 are reverse-scored so that SA = 0, A = 1, D = 2, SA = 3. The higher the score, the higher the self-esteem. The highest possible score is 30.

From Rosenberg M. *Society and the Adolescent Image*, rev ed. Middletown, CT: Wesleyan University Press; 1989.

BOX 4-2:   Self-Talk Questionnaire

Answer the following:

1. I sometimes talk to myself when I am working on a challenging problem.
2. I sometimes talk to myself when I am trying to remember information.
3. I sometimes talk to myself when I am trying to organize or plan something.
4. I sometimes talk to myself when I am assessing my performance.
5. I sometimes talk to myself when I am upset or angry.
6. I sometimes talk to myself when I am trying to encourage myself.
7. I sometimes talk to myself about persons I see or with whom I am talking.
8. I sometimes talk to myself when I am looking for information in a book or online.
9. I sometimes talk to myself when I am feeling physical discomfort.
10. I sometimes talk to myself when I am feeling lonely.

Adapted from Duncan RM, Cheyne A. Incidence and functions of self reported private speech in young adults: A self verbalization questionnaire. *Can J Behav Sci.* 1999;31(2):133-136.

Guiding Assumption #1: "The Map Is Not the Territory"[20]

One way to look at the collective components of internal communication is to consider them as our map of the world and thus the determinants of our reality. For example, the saying that a person can see a cup of fluid as either half empty or half full speaks to how inner perceptions guide our external outlook. Based on these perceptions (the map), we then use our internal communication to help us navigate through the events (the territory) of our lives. Obviously, the more realistically our map represents these events, the more successful we will be. If our map (our internal communication in this case) is distorted, it is likely that our reactions will be as well, with the result being a lack of success in our interactions.

Often, when there is a lack of understanding between two persons, it is because the meaning of the sender is filtered through the receiver's faulty internal map, resulting in a misinterpretation on the part of the latter. In turn, this may generate ineffective response. One example is when a constructive suggestion given in the spirit of collegial goodwill is interpreted as a hurtful criticism, causing the receiver to respond defensively.

Understanding that our internal map may not be an accurate representation of reality is an important first step in recognizing and changing counterproductive self-talk.[20] This premise suggests that our internal representation (the map created by our self-talk) is *merely our perception of what our collective thoughts, feelings, and attitudes tell us about the world* (which is the territory of real circumstances and events). Accordingly, we act on the basis of what we have told ourselves about the world. If you have ever tried to locate a destination using a faulty map, you can readily appreciate how such inaccuracies can lead one astray. The good news is that just as maps are often updated to reflect changes in the territory they represent (such as the addition of new roads), we can also change our internal maps (through the addition of empowering self-talk) to enhance our navigational effectiveness in our world. Some helpful strategies are explored further in this chapter.

Guiding Assumption #2: "Our Experiences Have a Mental Structure."[20]

This is another key premise of NLP, which states that our thoughts and memories have an accompanying sensory pattern in our minds that is narrated by self-talk. In other words, our memories include visual, auditory, and olfactory cues (as well as those from our other senses). These sensory cues are highlighted as stories that repeatedly unfold through our internal dialogue. For example, our memories of happy events, such as gatherings of loved ones, may be accompanied by sensations of warmth and lightness. In addition they may be illustrated by brighter colors and narrated with joyful and encouraging self-talk. In contrast, our sad memories are often accompanied by heavy sensations, darkness, and depressing self-talk. These sensory patterns tend to persist in our minds, and their accompanying narratives are often replayed when we are faced with new events of a similar nature. Thus, the persistent application of old patterns to new experiences may limit our potential for success.

For example, many people are fearful of public speaking, perhaps from one past experience that was not successful. Thus, every time such persons imagine themselves in front of an audience, the negative pattern of their inner dialogue and memories evokes feelings of anxiety, often accompanied by physical discomfort and greatly exaggerated by negative self-talk. This pattern of negativity is replayed in memory every time the person contemplates public speaking, and the unpleasant thoughts, feelings, and sensations keep them from enjoying this activity. As it turns out, we can "grade" the intensity of such negative experiences, using our score as a baseline against which to measure future progress.

Quantifying Our Mental Structures: Subjective Units of Discomfort (SUDS)

The internal maps we have created in our minds regarding the various persons, places, and things in our lives all have an emotional "valence," which is perceived as either an attraction, or aversion. Accordingly, maps with a positive emotional valence are accompanied by pleasant physiological sensations and encouraging self-talk, while those with a negative valence provoke painful feelings and negative internal dialogue.

Humans grow and make positive changes by stretching to meet new life goals. A great many of us have less than encouraging internal maps to empower us, and it is very common for feelings of anxiety to arise in the face of challenge. In order to measure positive change in our internal maps and the physiological sensations they produce, it is helpful to have a rating system to track our progress. A highly useful tool in this regard is the Subjective Units of Discomfort (SUDS) scale, which is the psychological variant of the 1-to-10 rating scale for physical pain that is widely used in clinical practice.[21]

The SUDS scale has been repeatedly determined to be a valid measure of the physiological manifestations of stress and relaxation.[22] The SUDS scale was developed by Joseph Wolpe in 1969 as an objective measure of anxiety for use in the treatment of phobias.[23] It is a simple subjective rating scale, as shown in **Figure 4-2.**

1	2	3	4	5	6	7	8	9	10
Completely relaxed, at ease			Alert, focused			Tense, anxious			Panic, sweating, dry mouth, racing thoughts, pounding heart

Figure 4–2. The Subject Units of Discomfort (SUDS) Scale (Wolpe, 1969). See reference 23. The SUDS scale provides an objective rating for the physiological indicators of complete relaxation (as shown on the left end of the scale), moving along a continuum toward extreme stress (as shown on the right end of the scale). The SUDS scale is helpful in providing a measure of progress when one is working to reduce the emotional valence of stressful life events.

Talking Points/Field Notes

Using Suds to Quantify the Emotions in Our Self-Talk

Part 1

In a small group and/or in your field notes, describe your self-talk and general feelings about the following activities. Give each one a SUDS rating using the scale below. Note also how past experiences affect your current attitude, and note the emotional climate that arises as you consider each of the following:

1. Giving a presentation to a group of peers (such as a staff in-service or class presentation)

2. Starting a conversation with a person you have never met before at a work related or professional gathering

3. Being interviewed for an important position

4. Asking a question or making a comment in class

Part 2

1. After discussing or writing about your perceptions, note any differences between your SUDS ratings and your self-talk. Is there a relationship between higher SUDS ratings and more negative self-talk?

2. Have you considered that all four activities are really the same (presenting yourself in front of an evaluative audience of one or more persons)?

3. Consider how past memories, old messages, and automatic emotional responses to different aspects of the same activity exemplify an inaccurate internal map.

4. Do you think the ability to present yourself to an audience of one or more persons is an important element of physical therapy practice?

5. How might you begin to change your internal map of this activity?

Guiding Assumption #3: "You Are ALWAYS Communicating"[20]

This supposition states that we are continuously communicating, even when we are not talking. Studies by Dr. Albert Mehrabian of UCLA indicate that in the majority of interactions, verbal communication contributes to only 7% of the meaning of our messages, followed by tone of voice and inflection (38%) and body language (55%).[24]

Mehrabian's findings suggest that our nonverbal communication is a highly potent modality that often reflects the honest nature of our self-talk and accompanying emotional overtones. Our posture, gestures, and facial expressions send powerful messages that can be stronger (and more reflective of our emotional state) than what is conveyed in our words. For example, it is not uncommon for persons who are depressed to walk with a stooped posture, eyes cast downward, and face expressionless. Even if they were to tell you that they were "completely fine," their nonverbal communication clearly suggests otherwise. On the other hand, we can also harness the power of positive body language to increase our confidence and outlook. There is, in fact, evidence to support the truth of the old adage, "fake it 'til you make it."[25,26] Most importantly, you can use your body language to facilitate positive responses from others in the service of desirable outcomes, as with a genuine smile to a patient as a form of encouragement. A genuine smile is known as a Duchenne smile and involves activity in the muscles around the eyes that produce "crow's feet."[27] Interestingly, Duchenne smiles have been shown to facilitate positive emotions in both the giver and the receiver.[28] In contrast, less genuine smiles (which do not involve activity of the eye muscles) are considered a form of social politeness and have no such positive impact.

Talking Points/Field Notes

The Impact of Incongruencies Between Words and Body Language

This is an activity for three persons that can be done in small groups or in front of the entire class:

1. **Person #1** writes several emotions, each on a separate index card. Suggestions: disinterested, impatient, sad, interested, defiant, disgusted.

2. **Person #1** then gives one of the cards to **Person #2**.

3. **Person #2** will then have a 1- to 2-minute conversation with **Person #3** while using *body language* to convey the *same emotion* written on their index card. However,

Person #2 should use *verbal communication* conveying a *different emotion* from the one on the card. Suggestions for conversational topics: a favorite hobby or interest, the last movie you've seen or book you've read.

4. Following the conversation, **Person #3** will try to identify differences between the emotional content of the verbal communication and the body language and discuss his or her perceptions of the conversation.

5. Person #1 **observes the conversation and provides feedback.**

Discuss the following questions and record your observations in your field notes:

1. How might you address a situation where the emotions conveyed in a person's body language are different from that conveyed in their words?

2. What have been your experiences with the deliberate use of body language to improve the effectiveness of your communication?

Guiding Assumption #4: "The Meaning of Your Communication Is the Response You Get"[20]

The cycle of "What goes around comes around" shown in Figure 4-1 speaks to the cyclic effect of our internal dialogue on both self and others. Since our first relationship is with self, it is helpful to understand how internal dialogue affects our sense of well-being.

To that end, it is likely that you have already observed the self-perpetuating impact of a consistent stream of either positive or negative self-talk within yourself. The powerful effects of such have been repeatedly documented in the area of mental health. One study of adolescents found that negative self-talk was a predictor of anxiety disorder.[29] Another study of college women found that negative self-talk was the major contributing factor to poor self-esteem and related depression.[30] Thus, these studies indicate that anxiety and depression are in part the physiological and mental consequences of our self-communication.

The persons with whom we interact also use their self-talk and internal maps to interpret your communication and respond accordingly. Thus, their responses provide feedback to you about how your communication was received. Skilled communicators are always carefully observing the responses to their communication, using the emotional intelligence elements of empathy and social expertness for cues about how these were interpreted. Obviously, it is most effective to identify any discrepancies immediately and to remedy these before they result in painful misunderstandings.

The relationship between ineffective self-talk and negative responses from others is a growing area of study in business, where it has been identified as a major barrier to employee engagement.[31] According to the Arbinger Institute, an international group of leadership consultants whose primary goal is to promote effective communication in business, community, and family settings,[32] faulty internal communication often originates from an inflated sense of one's importance, which is conveyed as the inability to treat others with genuine concern and kindness. When we treat those around us as means to our ends (e.g., consider the interactions of an employer who views workers solely as generators of profit), the response is returned in kind, often in the form of passive-aggressive behaviors. Arbinger calls the habitual use of such a self-serving point of view as "being in the box." Furthermore, interactions occurring from this position will have predictably negative results.

In order to observe others functioning "in the box," you do not have to look far. Behaviors such as aggressive driving or being impatient with salespersons who aren't fast enough for our liking are everyday examples. On a broader scale, the desire to meet personal needs at the expense of others can result in tremendous harm, as seen in the 2008 collapse of the U.S. housing market because of "predatory lending" by banking institutions. Thus, according to Arbinger, any lack of human civility begins with faulty internal maps and ego-driven self-talk.

Talking Points/Field Notes

The Effect of a Compassionate Internal Map

In the next few days, do this exercise at least once, then share your observations with a small group in class. You can also record your observations in your field notes.

This exercise will be most effective if it is a situation where the actions or lack of actions of others are preventing you from meeting your needs. Examples include being frustrated with other persons because of having to wait in a long line, or a delay in getting service in a busy establishment. This can also include your reactions to friends/loved ones who don't do something you want them to do because of their own needs (your spouse doesn't get up to feed your newborn because he is tired, your roommate is too slow at cleaning up, etc.).

Continued

Talking Points/Field Notes—cont'd ■ ▬▬▬▬▬▬▬▬▬▬▬

Pay attention to the self-talk around your frustration. You can use a SUDS rating to quantify these feelings. Note any self-talk suggesting that your needs are more important than those of the other persons in this situation. Such self-talk is often critical of others, overly self-sympathetic ("poor me"), and defensive.

Part 1: Monitoring My Self-Talk as It Normally Is

For the next 24 hours:

1. Pay attention to self-talk that negatively labels and judges others for getting in the way of your needs. What sort of messages arise?

2. Note any self-talk that places your needs and virtues above those of others. What does this look like?

3. Pay attention to self-talk suggesting that you act in a way that puts yourself before the others in this situation. Play out in your mind what the likely responses might be *if* you acted from this perspective.

Part 2: Consciously Changing My Self-Talk Toward Compassion for Others

For the next 24 hours:

1. Imagine yourself stepping back from your self-talk. Take the viewpoint of a casual, nonjudging observer.

2. Whenever you find yourself becoming frustrated in an interaction (presumably when others aren't meeting your needs), note any negative messages in your self-talk.

3. Change your self-talk to that of compassion and caring for those with whom you interact. Imagine their needs as even greater than yours. Imagine their frustrations around this situation.

4. Act with kindness and other-centered regard to one of the individuals. It can be something as simple as a genuine smile or asking another person in line "how is your day going?"

5. Note the reaction of others and changes in your own self-regard when your self-talk and inner map reflects a more compassionate view of others. How is a compassionate approach different from a self-centered one?

Implications for Physical Therapy Practice

As we engage with our patients in the course of carrying out our mission, we will find ourselves using our self-talk and internal maps with regard to a variety of issues, such as our sense of professional competence, our ability to interact effectively, and, most importantly, the level of genuine caring and unconditional positive regard we bring to the therapeutic partnership. Awareness and conscious change of internal dialogue that does not serve these therapeutic outcomes may be the single most important strategy for success in our various life roles. Maintaining this awareness will be a lifelong process that will enhance our engaged professionalism, the authenticity of our relationships, and our overall well-being.

▌Elements of Explanatory Style

The RIDE of Attributions

Our self-talk also involves the use of long-held internal maps to frame explanations for everything that happens to us. As we discussed early in this chapter, this process involves the use of *attributions*, through which we make sense of life events by assigning them a cause, purpose, and meaning (our collective explanatory style). As you will quickly discover in clinical practice, our patients will struggle with their own attributions when confronted with unexpected, seemingly senseless injuries or illnesses. The question "why me?" is a common reflection of this struggle.

Human attributions are complex and powerful, giving us an anchoring interpretation for our lives (again, viewed through the subjective lens of our internal map). As we have discussed, these interpretations give rise to a cascade of subsequent feelings, thoughts, and actions.

In order to modify our attributions and explanatory style toward a more optimistic outlook and greater personal empowerment, it is important to be aware of their specific components and how they contribute. These components can be explained by the acronym RIDE as follows:

1. Where *responsibility* for the situation lies

2. Where the emotional *impact* of the situation is felt

3. The *duration* of the emotional impact and outcome

4. The *extent* to which the emotional impact and outcome affect our lives

The elements of RIDE are presented briefly in the following section; you will have a chance to examine each of these as they pertain to your personal and professional experiences.

Responsibility: The Origin of Cause

Responsibility speaks to the element of ownership for the cause of the situation and its consequences. In other words, who gets the credit or the blame?

In a society that has long been based on individual rights, most of us have no difficulty accepting credit for positive outcomes. However, it is considerably more difficult to accept responsibility when outcomes are disappointing. Nevertheless, standards of ethical and moral conduct dictate that we take responsibility for our actions, regardless of the outcome.

Responsibility to others is a privilege that gives us the chance to follow through on our commitments and to act in accordance with societal expectations of our various life roles. However, because the acceptance of responsibility often involves a set of obligations, there may be a reluctance to follow through with these, especially if it involves admission of an undesirable behavior or the need for retribution. Thus, failure to acknowledge our responsibilities or meet our obligations can lead to a self-serving internal framework that may harm others. For example, a driver's license confers freedom of mobility along with the responsibility for driving safely. Should we happen to back into another person's car in a parking lot, our responsibility would be to initiate communication with the owner of the vehicle in order to arrange for any needed restitution. If we drive away instead, we burden an innocent person with the need to fix the car at his or her own expense.

Abdication of responsibility is likely a factor in the extensive use of the legal system in the United States. Accordingly, lawsuits are used to force acceptance of responsibility through sometimes bankrupting levels of monetary restitution. (Interestingly, the United States has 70% of the world's lawyers and only 5% of the world's population.[33]) Fear of such consequences has possibly been a factor in deterring some individuals from claiming ownership for their actions. Accordingly, in a chilling example, the numbers of fatal hit-and-run traffic accidents in the United States has increased by 20% since the year 2000, with 947 pedestrian deaths reported in 2005.[34]

Generally speaking, life makes more sense when we can identify who has responsibility for situations that have an impact on us. However, in most cases, we contribute to these events in some way through our own actions and behaviors. We are more likely to have a sense of empowerment when we accept responsibility for our role in these events and move forward to fix the problem. In contrast, blaming others does little to change an unwanted outcome. More importantly, by acknowledging our role in the little events of our lives (for example, accepting our responsibilities as physical therapy students), it becomes easier to assume greater levels of empowerment as our scope of influence widens (for example, as a physical therapist, one has responsibility for the development of potentially life-changing patient interventions). The important influence of responsibility on our self-esteem and empowerment is summarized in **Box 4-3**.

BOX 4-3

Accepting responsibility for our actions can *increase empowerment* and *self-esteem. Evading* responsibility for our actions can *lessen empowerment* and *self-esteem.*

Talking Points/Field Notes

Responsibility RoundUp

For each of the following examples, consider your typical self-talk related to your acceptance of responsibility for the following events. Feel free to add your own examples. Then discuss questions that follow and reflect on your observations in your field notes.

1. You oversleep and are late for a meeting.

2. You are not prepared for class and can't answer a professor's question.

3. You have a disagreement with someone you care about. You become upset and say something you regret.

4. You are driving to an important interview, run a red light, and get stopped by a police car.

5. You agree to do something you really don't want to do and fail to follow through when the time comes.

Questions:

1. Regarding the situations above, were you more likely to accept all or most of the responsibility? Why or why not?

2. Are you more or less likely to have a level of control over the outcomes for which you accept responsibility?

3. What is your self-talk like when you are evading responsibility for events such as these? Is it kind and empowering, or is it negative and critical?

4. What is your self-talk like when you are accepting responsibility for events such as these? Is it kind and empowering, or is it negative and critical?

5. How might your communication with the individuals in each of these situations differ depending on whether or not you accept responsibility?

Implications for Physical Therapy Practice

As a physical therapist, both your professional practice act and your code of ethics compel you to accept responsibility for the effective management of your patients. To help reinforce this, the American Physical Therapy Association (APTA) has a set of seven core values, one of which is *accountability*, which pertains to "*the active acceptance of the responsibility for the diverse roles, obligations and actions of the physical therapist including self-regulation and other behaviors that positively influence patient/client outcomes, the profession, and the health needs of society."*[35]

A Challenging Case of Patient Responsibility

Rena is a physical therapist in an acute trauma unit, having just returned to full-time practice after a 6-month maternity leave. She is preparing to conduct an initial examination on Mr. Piper, who sustained a closed femoral fracture in a rollover motor vehicle accident where he was the driver. His two passengers, Mr. Piper's 24-year-old daughter and 9-month-old grandson, were both killed. Mr. Piper's blood alcohol level at the scene of the accident was well over the 0.08% legal limit for driving under the influence (DUI). He was also driving without a license owing to several previous DUIs. As Rena finishes reading Mr. Piper's chart, one of the nurses working with him informs Rena that Mr. Piper has been complaining continuously about pain at the fracture site. The nurse expresses frustration with this behavior, since the fracture appears to be minor.

Once in Mr. Piper's room, Rena finds herself feeling very uncomfortable, wanting to get the examination over with as quickly as possible. Rena is surprised at her own feelings of rage toward Mr. Piper, since she is generally a compassionate therapist.

Questions to consider:

1. How might the events surrounding Mr. Piper's accident affect Rena's perceptions of his responsibility for the outcome? What might her self-talk look like?

2. How might Rena's judgment about Mr. Piper's responsibility affect her interactions with him?

3. What are Rena's responsibilities as a physical therapist in this situation?

4. How should physical therapists address the role of patient responsibility in the case of illnesses that are related in part to lifestyle choices, such as obesity, or addictions to alcohol or other substances?

5. What issues in Rena's own life might make her particularly sensitive to the effects of Mr. Piper's accident? How might she address these in order to carry out her responsibilities as his physical therapist?

Clinical Scenario

Impact: Who Is This About?

In our interactions with others, there is often an emotional residue of some magnitude; we probably don't notice its impact unless the feeling is strong. Whenever an event or interaction evokes a strong emotion (i.e., rage or joy), our self-talk compels us to locate these emotions either internally (personalizing) or externally (depersonalizing). The impact on our outlook also depends on whether the event is negative or positive. We shall first consider how self-talk related to impact affects us in negative situations.

Let us consider an example where during a study session with classmates, you are unable to remember an anatomic landmark. Your classmate Sue then says, "If you can't remember a simple fact like this, you are going to flunk this test!" Most likely, Sue's comment will provoke a negative emotion of sorts. If your self-talk leads you to internalize this feeling, it is likely that your self-messaging might include a statement like, "Yeah, I probably will flunk, because I'm not very good in this subject." With this message, you have personalized Sue's comment, internally translating the suggestion that you may flunk the test into a personal attribute ("I'm not very good at this subject"). In other words, Sue's comment is all about *you*. Obviously, this approach might escalate your feelings from mild irritation at Sue's thoughtless comment to feelings of worthlessness.

On the other hand, if your self-talk leads you to externalize Sue's comment and not take it to heart, you might say to yourself, "What's up with Sue? She must be stressed about this exam!" In this instance, you make Sue's comment all about *her*. Thus, any little irritation you might have felt with her comment is quickly dissipated, with no change in your sense of self.

As another example, Bob, a close friend, forgets your birthday. If you personalize (i.e., internalize) Bob's action, your self-talk would probably be something like, "Bob obviously doesn't care very much about me" or "I'm not really that important to Bob," and you might harbor growing feelings of hurt or resentment that play out in your next interaction with him.

On the other hand, if you choose to depersonalize Bob's action (externalize it), your self-talk might go like this: "Bob must have had a lot of things on his mind, I'm sure he didn't mean to forget." This reaction might lead you to make a casual joke about it with Bob or perhaps even to forget the incident.

As these examples suggest, our emotions will become more negative when we take life's disappointments personally. This is the core of a victim mentality, where every failure leads to self-talk that escalates feelings of worthlessness. Such dialogue can lead to habitual self-labeling, which can further erode self-esteem. As you will learn further on in this chapter, the type of self-label we tend to favor has a significant impact on our outlook on life.

Let us now consider the element of impact when a situation is positive. Going back to the study session, you answer a question with a brilliant explanation that clearly impresses everyone. Sue now says, "Wow, you really know this material! You are probably going to get the best score in the class!" If you were to internalize or personalize Sue's comment, your self-talk might include a statement such as, "Of course I am going to do well! I'm really smart at this subject!" Such self-talk would likely increase your feelings of worth and competence and might even motivate you to work harder in order to uphold this self-statement. In this case, the internalization of a positive comment leads to positive feelings and the enhancement of self-worth.

On the other hand, you might externalize Sue's comment and say to yourself, "Sue must be feeling very generous today!" and go back to your study with little change in your self-estimation. Accordingly, externalizing positive comments does not tend to increase positive feelings.

Let's also say that your friend Bob throws you a big surprise party in honor of your birthday. An internalized response to this might be, "I am important to my friends," while an externalized response might be, "Bob was looking for a reason to have a party." Obviously the perception of being important to one's friends is a more empowering sentiment than that of serving a friend's selfish interest (e.g., your birthday serving only as an excuse for Bob to have a party).

These examples suggest that internalizing positive events has a positive effect on outlook and self-worth, while externalizing them produces little change. Indeed, this finding has been well supported in the literature of positive psychology.[6,11,13]

The impact of the manner in which we internalize and externalize the events of our lives is summarized in **Box 4-4**.

BOX 4-4

Internalizing positive events or *externalizing negative* events can *improve* mood.
 Internalizing negative events or *externalizing positive* events can *worsen* mood.

Talking Points/Field Notes

Investigating the Impact of Emotions

Discuss the following questions and record your observations in your field notes:

1. Recall any situation where you personalized the negative actions of another individual. How did you address this and what was the outcome?

2. Recall any situation where you externalized the negative actions of another person. How did you address this and what was the outcome?

3. Are you more likely to internalize or externalize the feelings arising from positive interactions with others? What effect does this have for you?

4. Are you more likely to internalize or externalize the feelings arising from challenging interactions with others? What effect does this have for you?

Implications for Physical Therapy Practice

In clinical practice, the ability to appropriately manage the emotional impact of challenging interactions is an important skill that helps us to maintain our therapeutic effectiveness.

I will never forget my first patient on my first day as a graduate physical therapist. Bill was a young man recovering from a severe brain injury. When I nervously introduced myself to him and informed him of my intention to conduct a PT evaluation, Bill became agitated and started to swear at me. I became anxious and couldn't think what to do next, which led me to terminate our interaction (needless to say, my self-talk at that point was not very empowering). It took a reassuring conversation with an experienced colleague for me to understand that Bill was *not* reacting to my *obvious* lack of clinical expertise (the perception generated by my self-talk). Rather, it was the result of Bill's disorganized central nervous system processing, leading to confusion and agitation, which are common sequelae of serious brain injury. This new understanding was essential for my ability to treat Bill effectively. Although this example may seem extreme, many of our patients are under significant stress, leading to anger that is sometimes directed at their health-care providers. We need to understand the factors contributing to this reaction instead of personalizing it. This perspective will better enable us to be supportive and helpful in our therapeutic interactions.

Clinical Scenario

Don't Keep Me Waiting!

You are scheduled to see Mrs. Smith for an appointment at 9 a.m. at your outpatient clinic. Just as you are about to greet her in the waiting room, right on time, a physician returns an important phone call that lasts for 10 minutes. When you get to Mrs. Smith at 9:10, you offer an apology, but she is very irritated, saying, "I get so tired of sitting in waiting rooms! My doctor made me wait 45 minutes yesterday and I didn't expect to have to wait for you too!"

1. Where does the responsibility lie for your being late?

2. How might you frame this responsibility when you apologize to Mrs. Smith?

3. Consider how your response to Mrs. Smith's comments would differ depending on whether you took her comments personally versus externalizing them.

4. How can you use empathy to support Mrs. Smith in her frustration? What impact might this have on your own feelings?

Duration: Are Your Feelings Passing Through Town or Taking Up Residence?

As our self-talk system processes the daily events of our lives, assigning them ownership and directing their impact inwardly or externally, related emotions emerge and take hold of our attention.[6,11,13] Perhaps you have had the experience of going to class in a happy state of mind, then getting back an exam paper with an unexpectedly poor grade. In such an instance, this unwanted news may cause your mood to descend very quickly. Depending on the type of self-talk that arises (particularly whether you internalize or externalize your response), you may spend the rest of your day or even longer under a dark emotional cloud. Thus our emotional reaction to life events may be fleeting or persistent, and the nature of our self-talk while under its influence may further increase both the intensity and duration of these. If you encounter what you perceive to be other negative events as your day progresses, you may feel increasingly unhappy, and your subsequent interactions may be adversely affected.

On the other hand, what if your grade was much better than expected? You might enjoy some pleasant euphoria all day long, and this might compel you toward extra kindness to yourself and others.

We all know persons who react with extreme emotional intensity to the ups and downs of their lives and who spread this energy to everyone around them. Furthermore, workplace satisfaction can be greatly affected when persons who work closely together allow their ups and downs to color their interactions, as illustrated in the following example.

Moody Mike

You have just begun a private practice where you are the sole clinician. You have just hired Mike to be your office manager and have given him a 3-month probationary period. Mike's responsibilities include greeting patients when they arrive for appointments, patient scheduling, and working with your insurance companies for billing. From what you have observed during his first month with you, Mike is organized, efficient, and has great experience with billing, which saves you a lot of time. However, you've seen him be abrupt with patients a couple of times. You decide to confront Mike about this behavior, and he responds with "I know that I can be like that when I'm in a bad mood, but I'll try to change." Unfortunately things really don't get better in the next few weeks, and you even find yourself avoiding Mike when you sense that he's in a bad mood.

1. What are your concerns at this point regarding Mike's performance?

2. If you decide to keep Mike as your receptionist, what expectations do you put in place and how do you enforce them?

3. If you decide to terminate Mike, how would you explain this to him?

4. What are our professional responsibilities in terms of managing our moods and feelings at work? What strategies might be helpful?

Long-Duration Messages Can Become Self-Fulfilling Prophecies

The repetitive messages of our self-talk pertaining to related life events can begin to accumulate over time to the point of self-labeling.[6,11,13] In reality, such labels are nothing more than personalized, relatively permanent (long-duration) internal messages about our strengths and weaknesses. Obviously, depending on whether they are positive or negative, these labels can either empower or demean us.

Obsessive repetition of negative self-talk is known as *rumination*,[3] which has been shown to either bring on or maintain a depressive state—for example, after our anatomy exam is returned to us with a poor grade. As our mood descends with increasingly negative replays of this event, our self-talk might eventually suggest, "I will never pass this anatomy course." Thus, an isolated disappointment becomes a prediction for future ones of similar nature. Such pessimistic forecasts can diminish our sense of empowerment and contribute to a dismal self-fulfilling prophesy.

On the other hand, we might look at this poor test grade as an exception, perhaps even taking responsibility for the fact that we didn't study enough. In such a case, our self-talk might say "I simply didn't study enough. I will have to work harder next time." In such a case, we would quickly put an end to lingering unhappiness and thus feel empowered to improve the next time around.

When we are feeling discouraged, it can be very helpful to explore the self-talk behind our emotions. Which long-duration messages are behind these? Are we focusing on the positive or negative elements of our self-talk? The manner in which long-duration messages can affect self-esteem is summarized in **Box 4-5.**

BOX 4-5

Long-lasting positive messages can *enhance* self-esteem and mood.
Long-lasting, negative messages can *worsen* self-esteem and mood.

Talking Points/Field Notes

My Labels

Without thinking too much about it, generate a list of your labels (aim for 25). It might help you to fill in this sentence: "For the most part, I see myself as_____." Then discuss the questions below and reflect on your observations in your field notes.

1. Which labels are the most and least empowering?

2. As you examine each of your labels, reflect on which kinds of experiences have led you to form these perceptions of yourself.

3. If you have labels that are not helpful to your sense of emotional empowerment, how can you begin to change your self-talk around these?

Extent of Emotional Impact: Ripples or Tidal Waves?

Related to the duration of our feelings is the extent to which they affect our sense of self as a whole. We can either use self-talk that limits their impact to a discrete area or we can expand it to include other aspects of our lives. Again, depending on whether our perceptions are positive or negative, this can either empower or impair us.

Let's say that you have just been invited to Lauren's party and are very happy. You might give this happiness a prominent place in your life with self-talk that says, "I was invited to Lauren's party because I am popular." With such self-talk, you are likely to behave in ways that support this expansive view of yourself as being likeable in all areas of your life. On the other hand, if your self-talk was on the order of "I was invited to Lauren's party because I'm her lab partner," you have limited your explanation to a single, discrete aspect of your life (being a lab partner). With this attribution, you might not get as much emotional pleasure from Lauren's gesture.

Negative labels of an expansive nature do little in the way of self-empowerment and can even be destructive. For example, a student whose reaction to a poor grade on an anatomy test is "I'm totally stupid" will probably not feel strong confidence of his ability to succeed in other classes.

High self-esteem is related to the degree to which our self-talk focuses on positive attributes of an internal and expansive nature.[6,11,13] Statements such as "I'm smart," "I'm athletic," or "I'm funny," indicate that we see these attributes as elements of self that touch all aspects of our lives. Obviously such self-talk is empowering and enables us to more easily engage in behaviors that continue to promote these attributes. Evidence suggests that replacing negative self-talk with positive suggestions (known as self-affirmations) can enhance empowerment and positive lifestyle change.[36] The extent to which we allow our emotional self-talk to color our view of self is summarized in **Box 4-6**.

BOX 4-6

Self-esteem can be *enhanced* if we view *positive* events as *expansive elements* of self.
Self-esteem can be *worsened* if we view *negative* events as *expansive elements* of self.

Talking Points/Field Notes

Expanding Life Empowerment

One powerful way to strengthen our sense of personal empowerment is to incorporate healthy life behaviors into our daily lives.[36] In a small group, identify one goal for a positive change in your life. It can be a very small one. (For example, one student decided to spend at least 10 minutes outdoors each day.) Determine how you will measure your progress. Give yourself a time frame.

Consider how you can use self-talk to frame this change in the context of an expansive perception of yourself. Discuss what your life would be like if you were successful in achieving this goal and record your observations in your field notes.

Sample goal: "I will limit my junk food intake to one meal per week."

Expansive perception: "I take great care of my health and nutrition."

Life with this perception: This behavior would enhance my sense of self by...

Implications for Physical Therapy Practice

Much of our work as physical therapists involves the promotion of health-related behavior change in our patients. Effective lifestyle modification involves helping our patients to redesign their internal maps to promote the internal integration of positive, expansive self-perceptions. Our ability to help our patients in this manner involves encouraging them to discard expansive perceptions that no longer serve them. The process of positive behavior change involves the use of meaningful and achievable goals, tracking the patient's progress toward these, and encouraging every positive gain. It also involves limiting the extent and duration of stress related to setbacks and keeping a focus on long-term gains. Much of what we call quality of life involves this internal restructuring. Thus anything we can do to help our patients achieve this restructuring in a positive way can yield tremendous results in terms of treatment outcomes.

Promoting an Expansive Self-View for Our Patients

Sherry is a 40-year-old woman with a history of mild left knee pain due to osteoarthritis. Sherry is 30 pounds overweight and has been informed by her physician that a combination of weight loss and walking may prevent the need for surgery. Thus Sherry has come to you for an exercise program related to walking. Sherry is very motivated toward the walking program but says "I'm not exactly the exercising type, but I would like to change that!"

Discuss:

1. What questions do you have for Sherry that will allow you develop an enjoyable and realistic walking program?

2. What community resources might support Sherry's goals?

3. What suggestions might you have to promote Sherry's expansive self-perception as a person who exercises regularly?

4. What suggestions do you have for Sherry to monitor her progress?

Where Does Your Ride Take You? The Role of Self-Talk in the Development of Outlook

Winston Churchill once distinguished optimists and pessimists with the words "Optimists see the opportunity in every difficulty, while pessimists see the difficulty in every opportunity." In Churchill's time, his country was heavily involved in World War II and there were probably no scientific ways to distinguish between these traits. Thankfully this is no longer the case. One of the most important contributions in the field of positive psychology is the concept that our explanatory style directly affects our general life outlook in the direction of either optimism or pessimism.

If we tend to embrace life with a general sense of hope and self-efficacy, not letting setbacks discourage us, we are considered optimistic. On the other hand, if we see ourselves as generally powerless in the face of setbacks and tend to project the worst possible outcomes for our life situations, we can be considered pessimistic. Optimism and pessimism can be considered endpoints along a continuum. Most of us are probably somewhere in the middle, combining both elements in our day-to-day lives. However, research in health psychology and health promotion has provided compelling evidence linking optimism to improved outcomes and delayed progression of chronic diseases such as cancer, heart disease, and AIDS.[37,38] This research also suggests that persons who are optimistic have better support systems, are more likely to adhere to treatment regimens, and suffer significantly less depression and anxiety related to their conditions.

Thus interest in the elements of optimism and how these can be cultivated is an ongoing area of research in many health disciplines and may prove to be among the most important elements of patient self-efficacy. **Figure 4-3** illustrates the impact of RIDE on the outcomes of pessimism and optimism.

The most exciting research related to optimism has evolved from the work of Martin Seligman, author of *Learned Optimism: How to Change Your Mind and Your Life.*[13] Seligman has specifically identified the types of attributions that correlate with either optimism or pessimism. Furthermore, he has shown that one can deliberately change one's self-talk in order to promote a more optimistic outlook, a process he calls "learned optimism." **Table 4-1** details how the elements of RIDE are used differently depending on whether an individual is optimistic or pessimistic.

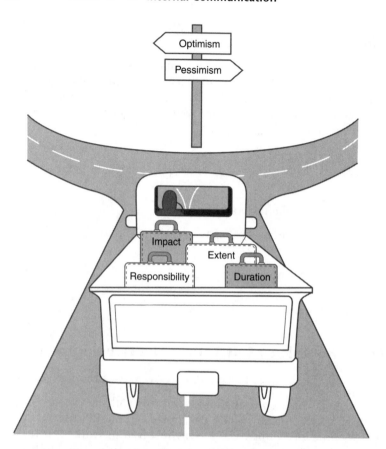

Figure 4–3. Where does your RIDE lead you? The impact of RIDE on the outcomes of pessimism or optimism.

Table 4–1.   Attributional RIDE Patterns in Optimists Versus Pessimists

	Optimists	Pessimists
Responsibility for actions with negative consequences	Always take responsibility for their actions. Avoid internalizing and self-blame. Engage in problem solving to find effective solutions. *"I made a mistake and I will correct it"*	Sometimes take responsibility for their actions. Internalize and self blame; may blame others. Negative self-talk may limit the problem-solving process and ability to find solutions. *"I was stupid to say that, it probably won't make a difference what I do now"*
Responsibility for actions with positive consequences	Internalize positive emotions from good outcomes. *"I really handled that "well because I'm a good listener"*	Externalize positive emotions from good outcomes. *"It went well because it was just my lucky day"*
Impact	Internalize and generalize positive emotions. *"I got a good grade because I'm smart"*	Externalize and specify positive emotions. *"I got a good grade because it was an easy test"*
	Externalize and specify negative emotions. *"I didn't get the job because I didn't have the skills they were looking for"*	Internalize and generalize negative emotions. *"I didn't get the job because I'm not smart enough"*

Table 4–1. Attributional RIDE Patterns in Optimists Versus Pessimists—cont'd

	Optimists	Pessimists
Duration	Assign positive outcomes a more permanent duration. *"I won the race because I'm a good athlete"*	Assign positive outcomes a limited duration. *"I won the race because I trained hard"*
	Assign negative outcomes a limited duration. *"I lost the race because I didn't train enough"*	Assign negative outcomes a more permanent duration. *"I lost the race because I'm a poor athlete"*
Extent	Assign wide expansiveness to positive events. *"I was elected class president because I'm a natural leader and others see that in me"*	Assign limited expansiveness to positive events. *"I was elected class president because I'm a hard worker"*
	Assign limited expansiveness to negative events. *"I got sick because I wasn't getting enough sleep"*	Assign wide expansiveness to negative events. *"I got sick because I'm in poor overall health to begin with"*

Adapted from Seligman, MEP. *Learned Optimism: How to Change Your Mind and Your Life.* New York: Pocket Books; 1992.

Conscious application of optimist strategies can help reduce the impact of negative self-talk.[13] For example, when we seek externalized attributions for the actions of others (i.e., "Mary must have forgotten to do the dishes" versus "Mary is a thoughtless slob who leaves everything to me"), we may find ourselves becoming more compassionate.

Optimists Stack the Self-Talk Deck in Their Favor

Optimists use self-talk strategies that externalize negative events so that their self-esteem remains protected. They also limit the duration and extent of negative events, using self-talk that makes these an exception to the rule for their normally happy lives. The saying that optimists see the glass as half full speaks to their natural predisposition to adapt their self-talk in ways that maintains hope, empowerment, and self-esteem. For optimists, the sun is always shining.

Talking Points/Field Notes

Developing Optimistic Self-Talk

Examine the following situations. First consider your normal RIDE and write it down. Now, if any elements of your RIDE were pessimistic, change them to reflect an optimistic outlook. Then discuss the questions that follow:

1. A friend fails to show up for a get-together.
2. A friend compliments you on your appearance.
3. You blow your diet or skip exercising.
4. You struggle to complete a patient evaluation or other class assignment.

Continued

Talking Points/Field Notes—cont'd

5. You give an excellent oral presentation to your class.

6. You greet a friend as you cross paths in the hallway or street, and the friend ignores you.

Now answer the following questions:

1. Were your original RIDEs to the above situations more optimistic or pessimistic?

2. What did it feel like to change your RIDE?

3. What effect would there be if you were more optimistic in your approaches to these situations? Do you think they would be less stressful?

4. Which element of your RIDE was most difficult to change?

Is There Any Value to Being Pessimistic?

A major premise of positive psychology is that an optimistic explanatory style can be harnessed to promote self-esteem, empowerment, and health. Thus it is important to distinguish optimism from ignorance or recklessness. Accordingly, the decision not to wear your seatbelt because of supposed optimism about your driving skills is plainly misguided. Optimism is also not denial, and this is something to keep in mind with our patients. Expressions of sadness, anger, and confusion are normal and healthy responses to traumatic life events; these must be experienced and processed if emotional healing is to occur.[39] Thus, the appropriate definition of optimism is an outlook that promotes conscious choices of self-talk and behaviors that promote happiness and well-being, including the use of all available resources.

In a similar vein, *defensive pessimism*[40] is an empowering strategy used by many successful and happy individuals, which involves visualizing the worst-case scenario as a motivator for planning and preparation. If you have ever studied diligently (and effectively) for a test out of fear that your lack of preparation might lead to a failing grade, you have probably used defensive pessimism to your advantage. However, if the same fear led to such severe anxiety that you were unable to study, this type of pessimism could not be defended as an empowering strategy.

The bottom line about the use of defensive pessimism is whether or not you are empowered by its use. For example, defensive pessimism in a new faculty member might compel them to type out lecture notes word for word as a measure of protection against inadequate preparation.

Implications for Physical Therapy

Illness or injury is a challenging life event that stresses coping methods. The elements of explanatory style are used by each of us, including our patients, in the face of such events in order to provide the sense of purpose and meaning from which hope can evolve.

Some of our patients will struggle for a considerable period of time with their attributions, particularly if the injury or illness is significant. In the meantime, they may experience a myriad of strong emotions such as anger, sadness, despair, and even guilt. It is our role to support our patients wherever they are in their process.

It is also important to understand that culture plays a significant role in the attribution process. In the western world, it is most common to attribute the cause of an illness to an organic or physiological process. Other cultures may have different explanations for illness, which could include the presence of evil spirits or retribution for bad deeds. For example, a Native American patient believes that her back pain is due to an evil curse. While this patient's physical therapist may not agree with or understand this perception, it is important to support this patient in her belief system. The following questions can be used to assist you in this process.

Useful Patient Interview Questions Related to Explanatory Style

1. What do you think contributed to or caused your pain or difficulty?
2. What do you think will help you get better?
3. What will need to happen for you in order for you to feel like you are getting better?
4. What treatments have been helpful in the past? (If problem is recurring or similar to previous ones.)
5. Which activities are you having problems with as a result of this problem? (What day-to-day things are hard for you right now?)
6. What would you like to be able to do better with PT?

Strategies for the Development of Happiness and Optimal Self-Talk

The Enhancement of Positive Emotion, Engagement, and Meaning

An important facet of positive psychology is the development and validation of interventions to increase optimism and happiness. In order to scientifically objectify the construct of happiness, Seligman has dissected this to include three specifically measurable components.[41,42] The first is *positive emotion*, the second is *engagement*, and the third is *meaning*. Recent research in positive psychology has demonstrated that an individual's outlook can be enhanced through guided questions that allow them to experience the elements of happiness described above.[42] For most of us, these elements exist in our day-to-day lives, but we are often too preoccupied to notice, much less to appreciate them. As we learn to be more mindful of even the smallest positive events, we can increase our happiness, which can become more permanently entrenched in our minds through our self-talk. As a beginning exercise, consider the following questions in the Talking Points listed below. You can also feel free to devise your own, as long as they enable you to uncover the gifts of your day.

Talking Points/Field Notes

Claiming the Happiness in Your Life

Every day for the next week, reflect on the following questions in your field notes. Take the time to enjoy the positive feelings that arise and jot these down too. At the end of the week, summarize the impact of this exercise in terms of positive feeling, engagement, and meaning. It can be helpful to rate your happiness on a scale of 1 to 10 (with 10 being the highest level) before and after the exercise each day. You can also share your observations with classmates during a discussion.

1. Gratitude list: What are you most grateful for today? Make your list as long as you can, not forgetting the little things that can make you happy.

2. Accomplishment of the day: What is one thing you did today that you are proud of or feel especially good about? What feelings does this bring forth for you?

3. Service of the day: In what way were you kind or helpful to another person today? (It doesn't matter how small the interaction.) What does this say about you?

Reinforcing Positive Outcomes Through Mental Practice and Affirmation

Once we begin the process of claiming the positive aspects of our lives, we can reinforce these through mental practice. Mental practice has long been recognized as an effective strategy for improving motor performance in both healthy individuals and those with brain dysfunction from disease or injury.[43,44] Imagery and visualization have been shown to activate the same neural and muscular structures as actual practice, as well as producing the same autonomic events.[45,46] Thus, mental visualizations of happy and positive events can enhance our outlook in much the same way as those in real time.

Accordingly, one effective way to change negative mental structures is to deliberately substitute positive and empowering self-talk (known as affirmations) along with mental visualizations of success. This strategy can be effective even under highly stressful conditions such as competitive athletic performance. One study of 17 national champion figure skaters found that 40% used positive self-talk and visualization of success as a strategy to enhance their performance.[47]

For example, let's say that you have a practical exam next week. As you study, the use of mental practice could involve visualization of an effective performance. Walk your mind through the exact skills over which you will be tested, visualizing yourself feeling confident and competent as you execute each one. Furthermore, your affirmations can include positive affirmations such as, "I am well prepared for this exams," "I am confident of my skills," and even, "I enjoy the learning process involved in practical exams." If this latter suggestion seems extreme, consider the impact of self-talk regarding dread, distaste, and lack of enjoyment of the same experience.

The saying "what your mind can perceive, you can achieve" speaks to the great potential that lies in the process of affirmation and visualization. **Box 4-7** contains exercises for enhancing outcomes through mental practice and positive self-talk.

BOX 4-7:   Exercise for the Enhancement of Outcomes Through Mental Practice and Positive Self-Talk

1. Take at least 10 minutes for this exercise, and do this when you can be relaxed and unhurried. Sit comfortably in a chair (lying down might result in your falling asleep).

2. Select an upcoming event or situation that is typically associated with negative self-talk. You might want to choose something relatively simple such as asking a question in class or making small talk at a party.

3. Imagine the setting where the event will take place, framing it as if you were making a movie. Make the setting bright and comfortable. You can even provide an enhancing music soundtrack.

4. As you prepare to enter this setting, create an affirmation for yourself. This is a positive statement suggesting that you have *already achieved the outcome you are working toward*. In the example of small talk, this could be, "I enjoy meeting new people and talk to them with ease." It can be very helpful to write down your affirmation.

5. Once you have developed your affirmation, close your eyes and imagine yourself in the actual situation, as if watching yourself in a movie in real time. Imagine the physical sensations associated with the event. Make it as real as possible, imagining your posture, your movement, your facial expressions, and your dialogue. As you view your performance, imagine feeling light, happy, on top of your game. You can also narrate the event with positive self-talk that highlights what you are experiencing, such as "I am relaxed, I am really enjoying myself."

BOX 4-7:   Exercise for The Enhancement of Outcomes Through Mental Practice and Positive Self-Talk—cont'd

6. You can reinforce the effect of this exercise by creating a written description of your visualization in your field notes. Your written description should reflect the event as realistically as *though it had already happened in the best way possible.*

7. Now that you have mentally created this experience for yourself, you can use all or part of it whenever you desire as a way to prepare. With practice, affirmations and visualizations can be a part of your strategy for success in anything you desire.

Implications for Physical Therapy: Practicing What You Preach

The ability to reframe one's self-talk in a more positive and empowering way has tremendous implications for health and healing. Most physical impairments are accompanied by psychological challenges that can become even more disabling than the original insult. For example, if a patient with stroke succumbs to a chronic sense of powerlessness because of a perception that he will never walk again, he may become depressed and have difficulty fully participating in his rehabilitation program.[48] Accordingly, his depression may prevent him from practicing the motor skills involved in walking, even in the presence of motor potential. The impact of depression is significant, as patients who are depressed are less likely to make functional progress in their rehabilitation programs.[45,46] They also have more difficulty with cognitive skills such as attention and memory.[46]

Although the comprehensive management of depression and other psychological impairments is beyond the scope of PT practice, our patients can benefit from our encouragement and coaching. We can guide them toward an optimistic view, and we can direct our interactions to promote a more empowering explanatory style. For example, it is not unusual for some patients to focus more on their deficits than on their potential. If they are discouraged, they may also fail to celebrate their progress. While we do not want to promote unrealistic expectations for our patients, we can certainly encourage them to aspire toward reasonable goals, helping them focus on their efforts and accomplishments, no matter how small. Much of this encouragement has the demonstrated potential to enhance our patients' outlook, and there are numerous studies supporting the relationship between a therapist's encouragement and positive patient health outcomes.[49]

As this chapter has demonstrated, such progress requires effort and the willingness to change less-than-helpful internal maps and obstructive self-talk. Perhaps by having a better appreciation of the effort involved in changing our own self-talk for the better and, in turn, experiencing first-hand the positive impact such change can have on our own lives and our interactions, we can enrich our patient communication with greater authenticity and compassion. Such communication can greatly increase the potential for healing at many levels for ourselves and those we are called to serve.

Stress Management: Managing the Physiological Sequelae of Negative Self-Talk

There is abundant evidence to support the effects of long-term stress on health and well-being. We now know that chronic stress results in a cascade of physiological responses that affect virtually all systems in the body. Stress is the emotional and physical strain caused by *our response* to pressure from the outside world.[49]

Our stress levels are significantly affected by our self-talk, particularly the attributions within our explanatory style. As an engaged professional, your ability to control your stress is an important tool for success. Further strategies for this are considered in the next chapter.

The 10 generic abilities for success in the physical therapy profession evolved from the work of Warren May and his colleagues at the University of Wisconsin.[50] Among these behaviors is stress management, which pertains to *the ability to identify sources of stress and to develop coping behaviors.* Obviously we are much more effective in all aspects of our lives when we are able to reduce our stress levels.

The fact that you are now in a demanding PT education program is an indication that you already have some effective stress management strategies in place. It can be very helpful to explicitly identify these. In addition, as the demands of life escalate, it is helpful to continue to develop your stress management skills. One important way of doing this is to harness the power of effective attributions.

Talking Points/Field Notes

Effective Self-Talk for Stress Management

Reflect on the following questions and discuss them in a small group. You can also reflect on your observations in your field notes.

1. Consider the last time you were in an unhappy mood over a specific event *that you were able to effectively resolve.*

2. What happened?

3. Where did the responsibility lie?

4. Where did you feel the impact (personally or externally)?

5. What self-talk strategies did you use to pull yourself out of your mood?

Implications for Physical Therapy Practice

Our patients face considerable emotional challenges, some of which involve the reconstruction of their lives after a serious injury or illness. Thus you may face patients who are depressed, angry, and frustrated for considerable periods of time. As mentioned in the previous section, you will be most helpful if you do not personalize their interactions with you. Furthermore, you will need to support them through their emotional challenges. This may involve enlisting the help of other professionals, such as psychologists or social workers.

The ability to manage our moods, emotions, and stress will be critical to our success as helping professionals. It takes considerable self-awareness and determination to move positively through the darker times of our lives; however, we must always remain mindful that our professional responsibilities involve the emotional encouragement and support of others. Therefore we must take care of ourselves, managing our stress effectively and seeking support when needed in order to be emotionally available to our patients.

Chapter Summary

1. Our self-talk directs our outlook and affects and thus influences our communication with others.

2. We assign meaning and purpose to our life events through our explanatory style and its component attributions.

3. The components of attributions are responsibility, impact, duration and extent (RIDE).

4. The nature of our RIDE may result in either an optimistic or pessimistic orientation to our life events. Learned optimism is the conscious selection of attributions that broaden the impact, duration, and extent of positive events.

5. Self-talk can be modified through interventions that increase the three elements of happiness—positive emotions, engagement, and meaning.

Take-Home Menu

1. For even more information and learning about positive psychology, the following website can be accessed for opportunities to participate in positive psychology research, for learning more about assessments for engagement, explanatory style, and other related areas:
   http://www.reflectivehappiness.com

2. More practice exercises to enhance your RIDE:
   a. For the next week, anytime you find yourself reacting negatively to an everyday life frustration, consciously reframe your RIDE toward an optimistic approach. Note any changes in your stress level and outlook.
   b. The next time you are confronted with a minor situation involving another person that causes you to feel a little upset, consciously externalize the impact. Note how this shift affects your subsequent communication with this individual.

3. Draw your internal map:
   a. This is not an art contest. The point of this map is to identify and represent the people, places, and things that are important to you and which have helped you become the person you are.
   b. Draw the borders of your territory, just as a map has borders. Use any shape you wish. Your territory will depict the elements of your usual day-to-day life, which can be depicted with stick figures or simple art.
   c. Make sure you have space in your territory for the important elements of your life. Who are the important people in your territory? What are the important places? What are your important experiences, related to your mission? You can simply put them in as they come to mind, representing them with words or symbols. If you feel especially creative, you can use colored markers.
   d. The borders around your territory represent the yet-to-be-reached destinations of your life, representing your life goals. As you label your borders, be sure to have one area that depicts your life mission (as defined in the previous chapter).

It can be great fun to share your map with classmates if you are comfortable doing so. This can be an enjoyable class session if everyone is open to it.

References

1. Verplanken B, Friborg O, Wang C, et al. Mental habits: Metacognitive reflection on negative self-thinking. *J Pers Soc Psychol.* 2007;92(3):526-541.

2. Ciesla JA, Roberts JE. Rumination, negative cognition and their interactive effects on depressed mood. *Emotion.* 2007;7(3):555-565.

3. Calvet E, Estevez A, Landin C, et al. Self-talk and affective problems in college students: Valence of thinking and cognitive content specificity. *Span J Psychol.* 8(1):56-67.

4. Treadwell KR, Kendall PC. Self-talk in youth with anxiety disorders: States of mind, content specificity, and treatment outcome. *J Consult Clin Psychol.* 1996;64(5):94-150.

5. Peterson C, Semmel A, VonBaeyer C, et al. The attributional style questionnaire. *Cogn Ther Res.* 1982;6:287-300.

6. Fitzpatrick MR, Stalikas A. Positive emotions as generators of therapeutic change. *J Pyschother Integr.* 2008;18(2):137-154.

7. Gebhauer JE, Broemer P, Haddock G, vonHocker U. Inclusion-exclusion of positive and negative past selves: Mood congruence as information. *J Pers Soc Psychol.* 2008;95(2):470-487.

8. Taylor SE, Kemeny ME, Reed GM, et al. Psychological resources, positive illusions and health. *Am Psychol.* 2000;55:99-109.

9. Swann WB, Chang-Schneider C, McClarty KL. Do people's self-views matter? Self concept and self esteem in everyday life. *Am Psychol.* 2007;62:84-94.

10. Siegrist M. Inner speech as a cognitive process mediating self consciousness and inhibiting self-deception. *Psychol Rep.* 1995;76:259-265.

11. Depape AMR, Hakim-Larson J, Voelker S, et al. Self-talk and emotional intelligence in university students. *Can J Behav Sci.* 2006;38(3):250-260.

12. Chi-ching Y, Wing-tung A, Ka-shing KC. Efficacy = endowment x efficiency: Revisiting efficacy and endowment effects in public goods dilemma. *J Pers Soc Psychol.* 2009;96(1):155-169.

13. Seligman MEP. *Learned Optimism: How to Change Your Mind and Your life.* New York: Simon and Schuster; 1998.

14. Rosenberg M. *Conceiving the Self.* Malabar, FL: Krieger; 1986.

15. Deci EL, Ryan RM. The "what" and "why" of goal pursuits: Human needs and the self-determination of behavior. *Psychol Inq.* 2000;11:227-268.

16. Ojanen T, Perry DG. Relational schemas and the developing self: Perceptions of mother and of self as joint predictors of early adolescents' self-esteem. *Dev Psychol.* 2007;43(6):1474-1483.

17. Stinson DA, Logel C, Zanna MP, et al. The cost of lower self esteem: Testing a self-and social-bonds model of health. *J Pers Soc Psychol.* 2008;94(3):412-428.

18. University of Maryland. Department of Sociology. *The Rosenberg Self-Esteem Scale:* http://www.bsos. umd. edu/socy/Research/rosenberg.htm. Accessed January 25, 2009.

19. Duncan RM, Cheyne A. Incidence and functions of self reported private speech in young adults: A self verbalization questionnaire. *Can J Behav Sci.* 1999;31(2):133-136.

20. The NLP comprehensive training team. Andreas S, Faulkner C, eds. *NLP: The New Technology of Achievement.* New York: Quill William Morrow; 1994.

21. Huskisson EC. Measurement of pain. *J Rheumatol.* 1982;9:768-769.

22. Kaplan DM, Smith T. A validity study of the subjective unit of discomfort (SUD) score. *Meas Eval Couns Devt.* 1995;27(4):195-200.

23. Wolpe J. *The Practice of Behavior Therapy.* New York: Pergamon; 1969.

24. Mehrabian A. *Nonverbal Communication.* Chicago: Aldine-Atherton; 1972.

25. The Positivity Blog. *6 Reasons to Improve Your Body Language:* http://www.positivityblog.com/index.php/2006/10/26/6-reasons-to-improve-your-body-language/. Accessed September 27, 2007.

26. The Positivity Blog. *18 Ways to Improve Your Body Language:* http://www.positivityblog.com/index.php/2006/10/27/18-ways-to-improve-your-body-language/. Accessed September 27, 2007.

27. Niedenthal PM. Embodying emotion. *Science.* 2007;316(5):1002-1005.

28. Papa A, Bonnano GA. Smiling in the face of adversity: The interpersonal and intrapersonal functions of smiling. *Emotion.* 2008;8(1):1-12.

29. Kendall PC, Treadwell KR. The role of self-statements as a mediator in treatment for youth with anxiety disorders. *J Consult Clin Psychol.* 2007;75(3):380-389.

30. Peden AR, Hall LA, Rayens MK, Beebe L. Negative thinking mediates the effect of self-esteem on depressive symptoms in college women. *Nurs Res.* 2000;49(4):201-207.

31. The Arbinger Institute. *Leadership and Self-Deception.* San Francisco: The Arbinger Institute; 2000.

32. The Arbinger Institute. http://www.arbinger.com/en/home.html. Accessed September 28, 2007.

33. Castagnera J. How many lawyers are enough lawyers? News of Delaware County, January 10, 2007: http://www.zwire.com/site/news.cfm?BRD=1725&dept_id=45406&newsid=17693500& PA%20G=461&rfi=9. Accessed October 2, 2007.

34. Heath B. Hit and run deaths see 20% increase. *USA Today,* October 17, 2006: http://www.usatoday.com/news/nation/2006-10-17-hit-and-run-deaths_x.htm. Accessed October 1, 2007.

35. Professionalism in Physical Therapy: Core Values Self Assessment: http://www.apta.org/AM/Template.cfm?Section=Policies_and_Bylaws&TEMPLATE=/CM/ContentDisplay.cfm&CONTENTID=36073. Accessed October 2, 2007.

36. Epton T, Harris PR. Self-affirmation promotes health behavior change. *Health Psychol.* 2008;27(6):746-752.

37. Mann T. Effects of future writing and optimism on health behaviors in HIV. *Ann Behav Med.* 2001;23(1): 26-33.

38. Deimling GT, Bowman KF, Sterns S, et al. Cancer related health worries and psychological distress among older adult, long term cancer survivors. *Psycho-Oncology.* 2006; 15(4):306-320.

39. City of Hope and American Association of Colleges of Nursing. End of Life Nursing Education Consortium (ELNEC) Core Training Program. Kansas City, MO, April 2006.

40. Norem K. *The Positive Power of Negative Thinking: Using Defensive Pessimism to Harness Anxiety and Perform at Your Peak.* New York: Basic Books; 2001.

41. Seligman S, Steen TA, Park N, Peterson C. Positive psychology progress: Empirical validation of interventions. *Am Psychol.* 2005;60(5):410-421.

42. Peterson C, Park N, Seligman ME. Orientations to happiness and life satisfaction: The full life versus the empty life. *J Happiness Studies.* 2005;6:25-41.

43. Page SJ, Levine P, Leonard A. Mental practice in chronic stroke: Results of randomize placebo controlled trial. *Stroke.* 2007;38(4):1293-1297.

44. Tamir R, Dickstein R, Huberman M. Integration of motor imagery and physical practice in group treatment applied to subjects with Parkinson's disease. *Neurorehabil Neural Repair.* 2007;21(1):68-75.

45. Chemerinski E, Robinson RG, Kosier JT. Improved recovery in activities of daily living associated with remission of post-stroke depression. *Stroke.* 2001;32(1): 113-117.

46. Saxena SK, Ng TP, Koh G, et al. Is improvement in impaired cognition and depressive symptoms in post-stroke patients associated with recovery in activities of daily living? *Acta Neurol Scand.* 2007;115(5):339-346.

47. Gould D, Finch LM, Jackson SA. Coping strategies used by national champion figure skaters. *Res Q Exerc Sport.* 1993;64(4):453-468.

48. Vickery CD, Seperhi A, Evans CC, Lee JE. The association of level and stability of self-esteem and depressive symptoms in the acute inpatient stroke rehabilitation setting. *Rehabil Psychol.* 2008;53(2):171-179.

49. Stress and how to manage it. E health MD: http://www.ehealthmd.com/library/stress/STR_whatis.html. Accessed October 8, 2007.

50. May WW, Morgan BJ, Lemke JC, et al. Model for ability based assessment in physical therapy education *J Phys Ther Educ.* 1995;9(1):3-6.

CHAPTER 5

Mindfulness: An Attentional Approach to Engaged Professionalism

"Most people treat the present moment as if it were an obstacle that they need to overcome. Since the present moment is Life itself, it is an insane way to live."

Eckhart Tolle

Chapter Overview

The extent to which we can give our full attention to interactions with others is perhaps the most direct measure of our compassion. Mindfulness is an attentional skill involving conscious awareness and full acceptance of the present moment, no matter what is occurring. A major theme of this chapter is that mindfulness is the most powerful form of therapeutic presence and one that must first be cultivated from within. This chapter explores the ways in which mindfulness can promote a more positive outlook, enhance professional engagement, and facilitate optimal health and well-being.

Mindfulness is a life skill that serves to benefit both health-care practitioners and the patients they serve. This chapter explores the value of mindfulness from both perspectives, providing practical suggestions for the development of this skill.

Key Terms

Mindfulness

Mindfulness-based stress reduction (MBSR)

Mindful practice

The Treasure of Your Attention

Along the spectrum of cognitive processes that promote responsiveness to the world around us, there are three overlapping levels. *Consciousness* is the cornerstone process, and relates to an appropriate level of arousal. *Awareness* is the process by which both internal and external sensory stimuli are monitored. Finally, *attention* is a process by which conscious awareness is focused on a specific sensory experience.[1] By consciously directing our attention, we can focus on the most important aspects of a sensory experience. Not surprisingly, an appropriate attention level is critical for learning.

In addition to learning challenges, persons with attentional deficits often struggle with appropriate social interactions because they have difficulty focusing on relevant sensory cues.[2]

In the case of our interactions, undistracted attention is required to accurately interpret and respond to the verbal and nonverbal components of language. If you have ever participated in a conversation with less than full attention, you likely know how this detracts from a genuine connection with the person involved. Divided attention (such as when having a conversation while watching television or while preoccupied with self-talk) detracts from the quality of our engagement in each activity.[1] Full attention is required for optimal awareness of both the content and meaning of our internal and external dialogue. Therefore the most important gift we can give to both self and others is our full attention. To use an analogy, our attention is like a high-energy light beam that can be focused on any object of interest, whether within or outside of self. The direction of focused attention is an amazing neurological feat, involving innumerable synaptic connections within the cerebral cortex. Accordingly, focused attention requires *conscious intention*, first to initiate and then to maintain. As you likely know, this is a challenge in our stimulus-intensive society. Furthermore, in addition to the typical distractions in our everyday environments, we now have a stunning array of wearable gadgets (cell phones, mp3 players, etc.) to further challenge our attention around the clock. Thus, we must constantly decide each waking moment where to focus our attention, and once we do, we must often struggle to maintain it in the midst of constant distractions.

The myth that people can multitask during their communication may be most damaging when it comes to human relationships, because multitasking actually requires the rapid alternation of attention *between* competing stimuli. For example, consider how it feels to talk to a friend who is constantly interrupting your conversation to answer his cell phone. Each interruption is, in reality, a withdrawal of his attention from your interaction, just as the energy from a flashlight must be withdrawn from one target in order to be directed to another. Most importantly, if such interruptions were a chronic feature of your interactions with this individual, you would likely interpret his inattention as a lack of interest in *being* with you. Such a realization might affect your relationship because the lack of another person's attention is emotionally painful.

As if the stimuli in our environment were not enough of a challenge, distractions can also arise from internal communication about the past or future (e.g., daydreams, worries, regrets, anticipation). This preoccupation further deprives us of full engagement with events as they unfold in the present. Perhaps you have had the experience of engaging in an activity with such inattention that when it was over, you were unable to remember what you did. In such instances, irretrievable moments of your life went by without your awareness, almost as if they had never happened. Optimal life engagement involves full attention to stimuli as they occur in the *present moment*.

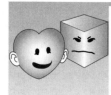

Champ and Blockhead

Champ and Blockhead Attend to Themselves

Champ and Blockhead are physical therapist supervisors in a large rehabilitation facility that is undergoing restructuring. In order to reduce administrative costs, the supervisory staff is being cut by 50%. When both Champ and Blockhead's supervisory positions are eliminated, they are told that they may retain their employment as staff members (with a corresponding reduction in pay).

Upon hearing the news, Blockhead is hurt and angry. She tries to ignore these feelings, numbing herself by overeating at lunch. Then, as the predictable midafternoon energy crash hits, Blockhead has a large cup of coffee with a candy bar. With her mental processes on caffeine-induced overdrive, she finds herself making several errors in her budget reports and snapping at staff. At the end of the day, Blockhead performs gait training with Mrs. Beans, a patient on the bariatric service who is regaining her mobility after gastric bypass surgery. By this time, Blockhead has a terrible headache and listlessly walks beside her patient as she counts down the minutes of their treatment session. Suddenly, Mrs. Beans loses her balance and begins to go down. Jolted from her mental fog, Blockhead grabs Mrs. Beans' gait belt at the last possible moment, breaking the fall. Unfortunately, because of her sudden jerky response, Blockhead fails to use optimal body mechanics in lowering Mrs. Beans to the floor. As a result, Blockhead injures her back and requires 1 month's disability leave.

Champ is also hurt and angry. She notices the negative self-talk that begins to arise and sits quietly at her desk for a few minutes, mentally observing her feelings and breathing slowly. Champ reminds herself that while it's okay to have these feelings, she still has immediate responsibilities to attend to. Thus, throughout the day, Champ continues to observe her self-talk with openness and without judgment while gently redirecting her focus on the task at hand. Thus it takes a little longer than usual for Champ to complete her budget report, but she is able to finish it without errors. When staff members come to her for help, Champ acknowledges the irritable feelings in her mind, but by keeping her focus on the staff members' needs, she is able to deal with them calmly. When Champ sees Mrs. Beans later in the day, she observes her closely during gait training while guarding her carefully. When Mrs. Beans suddenly turns pale, Champ is able to quickly summon a PT aide to bring her a chair, helping the Mrs. Beans to sit before she loses her balance.

Questions

1. Describe the attentional processes used by both Champ and Blockhead. How do these affect the quality of their experiences during their day?
2. Discuss how being mentally distracted and not focused on the present can lead to unfortunate mishaps such as those experienced by Blockhead.
3. Comment on the self-observation strategies Champ uses to maintain her focus on the present moment. How might this be helpful in reducing the intensity of negative feelings?

Narrow Attentional Focus, Task Accomplishment, and Stress

Attention is a basic unit of "cognitive currency," which is needed for all activities that involve learning and memory. As you likely know from your role as a physical therapy student, there are times when your attention must be narrowly focused in order to learn difficult material. We also use narrowly focused attention when the task at hand involves a high level of skill that is not yet completely learned (such as performing an examination technique on a patient for the first time) or where the possibility of danger exists (as when walking down a dark street in a crime-ridden part of town).

Narrowly focused attention is needed for high-demand task performance. Just as a magnifying glass focuses the sun so intensely on an object that it can make it burn, a high level of attentional focus can marshal all your cognitive resources toward a driving singular intent. As another example, consider your attentional focus while driving in a blizzard at night (which is a situation of some potential danger, requiring a high level of driving skill). In this instance, it is unlikely that you would be as relaxed as if you were driving on a clear day on a familiar highway with no traffic. Driving in the blizzard, you would sharpen and direct your attention to the greatest possible extent, rigidly focusing on the road directly in front of you. It is also unlikely that you would allow music from your car stereo, a lively conversation, or a cup of coffee on your dashboard to divert your attention.

While focused attention is an important skill in many situations, it does not generally serve us well in communication. The use of a narrow, task-oriented focus can lead us to miss many of the subtle nuances of human interaction that are important for genuine understanding. Furthermore, the chronic and inappropriate use of a narrow attentional focus is a major contributor to stress and anxiety. Accordingly, how are you likely to feel after driving in the blizzard? It is probable that most of your physiological systems would have reinforced your hypervigilant state. Accordingly, the muscles of your neck, shoulders, and jaw would have been excessively recruited to help you stabilize the steering wheel, resulting in tension and possible pain. Your heart rate and blood pressure would have increased as adrenaline coursed through your system to optimize alertness. Your self-talk would likely have been sharp and demanding, barking orders to yourself like an impatient drill sergeant. Most notably, once you arrive safely at your destination, you might feel uptight, stressed, and anxious, with this high state of arousal persisting long after it was no longer needed. Research in neuroscience suggests that chronic use of narrow focus is increasing in our society as a means of coping with the many converging demands in our lives.[3] Unfortunately, we can pay a high price for this in terms of stress, anxiety, and somatic distress.

With respect to communication, the chronic use of a narrow focus restricts our ability to perceive the wealth of inputs required for insightful interactions with both self and others. In essence, we become task-oriented and robotic. Responding to complex situations in with a rigid and narrow focus is the essence of *mindlessness*.[4]

Mindlessness: Disconnection From Self and Others

In the previous Champ and Blockhead example, Blockhead demonstrates many features of mindlessness, such as numbing her feelings, a preoccupation with negative thoughts, and a lack of attention to immediate responsibilities. She narrows her attentional focus to her agitated and negative internal state, thus failing to respond sensitively to those around her. This lack of full attention to the demands of her immediate situation is a hallmark of mindlessness. As the case of Blockhead illustrates, mindlessness involves a spectrum of automatic and subconscious behaviors that can limit personal and professional effectiveness.[4]

Mindlessness has its place in a specific context. With respect to the expression of motor behaviors, mindlessness can be a form of mental energy conservation. For example, in the realm of neurological rehabilitation, the ability to perform skilled functional movements without conscious thought (such as moving from sitting to standing) is a desirable outcome that leaves higher-level attentional resources available for other activities. Accordingly, all of us have enjoyed experience of mindlessly performing familiar and well-practiced skills such as sports, musical performance, or conversing in our native language.

Difficulties can arise, however, when we default to mindlessness in both our actions and interactions. Thus we may spend our days having entire conversations with our minds somewhere else, or—if we are confronted with boring routine daily activities (i.e., folding the laundry or doing the dishes)—we may do these with irritability and impatience (a form of mental resistance). If the tasks are demanding, we may make more mistakes (as Blockhead did with her budget). Unfortunately, many of us may spend entire days in mindless resistance, hurrying through daily routines as our irritation builds. To that end, consider your state of mind when you are confronted with a day of routine chores.

When mindlessness is used as a cognitive strategy, it causes us to filter new experiences through the lens of past ones in order to direct what is often an automatic response. Accordingly, mindlessness is characterized by a rigid and inflexible approach to new information and experience.[4] For example, in clinical practice, mindlessness may compel us to categorize patients with sweeping generalities in the manner of "all total hips are the same." Although such mental classification can be useful in guiding our treatment decisions, the failure to recognize important differences can impair our clinical effectiveness. Furthermore, the failure to appreciate the unique elements of human diversity contributes to stereotyping, labeling, and discrimination.[5]

Mindlessness can also involve the use of strategies to avoid or suppress negative emotions or unwanted somatic sensations. When our feelings make us uncomfortable, it is natural to seek relief. One quick and common approach is to reduce the intensity of noxious input (i.e., to numb our pain). Examples of such strategies include overeating as well as alcohol and drug abuse. Another approach is to divert our attention through distraction. Thus we may obsessively engage in common diversions such as shopping or gambling, or we may even work compulsively. Unfortunately, consistent use of these strategies can lead to addiction. We can also use mentally generated avoidance strategies, including denial, thought suppression, and emotional distancing.[6] Each of these strategies can keep self-reflection at bay and prevent us from solving our problems.

When mindlessness is used consistently to ignore painful emotions, the result is internal dysregulation, which can lead to psychosomatic complaints and the development of distorted emotional states, such as panic.[3] Effective treatment of these disorders often involves the use of mindful attention, which allows suppressed elements to be brought to conscious and nonjudging attention. This is the first step in establishing the self-regulation needed to make deliberate life choices that are "consistent with one's needs, values, and interests."[7]

Biofeedback has also been used to restore attention and awareness to one's internal processes in order to reduce unhealthy psychosomatic complaints.[8] Today, many computer-based biofeedback systems are available for reducing stress and related complaints. These are listed at the end of this chapter in the "Take-Home Menu."

In the Champ and Blockhead example above, Blockhead uses avoidance strategies to cope with her emotional discomfort. She numbs herself with excessive food and caffeine. Unfortunately, this leads to a headache, which creates an added distraction. Thus, she is unable to focus on the needs of her patient, jeopardizing her safety and injuring herself in the process. Needless to say, her work day is not one of high engagement. Furthermore, if Blockhead routinely deals with work-life challenges in this manner, her outlook and work performance are likely to suffer.

How Mindlessness Can Impair Clinical Practice

A lack of mindfulness in practice may lead clinicians to frame patient care into a narrow, task-oriented focus. Failing to consider all aspects of the *person* with the illness, they may approach patients with a checklist of symptoms that they use only to confirm what they already think is the problem ("it *must* be diagnosis X, and I will use my test and measures to confirm my thinking").

In the absence of complicating factors, this approach can often result in appropriate patient management. However, the clinician's lack of authentic presence is likely to be perceived by the patient and may impair treatment outcomes. In the worst-case scenario, clinicians who "don't know what they don't know" may take an inflexible approach to their evaluations, resulting in incorrect diagnoses and inappropriate management. Thus, rather than being comfortable with the many ambiguities that can arise in the course of patient care, mindless clinicians hold onto their own views and seek to "fix" their patients' problems. With such an approach, the focus is on maintaining the practitioner's sense of competence at the expense of the patient. Perhaps you have had the experience of receiving services from such an individual. Quite possibly, you were able to perceive this narrow-focus approach, and this may have led you to look for another practitioner.

Clinical Scenario

A Case of Mindlessness in Physical Therapy Practice

Darren is a physical therapist in a busy outpatient orthopedic practice. His productivity requirements involve seeing four patients an hour, and Darren prides himself on his ability to complete a quick orthopedic screening. One morning, Mr. Lahey, a fit-looking, well-dressed 60-year-old, arrives for a shoulder evaluation. Before the appointment, Mr. Lahey fills out a form describing his medical history. As Darren quickly glances over the history form, he notes that Mr. Lahey has indicated a history of hypertension. Mr. Lahey also reports that his doctor has prescribed medication for this condition. Quickly assessing Mr. Lahey's expensive clothing and healthy physique, Darren assumes that he has the resources to manage his blood pressure. Thus, Darren begins his shoulder assessment. At the end of this, Darren determines that Mr. Lahey needs stretching of the pectoral muscles and gives Mr. Lahey a few exercises to do under the supervision of Paul, one of the athletic trainers at the facility. When Paul greets Mr. Lahey, he gets the strong sense that the patient seems stressed. He looks at Mr. Lahey's chart, noting the hypertension and medications listed in the history intake. When Paul asks Mr. Lahey if he has taken his blood pressure medication, Mr. Lahey replies that he quit taking it a month earlier because it was too expensive. Mr. Lahey also shares that he was just laid off from his job as a civil engineer and will be losing his health-care coverage. At that point, Paul measures Mr. Lahey's blood pressure and is shocked to see that it is 210/150. Paul informs Darren of this and together they tell Mr. Lahey to report immediately to the emergency department of the local hospital.

Questions:

1. How did Darren's assumptions limit his ability to provide effective care?

2. How do assumptions about our patients lead to mindlessness in practice?

3. How might productivity requirements lead to mindlessness in practice?

4. How does mindlessness in practice contribute to errors or substandard care?

Mindfulness: Living With Conscious Intention

Mindfulness is the purposeful direction of conscious awareness to the internal and external experiences of our lives. It is a quality of consciousness that promotes "vivid clarity" in our current experience, thus enabling us to disengage from automatic and negative thoughts, habits, and behaviors.[1] As the benefits of mindfulness become more thoroughly understood, it is gaining recognition as a powerful tool for self-regulation, the development of healthy behaviors, and optimal well-being. The consistent use of mindfulness is associated with greater levels of happiness and feelings of enjoyment, along with more consistent states of peace, tranquility, and understanding.[9] Even more interestingly, high levels of mindfulness have been shown to enhance important emotional intelligence skills such as self-awareness, self-control, and empathy.[3]

Mindfulness involves several key components, which include conscious intention, a present-moment focus, and acceptance of all that arises. When we greet our internal and external experiences with an open and receiving mind, we are more likely to be perceptive and thoughtful. In turn, we can then utilize this information to generate the most appropriate and effective responses. For example, because Champ maintained undistracted focus on her patient, she was able to notice when Mrs. Beans suddenly turned pale. This observation allowed Champ to quickly assist her patient to sitting, preventing a potentially serious mishap.

Not surprisingly, mindful attention is required for the authentic internal communication that facilitates effective communication with others. When we are fully attentive and accepting of our own feelings as they arise in the moment, it is much easier to be emotionally available to others. Thus, mindful attention is an important prerequisite for our authentic therapeutic interactions as physical therapist. As a starting point, you might find it helpful to explore your own levels of this important skill.

The Assessment of Mindfulness

There are several mindfulness assessment scales in clinical use that assess various elements of present-moment experience.[10] One of these is the *Acceptance and Action Questionnaire* (AAQ).[11] It measures the degree to which one is willing to experience negative thoughts and feelings without having to avoid them *(acceptance)* or have them affect one's responsibilities *(action)*. Several studies (including one involving 12 physical therapists) have demonstrated the relationship between low levels of acceptance (i.e., heavy use of avoidance strategies) and decreased work productivity, lowered job satisfaction, and burnout.[11,12] The AAQ is a valid and reliable 19-item self-report questionnaire that uses a 7-point Likert scale. It is shown in **Figure 5-1**.

A History of Mindfulness

The concept of mindfulness in its broadest form is defined as "observation of the elements of one's inner landscape without evaluating, judging or participating."[1] Epstein[13] further describes mindfulness as "a state of mind that permits insight, presence and reflection." The roots of mindfulness practice can be traced to 1500 BCE* as an element of Hindu contemplative spirituality. Mindfulness is also a prominent approach in other spiritual traditions, such as Buddhism, Christianity, Judaism, Yoga, and Islam.[14,15] A prominent form of Buddhist meditation known as Vipassanna (Vih-**pah**-senna) has been practiced for over 2,500 years as a means of enhancing self-awareness and insight.[14] In this context, mindfulness has been translated as "seeing with discernment."

Although mindfulness has typically been linked with religious practices such as prayer and contemplation of the scriptures, *mindfulness in itself is not a religious practice.* Moreover,

---

*BCE stands for "before the common era" and is equivalent in meaning to BC, "Before Christ. Both terms pertain to year 1 of the Gregorian calendar.

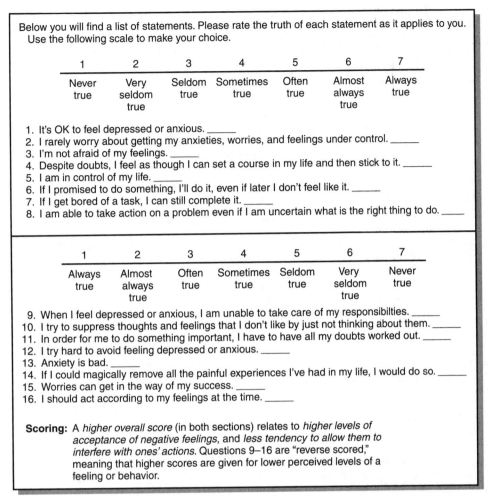

Figure 5–1. Acceptance and Action Questionnaire. *(From Bond FW, Bunce D. The role of acceptance and job control in mental health, job satisfaction and work performance. J Applied Psychol. 2003;88(6):1057-1060. Used with permission of the American Psychological Association.)*

Talking Points/Field Notes

My AAQ

Take the AAQ assessment shown in **Figure 5-1**. Then discuss your findings with your classmates and reflect on your observations in your field notes. Remember to share at your comfort level.

1. What factors might lead to difficulty accepting one's negative feelings? How might societal and cultural influences affect one's level of acceptance?

2. What happens if we accept negative feelings as they are without judging them as bad or getting stirred up by them?

3. How can self-talk help with accepting ones feelings and moving forward with the tasks of our lives even in their presence?

4. Must one always feel confident to be successful? Think of a time when you accomplished something meaningful even in the presence of fear or doubt?

Continued

Talking Points/Field Notes—cont'd ■▬▬▬▬▬▬▬

The *Mindful Attention and Awareness Scale* (MAAS)[1] assesses the levels of attention to and awareness of present-moment experiences. It is a 15-item self-report questionnaire graded on a 6-point Likert scale. The MAAS is illustrated in **Figure 5-2**.

Instructions: Below is a collection of statements about your everyday experiences. Using the scale below, please indicate how frequently or infrequently you currently have each experience. Please answer according to what really reflects your experience rather than what you think your experience should be. Please treat each item separately from every other item.

1	2	3	4	5	6
Almost always	Very frequently	Somewhat frequently	Somewhat infrequently	Very infrequently	Almost never

I could be experiencing some emotion and not be conscious of it until some time later.	1 2 3 4 5 6
I break or spill things because of carelessness, not paying attention, or thinking of something else.	1 2 3 4 5 6
I find it difficult to stay focused on what's happening in the present.	1 2 3 4 5 6
I tend to walk quickly to get where I'm going without paying attention to what I experience along the way.	1 2 3 4 5 6
I tend not to notice feelings of physical tension or discomfort until they really grab my attention.	1 2 3 4 5 6
I forget a person's name almost as soon as I've been told it for the first time.	1 2 3 4 5 6
It seems I am "running on automatic," without much awareness of what I'm doing.	1 2 3 4 5 6
I rush through activities without being really attentive to them.	1 2 3 4 5 6
I get so focused on the goal I want to achieve that I lose touch with what I'm doing right now to get there.	1 2 3 4 5 6
I do jobs or tasks automatically without being aware of what I'm doing.	1 2 3 4 5 6
I find myself listening to someone with one ear, doing something else at the same time.	1 2 3 4 5 6
I drive places on "automatic pilot" and then wonder why I went there.	1 2 3 4 5 6
I find myself preoccupied with the future or the past.	1 2 3 4 5 6
I find myself doing things without paying attention.	1 2 3 4 5 6
I snack without being aware that I'm eating.	1 2 3 4 5 6

Scoring information:
To score the scale, simply compute a mean of the 15 items. Higher scores reflect higher levels of dispositional mindfulness.

Figure 5–2. Mindful Attention and Awareness Scale. *(From Brown KW, Ryan RM. The benefits of being present: The role of mindfulness in psychological well-being. (From J Pers Soc Psychol. 2003;84:822-848. Used with permission of the American Psychological Association.)*

You are encouraged to take the MAAS now, and continue to use this as a measure of progress if you begin a mindfulness practice as suggested further on in the chapter.

a rapidly expanding body of evidence has demonstrated the value of consistent mindfulness practice as a *health-promoting behavior*. Furthermore, studies on the effects of mindfulness training have demonstrated that it can ameliorate a host of conditions including depression, anxiety, and chronic conditions such as psoriasis and fibromyalgia.[16] The consistent practice of mindfulness has also been shown to improve quality of life in other important ways, including enhanced work satisfaction, enjoyment, and productivity.[1,13–16] In reality, mindfulness is a powerful health-enhancing practice that can be useful to everyone.

There are two important ways to use mindfulness to enhance the self-understanding needed for effective communication. They are mindfulness meditation and mindfulness in action. Because mindfulness meditation enhances mindfulness in action, we explore this application first.

Developing Mindfulness Through the Practice of Meditation

Meditation is a mental discipline that involves directing attention away from the thinking mind and all of its distracting past- and future-oriented chatter. It involves concentrating one's attention on a single point of focus, which may be a sound, an object, or a body process such as breathing. By removing one's attention from the distractions of thoughts and other stimuli, meditation has long been used to increase awareness of the present moment, promote relaxation, and enhance personal growth.[17] The word *meditation* is derived from the Latin term *meditatio,* which refers to any form of physical or intellectual exercise.[18] Like mindfulness, meditation has been associated with various religious spiritual practices for many centuries.[17] However, as the numerous health benefits of meditation have become better understood, it is now considered a valuable health-enhancing behavior that can be used by anyone regardless of whether or not it is part of a spiritual practice. Thus meditation is simply another tool that can be used to reduce stress or pain, to promote greater awareness and concentration, and to enhance a host of physiological functions.[16]

In this health-promoting context, mindfulness meditation involves nothing more than inwardly directed awareness of the breathing process. The following sections describe the practice of mindfulness meditation and offer you guided instructions to try this for yourself.

An Overview of Mindfulness Meditation

In mindfulness meditation, one sits comfortably and quietly (lying down is not helpful, as it often results in falling asleep). With eyes closed, the meditator is asked to do nothing more than gently direct his or her attention to their breath, noting the rising and falling of the chest and abdomen. It can be helpful to note the cycle of inspiration with the inward speaking of the word *rising* and the cycle of expiration with the inward word *falling.*

Thus, the mind attends to the physical sensations of breathing, which are reinforced by the gentle inner repetition of "rising, falling, rising, falling" as the belly moves up and down. This brief description can best be understood through direct experience of the meditation process, a guide to which follows.

Mindfulness Meditation as a Form of Active Listening to Self

Given the busy nature of the human mind, distractions by thoughts, feelings, and sensations are a near certainty in mindfulness meditation. As you have probably already noted, the mind can be very persistent in its attempts to divert your attention from the natural and elegantly simple process of breathing. This can be frustrating, especially if you are new to meditation. You might even feel as though you would never succeed at simply being quiet and observing. In many ways, mindfulness meditation is a form of communication (active listening, in particular) to a quiet state of "just being." As with active listening, you must give this experience your full nonjudging attention in order to detect the

Talking Points/Field Notes

Settling in for Mindfulness Meditation: A 10-Minute Introduction

Directions: This activity can be done in or outside of class, in groups, pairs, or by yourself. You can set a timer for 10 minutes so that you are free to experience the elements described below. If you are in a group, a person can direct you through the following guidelines for mindfulness meditation.

- Sit comfortably with your back and neck upright and straight, either cross-legged, on the floor, or in a chair without head support. Close your eyes gently.

- Direct your awareness to your breathing. Note the gentle rising of your belly as you breathe in slowly and steadily through your nose. Gently focus on bringing your breath first into your belly, noting it moving upward to your abdomen and chest as your inhalation continues.

- As your inhalation reaches a comfortable end, note this feeling briefly, then slowly exhale through your mouth. Notice the gentle falling of your chest, abdomen, and belly as your breath moves outward.

- As you note the rising and falling of your belly, inwardly note your inhalation with the words "rising . . . rising," and your exhalation with the words, "falling . . . falling."

- You may become distracted by thoughts, feelings, or sensations. Simply observe their presence, much as you might note the passing of clouds. You can help maintain a detached, mindful presence by noting them with inner words such as "thinking," "sadness," or "itching." Noting these distractions makes it easier to move your attention back to your breathing.

- Do not measure the success or failure of your meditation by the number of times you become aware of distractions. This awareness alone is the beginning of mindfulnes. Each time you bring your attention back to your breathing, you enhance your mindfulness.

- If it is difficult to bring your attention back to your breathing, be present to your distractions, noting their coming and going while you continue to breathe slowly. Remember that awareness of things as they are, regardless of our liking, is the essence of mindfulness.

- You can remain in this meditation for as long as you like. Twenty minutes to an hour each day is ideal.

Once you have completed your 10 minutes of meditation, reflect on the following and record your observations in your field notes.

1. What was it like to maintain your attention to your breathing?

2. Did you note any feelings of physical discomfort? What were they? Were you able to note them without giving them more attention?

3. Did you become aware of any emotions? What were they? Were you able to note them without getting carried away by their content?

4. Did you become aware of any thoughts? What were they? Were you able to note them without getting carried away by their content?

5. Were you aware of any time when you were able to redirect your attention to your breathing in the midst of a distraction?

subtleties of communication. Thus, when we learn to quiet our minds and attend to our breathing, we become more aware of any stress and tension that our bodies communicate to us. Once these sensations are brought to conscious attention, they can be released through the meditative process.[1,16,19]

When we actively listen, we listen with our whole bodies, letting nothing distract us. We also suspend judgment and note the thoughts and feelings that are communicated to us. As with active listening, mindfulness meditation takes committed and consistent practice. In both our everyday lives and in our meditative practice, we can easily revert to old habits of distracted listening (especially when we are under stress). As a result, we can quickly fall out of the habit of a meditation practice, especially when we are busy. Unfortunately, when we stop actively listening to others and ourselves, we may bury emotions and tensions until they escalate to an interpersonal conflict or a somatic complaint.

Attending to Distractions

Distractions, when mindfully noted, are an integral part of mindfulness meditation practice because they demonstrate that we are engaged in the process of actively listening to our bodies. Consider the experience you just had practicing mindfulness meditation. In the short time in which you focused on your breathing, it probably did not take long for your attention to wander to any number of distractions. Perhaps you were surprised at their variety: memories, daydreams, feelings, physical sensations. You might have noticed these distractions immediately, after a few minutes, or toward the end of the session. Thus, if you are like the majority of meditators (regardless of experience), off your thoughts went without your awareness, until you suddenly realized that you were no longer attending to the rising and falling of your breath.

Although you might have felt frustrated upon discovering this lack of focus, maybe even further increasing your dissatisfaction with judging self-talk such as, "I'll never be good at this, I'm not cut out for this," *it is important to not be attached to any particular outcome.* In other words, there is no "right" way to engage in mindfulness meditation. Your meditation *will be as it is*, and nothing can be gained by wishing it to be anything otherwise. Accordingly, Eckhart Tolle states, "*We should regard every situation in which we find ourselves as though we had chosen it.*"[19] This *acceptance* of your meditation process, no matter what happens, is an element of the nonjudging and nonresisting elements of mindfulness. Rather than fighting your distractions, consider them an invitation for the practice of these important skills. Even more importantly, as you learn to offer yourself the gifts of nonjudging and nonresisting in your meditation practice, you are more likely to find yourself offering these to others in the course of your interactions. Through these practices, we can enhance empathy with self and others— a valuable communication skill that greatly enhances relationships.

In addition to nonjudging acceptance of distractions, we also make the mindful choice to invite them no further into our consciousness. In other words, if we note the presence of anger during our meditation, we mentally walk past it, just as we would step over a twig on our path during a leisurely stroll. In the manner in which we note the presence of the twig without further examination, in meditation, we resume attention to our breathing without allowing emotions to escalate and divert us from our active listening to breath. This is *the nonparticipation* element of mindfulness. As soon as you become aware of a distraction, you simply name whatever it is, saying it once or twice to yourself (thinking, feeling, itching, restless); then you return to awareness of your breath. Thus, no matter what your 10-minute mindfulness meditation experience was like, you gained the opportunity for practicing all of the important elements of mindfulness meditation.

The Analogy of the Wandering Puppy

Distractions that occur during mindfulness meditation can be likened to what you would probably experience if you were training a young puppy in a busy park. In such an instance, the puppy might obey your command once or twice and then wander off, his attention suddenly diverted by a squirrel, another dog, or children playing in the grass. If you were a mindful dog trainer, you would simply observe your happy puppy running off, perhaps even smiling to yourself and thinking "there he goes again!" Then, without getting angry or becoming frustrated, you would gently bring the puppy back to your training site and begin once again. If you have ever trained a puppy, you have probably had to repeat this process of redirection over and over again. It is nothing more than a natural learning process.

In mindfulness meditation, your attention is like the puppy, constantly wandering off to engage in a thought, memory, feeling, or sensation. Your conscious mind, which directs all attention, is the benevolent trainer, gently returning attention to the task at hand. By using the mindfulness training tools of awareness, acceptance, nonjudging, nonresistance, and nonparticipation, you will eventually be able to maintain your focus on the act of breathing for increasingly long periods of time. As you accomplish this, you will also note increasing times of calm focus, not only during your meditation but also in your everyday interactions.

Talking Points/Field Notes

Working With Distractions During Mindfulness Meditation

Directions: Repeat the mindfulness meditation practice as described above, increasing the time to 20 minutes. This time, consider that your mind's role is to simply observe everything that arises with *detached interest*. Each time you become aware of a distraction, observe it, gently name it, and redirect your attention to your breathing. If you find yourself becoming frustrated or restless, simply observe this feeling as it occurs and then name it if that is helpful ("I'm frustrated"). Then, when it feels right, redirect your attention to your breath without judgment. If you find yourself wanting to move or scratch an itch, observe and note this desire in your mind ("wanting to scratch," "wanting to move") without acting on it at first. You might observe that the urge diminishes or even disappears. If this happens, return your awareness to your breathing. You also might notice that your desire to act stays the same or increases, and if this happens, simply observe this and name your action while giving full awareness to it. "I am scratching, I am moving." At the end of 20 minutes, discuss or record your experience.

Perhaps the prospect of developing a regular mindfulness meditation practice is not of interest to you right now. Maybe you will explore it at a later point in your life. Nevertheless, the choice to include mindfulness meditation in your repertoire of health-enhancing behaviors is one worth making, even if you find yourself repeatedly coming and going from regular practice as your future unfolds. As the next section will show you, any time invested in the development of this health-enhancing skill is valuable, with increasing benefits accruing with consistent practice over time.

The Benefits of Mindfulness Meditation

Development of Stronger Focus and Attention

Although it might be hard to imagine, with practice, you may find that physical sensations and powerful emotions diminish just by bringing them to conscious awareness and moving back to your breathing. Persons who are highly skilled in mindfulness meditation, such as the Buddhist monks whom I met in Thailand in 2006, are able to sit cross-legged and fully erect without back support, unmoving, for hours at a time. These monks live very simply, in a manner that most Americans would consider close to poverty. Most remarkably, because they are content with whatever occurs in the present moment, they do not seek material distractions to occupy their attention and divert their self-awareness. Rather, they are extensively involved in writing, teaching, and service to their communities.

Enhancement of Brain Function

The benefits of mindfulness meditation on brain function are an ongoing area of research. A 2004 study at the University of Wisconsin-Madison found that monks with over 10,000 hours of meditation practice showed dramatic increases in high-frequency brain, activity (known as gamma waves), which underlies increased levels of consciousness and focus. The researchers in this study found that such increases were at a level never before reported in the neuroscience literature. They went on to suggest that meditation was a valuable tool in stimulating the development of structural changes in the brain, resulting in improved cognitive function.[20]

Another brain scan study of long-term practitioners of mindfulness meditation (where the subjects meditated for 40 minutes a day) demonstrated increases in the thickness of cortical regions related to improved attention as well as enhanced visual, auditory, and sensory perception.[21] This study suggested that meditation may slow age-related loss of cortical gray matter.

Decreased Pain and Stress

One of the first mindfulness-based stress reduction (MBSR) programs began in the 1980s at the University of Massachusetts Medical Center under the direction of psychologist Jon Kabat-Zinn. As a result of working with leading practitioners of mindfulness meditation, Kabat-Zinn was one of the first researchers to incorporate mindfulness meditation as a part of a therapeutic intervention program for surgical patients and persons with chronic pain, long-term illness, and emotional distress.

In discussing the benefits of mindfulness meditation as a means of enhancing one's quality of life, Kabat-Zinn uses the term "full-catastrophe living" to describe the richness of life experiences that can be enhanced by the nonjudging acceptance that results from the practice of mindfulness meditation.[16] Accordingly, Kabat-Zinn defines *catastrophe* as "the poignant enormity of life experience . . . the little things that go wrong and add up. Life is always in a flux and everything we think is permanent is only temporary and constantly changing. That includes our jobs, our possessions, our bodies, everything."

Increased comfort with constant change, or impermanence, is another benefit of mindfulness meditation. When we realize that everything is fleeting, we are even less likely to become attached to things that distract us from being present to our lives in the moment.

There is a growing body of evidence supporting the value of mindfulness meditation as a method of stress reduction. A recent randomized controlled study of 25 persons who participated in an 8-week mindfulness meditation program (involving 1 hour of meditation daily, 6 days a week) demonstrated significant increases in left-side anterior brain activation, the area associated with improved mood and reduced anxiety (this outcome was also clinically correlated with standardized test scores of these traits). These subjects also demonstrated improved antibody titers in response to an influenza vaccine given at the start of the study in order to assess the effect of meditation on immune function.[22] Other studies have demonstrated that mindfulness meditation can result in significant and sustained decreases in pain, anxiety, and depression in conditions such as fibromyalgia,[23] cancer,[24] and recovery from organ transplantation.[25]

Two major sources of emotional distress for many persons are anxiety and depression. Mindfulness-based treatment approaches are receiving increasing attention as an effective therapeutic intervention for these conditions. One particular approach, known as mindfulness-based cognitive therapy (MBCT), has shown promise in significantly reducing the rate of relapse for patients with a history of severe, chronic depression.[26] In conjunction with MBCT, mindfulness meditation practice has also been shown to reduce the severity of psychiatric symptoms among patients with severe chronic pain.[26]

It is important to note that in all of these studies, the basis of the meditation process used was mindful awareness of breathing, as described previously. As previously noted, the clinical term for this training—as originally described by Kabat-Zinn[16] and currently in use at the University of Massachusetts Medical School Center for Mindfulness in Medicine, Healthcare and Society—is Mindfulness Based Stress Reduction (MBSR).[26] Thus, in clinical practice, you may choose to use the term *MBSR* in place of *mindfulness meditation*. This term is used in the remainder of the chapter.

Clinical Applications of Mindfulness-Based Stress Reduction

Interventions Related to the Improvement of Quality of Life Are Important Aspects of Our Practice

Living with an illness or injury is stressful and often painful. As physical therapists, it is our responsibility to utilize interventions within our scope of practice to reduce related impairments in order to promote function and quality of life. Breathing is the only physiological activity that is under both voluntary and involuntary control. By voluntarily learning to monitor and slow our breathing, we can influence other physiological processes (such as postural muscle tension, heart rate, and blood pressure) in a manner that promotes homeostasis and optimal function.[27]

As physical therapists, we often work with our patients' breathing to promote relaxation and reduction of excessive effort. This can reduce anxiety from air hunger, which can restrict the functional performance of patients with severe heart disease or abdominal cancers.[28,29]

Even when healthier patients hold their breath during exercise, we provide suggestions for relaxation, perhaps suggesting that they inhale during an effortful movement. We also strengthen the muscles of breathing in patients with neuromuscular impairments such as spinal cord injury and stroke. Furthermore, in patients whose function is compromised primarily by respiratory distress, such as those with chronic obstructive respiratory disease (COPD), breath training often becomes the central focus of our intervention. As stated previously, breathing is one of the few vegetative functions served by both conscious and unconscious control mechanisms. When we are under stress or in pain, unconscious mechanisms prepare us for flight by short, rapid respirations. In the presence of real danger, these responses can help us escape. Thankfully, most of us go through our days without confronting true life-threatening danger, but our overstimulated nervous systems often act as if we were. Thus rapid, shallow, and irregular breathing patterns become a conditioned response to any perceived stress. Unfortunately, breathing in this manner maintains a high level of tension and may produce anxiety. Conversely, pain and anxiety can be reduced by increasing the depth of respiration while decreasing its rate.[30] In MBSR, attention to breathing in this manner (slower, deeper, and more regular) produces this effect. Accordingly, there may be times when instruction in MBSR can be a useful adjunct for pain control and stress reduction in a clinical context, particularly with respect to the promotion of overall health and wellness.

MBSR is an Element of Health Promotion and Wellness

The promotion of health and wellness is an emerging and vitally important element of PT management. A significant component of health promotion involves patient education and coaching for behavioral change.

According to the *Guide to Physical Therapist Practice*,[31] patient/client-related education is the process of informing, educating, and training patients with the intent of promoting and optimizing PT services. Such instruction may be related to the reduction of impairments, performance enhancement, or prevention of disease and injury. One of the expected outcomes from these interventions (such as MSBR) is *that "behaviors that foster healthy habits, wellness and prevention are acquired."*[31] The evidence in favor of MBSR suggests that it is a valuable health skill (along with diet, exercise, and weight control) that can improve the quality of life for all persons regardless of their health status. The following vignette is an example.

Clinical Scenario

The Use of MBSR in PT Practice

Susan is a physical therapist working in home health. She receives orders for a PT consult on Mr. Anderson, who has moderate back pain and shortness of breath from end-stage Hodgkin's lymphoma. Mr. Anderson is no longer ambulatory, and the consult is for "patient and family education for bed mobility, transfers, and pain control to optimize quality of life." When Susan meets Mr. Anderson, he states that he would like to be able to reduce his pain medication so he can enjoy more quality time sitting up with his wife and family. Mr. Anderson complains that the medication makes him very sleepy. However, he states that without it, his pain increases, making him anxious and even more short of breath. Susan's examination reveals range-of-motion limitations in the thoracic and lumbar spine and decreased lateral chest excursion during breathing. Susan decides to instruct Mr. Anderson and his wife in gentle stretching exercises that can be done in bed and while sitting. She also decides that he would benefit from MBSR as a nonpharmacological strategy for pain control, anxiety reduction, and to enhance the effectiveness of his stretching exercises.

Discuss:

1. How might you broach the subject of MBSR in the context of Mr. Anderson's pain and stress?

2. Role-play your instructions to Mr. Anderson. What do you include in your instructions with respect to the process, frequency, and duration of MBSR?

3. What instructions might you give in order for Mr. Anderson or his wife to measure the effectiveness of this training?

Personal/Professional Benefits of MBSR

To be an effective health-care provider in today's system is to truly face the "full catastrophe" of our patients' needs, challenges, and goals. In addition, family members, colleagues from other disciplines, case managers, and insurance payors also bring their needs and concerns to bear upon our efforts. In order to give these individuals our complete and compassionate attention, we must be well centered and capable of responding with compassion and equanimity. This is impossible if we are distracted, stressed, and out of touch with ourselves.

MBSR is gaining increasing attention as a valuable personal resource for health-care providers. The University of Maryland Medical School currently offers MBSR to their first- and second-year medical students as a means of *"developing intrinsic resources as non-judgmental awareness, concentration, openness, flexibility, equanimity, wisdom, warmth and compassion for self and others leading to a deeper appreciation of interdependence, and connectedness"*[26] Thus, the clear suggestion of this course is that mindfulness meditation training can be an important tool with which health-care providers can enhance the quality of patient care.

This suggestion has, in fact, been validated in one randomized double-blind controlled study of German psychotherapists in training (PiTs), which compared the patient treatment results obtained between those PiTs who practiced MBSR and those who did not. In this study, the PiTs who practiced MBSR were significantly more effective in reducing their patients' symptoms of anxiety, anger, and somatization (as measured by objective patient outcome measures).[32] This study raises interesting questions about the impact of MBSR on patient–practitioner communication, and implies that the virtues of mindfulness training are somehow conveyed to the patient in this process. Accordingly, placed in the context of strategies to enhance internal communication, MBSR appears to be highly beneficial. To that end, the impact of MBSR has been examined in a randomized clinical trial involving 98 rehabilitation workers in Singapore (including 12 physical therapists).[12] Interestingly, the authors cite evidence suggesting that physical therapists experienced greater burnout and stress than either physicians or technicians. The results of this study found significant increases in the subjects' perception of improved social and emotional functioning.

Developing Your Own MBSR Program

As you are no doubt learning, being a physical therapy student involves challenges and stresses. You are probably already finding ways to promote your own work-life balance through various stress-reduction approaches, some of which may be healthy and perhaps others that are not. The consistent use of healthy stress reduction approaches is a valuable life skill. If you do not already have a regular form of mindfulness meditation practice, you are encouraged to develop one now.

Although it is not necessary to have formal instruction in MBSR, it is highly beneficial to receive the support and encouragement that formal instruction can provide. There are numerous resources available; these are listed in the "Take-Home Menu" and references at the end of this chapter. In addition, courses in mindfulness meditation training are frequently offered at many universities and community colleges. You might find it enjoyable to pursue MBSR training with a classmate, where you could support each other in this valuable process.

Broadening and Building: The Social and Emotional Benefits of Mindfulness Meditation

One of the many benefits of mindfulness meditation is the increased acceptance of whatever occurs in the present moment. In other words, when we allow things to "be as they are" without resistance or judgment, we increase our capacity to experience positive, approach-related states of mind.[33] Evidence from the electroencephalograms of persons engaged in mindfulness meditation demonstrates increased left-sided anterior brain activation, which has been linked to the experience of positive emotions.[34]

Broadening and building theory suggests that mindfulness meditation promotes positive emotions which first *broaden* attention, thereby promoting openness to new experiences and increasing cognitive resources such as problem solving.[33,35] In clinical practice, this broadened state is a hallmark of what Epstein calls "mindful practice,"[13,36] which is a constellation of behaviors including attentiveness, curiosity, presence, and compassion.

In broadening and building theory, the cultivation of positive emotions has also been shown to *build* personal, cognitive, and psychological resources such as enhanced mastery, well-being, and life satisfaction.[33,36] Perhaps you have experienced such heightened levels of function in your own life when things have been going particularly well.

Another form of mindfulness meditation, known as loving-kindness meditation (LKM), has been shown to enhance *both* the broadening and building elements described above. In this form of practice, the meditator intentionally cultivates feelings of warmth and kindness in an open-hearted way.[33] In order to generate these emotions, meditators are directed to focus on the heart region, extending feelings of loving-kindness first to themselves, then to close friends and family members. As the LKM session progresses, the meditators extend their warmth and tenderness to an ever-widening circle of persons, finally moving on to all humans. A recent randomized study explored the benefits of a daily 7-week-long practice of LKM in 67 adults.[33] Compared with a group of control subjects, the LKM group experienced an increase in positive emotions (related to broadening). In turn, these positive emotions resulted in a perceived increase (i.e., building) of several personal resources, which included greater self-acceptance, enhanced personal relationships, and improved health. This study suggests that the benefits of mindfulness meditation extend to the elements of internal communication, which affect outlook and thus our interpersonal effectiveness.

More recently, Barbara Frederickson, the psychologist who developed and researched broadening and building theory, has presented evidence demonstrating that the cultivation of positive emotions at a 3:1 ratio leads people to become more resilient in the face of stress.[37] According to Frederickson, the spectrum of positive emotions is large, including awe, playfulness, contentment, inspiration, and gratitude. The more often we experience these feelings, the more able we are to build helpful resources (supportive relationships, increased empowerment) that enhance work-life satisfaction.[33,36,37]

We can continue to broaden and build these resources not only through the development of a mindfulness meditation practice but also by bringing mindful attention to the positive events of our daily lives.

Mindfulness in Action

The Cultivation of Mindful Attention in Daily Life

Mindfulness in action, in the full throttle of everyday life, is simply a way of paying attention to the way we interact with ourselves and others. As we discussed in the first sections of this chapter, we often pay attention in a narrow, hypervigilant manner that limits our ability to interact flexibly and openly.

We can certainly bring mindfulness to a narrow attentional focus, and this can be helpful in promoting learning and the completion of tasks. However, we should also realize that human interaction, particularly in a clinical context, requires attention to a broad scope of inputs. Fortunately, we can learn to mindfully broaden our attention in order to be fully present to these nuances.

New research in the areas of neurofeedback and psychology suggests that optimal human performance as well as health and well-being are largely related to the way we pay attention.[3,38,39] This research suggests that, as a society, we tend to spend most of our time in the state of narrow-focus attention described at the beginning of the chapter. The overuse of this attentional style contributes to a host of emotional, physiological, and relational problems. With respect to our discussion of mindfulness in action, many of us do not realize our tendency to go through our days in such an aroused, narrow state, blindly moving from one task to the next, driven to get things done with little awareness of anything else.

Thus, the first step of mindfulness in action is simply to be aware of how we are attending in the moment, then to gently broaden our attentional scope if it is too rigid. The goal is to move our attention from a narrow to a broad focus, bringing along the mindful elements of nonjudgment and acceptance of what is happening in the moment. In the manner of the "broaden and build" theory, by reaping the benefits of broadened attention (which include a greater sense of calm, well-being, and the experience of positive emotions),[33,35,36] we can build the communication skills that enhance engagement, strengthen our relationships, and empower our actions.

Using Mindfulness to Broaden Our Attention and Increase Positive Affect

Open Focus[3] attention is a concept developed by Lester Fehmi, director of the Princeton Biofeedback Center, based on years of neurofeedback research related to attention. Simply put, it involves broadening the scope of our attention beyond the immediate demands of the task at hand, including awareness of the surrounding environmental, sensory, and emotional landscape as well. For example, as you read this text, you are likely devoting a significant portion of your attention to the printed words you see in front of you. As you read, see if you can widen your attention to the spaces between the pages of this text, then to the space between the book and its support surface, then to the space between your body and the book, and finally to the space between your body and the room you are in. Like LKM, Open Focus attention involves progressively extending your awareness of space from your immediate environment to the vast expanse of the world around you. For example, as your attention broadens to the space between you and the room you are in, can you begin to perceive the space between the room and the building in which the room is housed? Can you broaden your awareness even more, perceiving yourself in aerial view?

This broadened attentional perspective (which includes perceptions of space and "nothingness") has been correlated with a shift in brain waves from the vigilant and rigid beta type (the fastest brain waves) to the alert but relaxed and spontaneous alpha type (a little slower), which promotes effective and enjoyable task performance.[3] Obviously, whenever we are able to be more relaxed and free from negative emotions and negative self-talk, we can become more receptive to positive emotions. More importantly, we can convey this positive affect in our communication with others. **Figure 5-3** illustrates the differences between a narrow and a broad attentional focus.

If these examples of broadened attention seem difficult to understand, you might consider how you feel when you are having a great time with friends at a party or when you are outdoors on a beautiful day. Although you might not realize it, your attention is relaxed and diffused and you are fully in the moment, taking everything in. Your attention is flexible, allowing you to move easily between conversations at the party or to appreciate the whole landscape, including the trees, clouds, and sky. Such attention is associated with an alert but relaxed state as well as increased receptivity to positive emotions, and it fosters high levels of capability.[3,37,39,40] Studies of broad-focus attention have

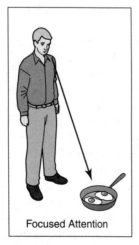
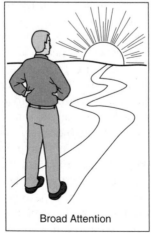

Focused Attention   Broad Attention

Figure 5–3. Narrowed attention directs focus on a specific task or thought, much in the same way that intensely focused light can fry an egg. Broadened attention allows focus on a wider expanse of inputs in a gentler, more relaxed manner, much as when one is watching a sunset.

shown that it is associated with increased athletic performance, reduced "stage fright," and more creative spontaneous interpersonal interactions.[3] With respect to physiological changes, broadly focused attention is related to decreased muscle tension, heart rate, and perceptions of stress. In order to utilize the benefits of broad focus attention, we must first become mindful of the way we are paying attention and the way our attentional style resonates in our bodies and emotional outlook.

Talking Points/Field Notes

Mindfulness of Attention

The following exercises are intended to provide an introductory experience of the concepts of broadened attentional focus. Suggestions for specific training in Open Focus attention are listed in the "Take-Home Menu."

Try to do these as much as possible for the next 48 hours, then discuss the reflective questions that follow the exercises with a classmate. You can also record your observations in your field notes.

1. Mindful attention check: Several times during your day, ask yourself, "how am I paying attention right now?" Then consider:

   a. Is my attention narrowly focused on a specific task, or is my attention broad and inclusive?

   b. Am I feeling stress in any level (you can use the SUDS scale to quantify this)? If you are feeling stress, practice accepting it fully, making no attempt to push it away.

   c. Where is the stress located and what does it feel like? Gently explore this in a nonjudging and fully accepting manner.

   d. Am I feeling a sense of urgency about what I am doing?

   e. What thoughts and self-talk are going through my mind?

2. Broadening your attentional focus: Just as light energy can be narrowly directed (like the intense light of a laser pointer), it can also be broadened and diffused (like sunshine filling a room). Practice these exercises, which relate to broad-focus attention.

   a. While sitting in class and listening to a lecture, see if you can keep a part of your attention to what is being said while broadening your attention to include not only the speaker at the front of the room but also the space around the speaker and then the space between the speaker and other objects at the front of the room. Broaden your awareness to include the objects and space around you. How does this affect your listening experience?

   b. While walking on campus or anywhere outside, broaden your focus to include not only the direct path in front of you but also the objects, people, and spaces between these. How widely can you "pan out" to include both awareness of yourself and the vast expanse of everything around you?

   c. The next time you find yourself feeling anxious or stressed, do the attention check described above, then mindfully work to broaden your attention to objects and spaces between the objects. See if you can hold onto this expanded view gently and simultaneously.

   d. If you are practicing MBSR, you can also expand your attention to include your inhalations–exhalations as well as the spaces between these. Imagine your breath flowing to all parts of your body (bones, muscles, organs) as well as the spaces between them.

   e. As you move into broad focus, note the thoughts and self-talk that emerge from within.

Reflective Questions

Question 1: Mindful Attention Check

a. How did the mindful attention check change your awareness about your attentional style?

b. Did you find yourself using narrowly focused attention more than was necessary?

c. How did the mindful attention check affect your awareness of stress and negative thoughts/self-talk?

d. How can you continue to develop your ability to be mindful of your attentional style? What benefits might result from this mindfulness?

Question 2: Broadening Your Attentional Focus

a. How easily were you able to move to a broader attentional focus?

b. What effect did the broadened focus have on your level of stress?

c. What effect did the broadened focus have on your ability to complete the task in which you were engaged?

Keep Breathing

Through the conscious regulation of our breath, we can carry the benefits of formal MBSR practice into our daily lives, no matter where we are. Making your breath slower, deeper, quieter, and more regular is associated with an increased sense of calm.[30] Even practicing this technique for 2 or 3 minutes can greatly induce a sense of calm before a presentation or other potentially stressful event. Andrew Weil also describes a mindfulness breathing technique called the 4-7-8 breath. This involves breathing in through the nose for a count of 4, holding the breath for a count of 7, and exhaling through the mouth for a count of 8. A cycle of three such breaths is also a quick mindfulness reinforcement and a valuable tool for producing a state of calm.[41]

Mindfulness in Clinical Practice

Mindfulness and Optimal Performance

Each of us has undoubtedly experienced the exhilaration of a brilliant performance; perhaps a virtuoso musical recital, a flawless athletic performance, or a dazzling oral presentation. Exhilaration of this nature can also occur in a learning environment (and hopefully this has been a regular feature of your graduate education), where you are so immersed in the material that your learning occurs rapidly and with great pleasure.

In the realm of human performance, such events are indicators of "peak performance," and significant attention has been directed at determining their elements. Not surprisingly, focused attention is a critical component of peak performance; however, the level of attention is not so rigid as to result in feelings of stress. Peak performance involves a sense of full immersion in the moment, where all cognitive resources are directed at the task at hand. Finally there is a positive emotional climate, including feelings of competence, joy, and excitement.[39,40]

In the realm of positive psychology, the experience of peak performance is conceptualized with the term *flow*, which has been described as "a short-term peak experience that is characterized by absorption, total concentration and immersion in the activity, and enjoyment."[39] Another critical element of flow is the matching of appropriate levels of situational challenge with personal competence. In other words, we are most likely to find flow in situations where the challenge is high but within our scope of competence. In many ways, flow, engagement, and broad-focus attention are thus related constructs. With respect to mindfulness, flow is the best-case scenario, as it is easy and enjoyable to be fully present to the satisfying and engrossing elements of our lives. Not surprisingly, most expert physical therapy clinicians find flow in their work on a regular basis.

However, what might be surprising is that these clinicians have also learned to use mindfulness to sustain their flow even when the conditions are less than ideal. The means through which they accomplish this are discussed a little further on in the chapter.

Talking Point/Field Notes

Finding the Flow in Your Life

Discuss the following with classmates and record your observations in your field notes.

1. Which activities are so enjoyable for you that you try to do them as much as possible? How long have you been doing these and why?

2. How would you describe your level of attention, awareness, and self-talk during your high-flow activities?

3. Which elements of these activities are the most satisfying and enjoyable?

4. Which elements of these activities are challenging for you?

5. Where have you found flow in your PT educational process?

6. What elements of your future practice are likely to produce flow for you?

With respect to the attentional demands of peak experiences, there is an elegant and well-choreographed dance between your central and autonomic nervous systems. These interact to enhance your capabilities in a way that can be described in the following scenario.

Clinical Scenario

The Experience of Peak Performance

It is your first day in the clinic and your first patient sits expectantly before you. You have read her chart and know that her chief complaint involves knee pain, a recent focus of study in your orthopedics class that you greatly enjoyed. Thus you are excited and feeling relatively confident, what you might describe as "psyched," "jazzed," or "running on all cylinders."

In attentional terms, this would also be described as a level of heightened cognitive arousal, which might be accompanied by slight feelings of "butterflies in the stomach" and perhaps a moderate increase in heart rate and blood pressure. Your hands might be cool to the touch, but being aware of this, you would be prepared to use humor to defuse any awkwardness with a witty comment. Most of all, you would feel an eager readiness to engage with the patient and to put your newly learned knee examination skills to work. If asked to rate your SUDS level, you would likely say somewhere in the midrange, perhaps between 3 and 5.

These cognitive and physiological indicators of increased arousal would allow you to function at your highest perceptual level, enabling you to receive and interpret both the overt and subtle

Continued

aspects of your patient's verbal and nonverbal communications, including her posture, gestures, and affective demeanor. Your communication would flow easily and confidently. You would be able to convey warmth and reassurance while effectively performing your examination, flexibly adapting the sequence of tests and measures to meet the needs of your patient. Most importantly, you would feel fully present to yourself and the patient throughout your interaction, watching yourself in action and using empowering self-talk in order to coach yourself toward the most beneficial communication approach.

As this scenario illustrates, peak performance involves a level of cognitive and physiological augmentation where all systems are primed for optimal function. As the next section shows, there is a certain level of arousal where this occurs.

Questions: Self-talk and mindfulness are important tools to modulate your level of arousal and attention for optimal performance. With this in mind, answer the following in a group and/or in your field notes.

1. How can you use mindfulness before and during the clinical encounter to facilitate an optimal interaction with your patient?

2. How can you effectively use self-talk before and during the clinical encounter to facilitate an optimal interaction with your patient?

3. What other stress-control strategies can you use before and during the clinical encounter to facilitate an optimal encounter with your patient?

4. The preceding description of optimal performance suggests that there is a small degree of stress, which is perceived as being "psyched." How do you tend to feel when you are keyed up to perform optimally?

5. Do you think it would be better to be completely relaxed in a challenging performance situation? Why or why not?

The Relationship Between Attention, Arousal, and Optimal Performance

The relationship between arousal and performance is a neurobiological concept developed in 1908 by Robert Yerkes and John Dodson;[42] it is best illustrated by a bell curve, as illustrated in **Figure 5-4**.

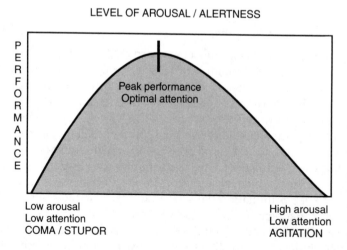

LEVEL OF AROUSAL / ALERTNESS

P
E
R
F
O
R
M
A
N
C
E

Peak performance
Optimal attention

Low arousal
Low attention
COMA / STUPOR

High arousal
Low attention
AGITATION

Figure 5–4. Adaptation of the Yerkes-Dodson curve. Arousal is shown as a continuum between the lowest and highest clinical levels (coma–agitation). As arousal increases, so do attention and performance up to a certain point, noted at the height of the curve. As arousal continues to increase, the person becomes overwhelmed by internal or external stimuli, resulting in agitation and decreased performance.

The arousal/performance curve suggests that both the lowest and highest levels of arousal/attention are associated with poor performance on tasks requiring high-level cognitive skills (i.e., those related to learning, memory, and motor performance). At the lowest end, when arousal is insufficient, the presence of boredom and apathy is likely to prevent the level of engagement needed for optimal performance.

At the highest level of arousal, engagement is prevented by increased stress, which generally occurs when the demands of the situation are greater than our perception of competence. When this occurs, our clearly focused attention is sabotaged by the onslaught of stress-related neurochemicals such as cortisol and norepinephrine, plunging us squarely into a flight-or-flight reaction.[40] The attentional effect of such a reaction is known as "frazzle" because of the significant cognitive deterioration that occurs in the midst of the feeling of being overwhelmed.[38,40] When we are frazzled, our highest-order cognitive functions such as insightfulness, creativity, and flexibility are replaced by reflexive, knee-jerk reactions that are largely in response to our inner turmoil. Furthermore, at the point of frazzle, the intense feelings of stress literally create a "fear of the fear," which further escalates our anxiety with negative, critical self-talk ("you're really going to mess up now!"). We might also attempt the stoic route, using distracting strategies to remove our attentional focus from our discomfort. Sadly, this is about as effective as adding condiments to a thoroughly burnt steak to make it palatable.

Implications for Physical Therapy Practice

Most of us experience an occasional bout of frazzle; failing to mindfully acknowledge it, we are likely to go about our interactions on a level of autopilot, which impairs our ability to be fully present to our patients. When we fail to be mindful of our internal emotional climate, our irritability, impatience, or anxiety will often be conveyed through our interactions. Should we then be confronted about this behavior, our lack of mindfulness may compel us to minimize or deny it, which can have a negative effect on our colleagues and patients.

Mindfulness is thus an important tool, not only during times of peak performance or quiet breathing but particularly in the midst of our "full catastrophe" spectrum of experiences. In order to apply mindfulness to all aspects of our lives, we must apply the concepts of detached observation, nonjudging acceptance, and nonresistance to every feeling that arises. The more we do this for ourselves, the more easily we can offer this to those we serve.

Every physical therapist has had a clinical experience where the needs of the patient were not within his or her area of comfortable competence. In rare instances, crisis situations can occur in a PT clinical setting: a patient collapses unexpectedly or a family member becomes verbally aggressive. Expert clinicians rarely succumb to frazzle in such situations and are able to stay present and engaged in the situation in order to address it effectively. They accomplish this through mindful awareness and acceptance of self and patient, which are a backdrop of the clinical encounter. Thus, the application of mindfulness to the patient interaction is known as *mindful practice.*[36]

Mindful Practice

The application of mindfulness concepts to clinical practice is receiving increasing attention in both medicine and PT.[36,43,44] Mindfulness has been identified as a critical element of expert PT practice, enabling such clinicians to attend to patients without predetermined biases or judgment. Furthermore, expert clinicians remain in touch with their own cognitive processes though consistent and ongoing self-monitoring, using all aspects of their sensory awareness, particularly active listening, to gain information.

The mindful practitioner enters each interaction with curiosity, comfort with ambiguity, and thus a more flexible approach (it *might* be diagnosis X, but I will explore other options with the patient as well). Using such a flexible, patient-centered approach, such clinicians are more likely to make decisions based on a variety of sources of evidence, including their own practical experience and the specific context of their patient's/family's situation.[13,36,43,44] Epstein describes mindfulness a characteristic of good clinical practice and states that mindfulness helps physicians to examine their own values and belief systems, to cope effectively with strong emotions, and to resolve conflict. Epstein further states that *"exemplary physicians seem to have a capacity for critical self-reflection that pervades all aspects of practice, including being present with the patient, eliciting and transmitting information and solving problems."*[36]

Self-reflection involves the ongoing awareness of one's emotional biases and tender spots and, most importantly, how these might affect the delivery of care. The ability to recognize these areas can prevent us from withdrawing from the patient or acting in ways that are detrimental to the therapeutic relationship. The following example was shared by an academic coordinator of clinical education (ACCE) and illustrates how mindfulness in both a physical therapy student and a clinical instructor affected an important clinical decision.

An Example of Mindful PT Practice

Richard was a physical therapy student doing an internship in a critical care trauma unit. Three months prior, Richard's older brother David, 28 years old, died in such a setting 3 days after sustaining severe multiple injuries in a rock-climbing accident.

One week into his internship, Richard received a consult to see Patrick, a young man who was admitted the previous day with severe multiple traumas from a rock-climbing accident. Upon reading Patrick's chart, Richard found himself becoming overwhelmed with sadness and began to cry. Before going to see Patrick, Richard sought out Sherry, his clinical instructor, and asked that he be assigned a different patient. Richard also explained the reasons for his request.

Sherry listened carefully to Richard's concerns. She expressed sincere empathy to Richard, while internally weighing the implications of not following her department's policy, which stated that therapists could not refuse patient assignments. She agreed to see Patrick that day, and recognizing the need for support for both herself and Richard, she asked him to discuss the matter with his school ACCE. There, it was decided that it would be in the best interests of all parties for Richard to be assigned a different patient. Although it might at first seem that Richard was allowed to avoid a challenging situation, mindful awareness by all parties brought several issues to light.

First, was Richard's own awareness of his emotional vulnerability in this unique situation. Knowledge of one's limitations is a critical aspect of mindful practice.[11] Such awareness can be critical in the promotion of effective patient safety. Physical therapy students and clinicians who lack insight into their limitations can place themselves and their patients at risk.

Second, Sherry, the Clinical Instructor, also showed mindfulness in the form of empathic presence to Richard and tolerance for the possible exception of this situation with respect to a strict department standard. Rather than framing Richard's request in black and white terms that would clearly indicate a deviation from policy (in which case she may have insisted that he see Patrick), Sherry mindfully noted that Richard's situation was not a simple case of "refusing a patient assignment". She was able to confront this ambiguity and request input from the school to assist her.

Third was the ACCE's awareness that Richard was an enthusiastic, hardworking student who had never demonstrated any behaviors that indicated an unwillingness to challenge himself appropriately. This mindful awareness of Richard's overall performance was helpful in reinforcing

Clinical Scenario

the sincerity and validity of his request. More importantly, while acknowledging the clinical education program goals related to unconditional positive regard of all patients, the ACCE also recognized the school's role in promoting the overall welfare of its students. The ACCE realized that both Richard and the patient could be negatively affected by working together. Thus, the decision to allow Richard to be reassigned to a different patient was made. This decision served to promote the best interests of both student and patient.

This mindful gesture of compassion resulted in an important decision for Richard. Shortly after this experience, he called his ACCE once again and shared that he needed further emotional support for his grief process. It was suggested that he explore family services at his local hospice. As a result, Richard began to attend a bereavement support program.

A major take-home point of this scenario is that mindful practice promotes compassionate and ethical professional behavior. Failure to acknowledge the unique details of certain situations can result in decisions with far-reaching undesired consequences, even if that decision is supported by legal guidelines. In this scenario, insisting that Richard follow a specific departmental policy could certainly be defended in terms of adherence to standards; however, the ultimate decision upheld important professional core values of altruism, caring, and compassion.

Core Elements of Mindful Practice: "Habits of Mind"

As you prepare for your journey as an engaged professional, you will be well served by a mindful approach to all that you do. As opposed to viewing mindfulness as something you practice only when necessary, you are encouraged to integrate it into your life as a way of living, or as what Purtillo calls a "habit of mind."[44] These are illustrated in Figure 5-5.

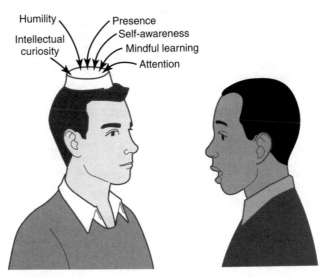

Figure 5–5. Habits for mindful practice.

Talking Points/Field Notes

Exercises for Developing Mindfulness

Self-awareness appears to be the foundation of mindful practice. If we are able to observe ourselves in action, without judgment, we are much better prepared to observe our interactions in a clinical context. The following exercises may be helpful in reinforcing these skills as part of your personal and professional life. After you have completed these exercises, you can discuss them with classmates and record your observations in your field notes.

Exercise 1: Your Internal Anthropologist (A Field Notes Exercise)

Anthropology is the study of humanity, derived from the Greek terms *anthropos* ("human being") and *pology* ("to talk about").[45]

One of the most important approaches to the study of humans is known as "participant observation," where the scientist objectively notes and records the actions of the persons of interest.

Directions:

For the next 48 hours, you will be your own internal anthropologist, stepping outside of yourself to observe your thoughts, feelings, impulses, ideas, sensations, and interactions with others. Try to note not only the types of feelings or thoughts but also their sensory quality in your body. In the spirit of anthropological study, you do not need to intervene or try to change what you observe, *only note it to yourself with full acceptance*. On the other hand, you may note occasions when self-observation helps you mindfully choose a different way of being in that particular moment (for example, if you become aware of being frustrated in a traffic jam, the awareness of this may help you to use mindful breathing to promote calmness). It will help you to read the reflection questions below before doing the exercise.

Reflect on the following:

1. How easy or difficult was it to be mindfully aware of your thoughts? What was the nature of these? How did they vary depending on your situation?

2. How easy or difficult was it to be mindfully aware of your feelings and their sensory presence in your body?

3. What was it like to simply observe and just accept what you observed?

4. How often did you find yourself resisting the situation of your present moment? What happened when you became aware of your resistance?

5. What thoughts, feelings, and sensations did you note in your observations of your interactions with others?

6. What did you learn from this experience?

Exercise 2: Talking Point: Developing Mindful Habits

Discuss the following with classmates: Refer to **Figure 5-6** for the list of behaviors you will be asked to reflect upon in this exercise.

When it comes to defending a strongly held point in the face of lacking or contradictory evidence, one question is, "Would you rather be right or happy?" Can you think of an example of this in your own life?

1. What does this mean to you in terms of defending your knowledge in order to meet an expectation? How can not knowing the answer lead to being more content in the long run?

2. How do you tend to react (in terms of self-talk thoughts, feelings, and actions) when you feel compelled to make a decision in situations where there doesn't appear to be one right answer (perhaps this has happened in some of your classes)? Which examples come to mind?

3. How might a mindful awareness of this ambiguity direct your course of action?

Talking Points/Field Notes—cont'd ▬▬▬▬▬▬▬

Exercise 3: Talking Point/ Field Notes : Self-Reflection in the Clinical Encounter

Note: This exercise can be done in conjunction with a patient case study presented in class or following a patient encounter. Refer to Figure 5-6 for the list of behaviors that you will be asked to reflect upon in this exercise.
   Reflect on the following in your field notes and discuss with classmates:

1. Where did you use mindfulness skills in this encounter? What did you pay attention to?

2. Which elements of the encounter went well for you and why? What sort of self-talk did you note?

3. Which elements of the encounter were ambiguous or unclear to you? What sort of self-talk did you note? How did you react to this in terms of your thoughts, feelings, and actions?

4. How did you demonstrate the skills of intellectual curiosity and intellectual humility in your encounter? What were the results?

Implications for PT Practice

The regular practice of mindfulness (both in action and during meditation) has profound implications for an enhanced quality of life and work. As PTs, we must realize that a mindful approach to our work can optimize our clinical skills. Furthermore this practice can reduce the stress of providing health care in today's struggling delivery system and keep us positively engaged in all that we do. As a therapeutic approach, the integration of MBSR as an intervention can enhance patient empowerment by reducing pain and stress. Finally, by situating all contexts of our lives in a mindful perspective, we can broaden our experience of positive states, both for the benefit of those we care about and those we care for.

Chapter Summary

1. This chapter has explored mindfulness as a life skill that will enhance your internal communication through improved self awareness, presence, and self-acceptance. These skills can have a strong positive impact on your interactions with others in everyday and professional contexts.

2. Attention is the foundational cognitive resource for mindfulness. The continual use of a task-oriented, narrow focus of attention can lead to stress. We can adapt our attentional approach toward a broader focus that allows us to consider both the overt and subtle aspects of communication. Mindfulness-based stress reduction (MBSR) uses attention to breathing in a quiet environment as a potent means to decrease tension and broaden awareness.

3. Broadening and building theory suggests that mindfulness can broaden our receptivity to positive emotional states, which in turn allow us to build resources that enhance life and work.

4. "Habits of mind" for mindful clinical practice include self-awareness, being present in the moment, full attention, intellectual humility, and curiosity.

5. By fully accepting everything in the moment as if we "deliberately chose it for ourselves,"[19] we are more likely to be thoughtful and thorough in our interactions with patients and choices of interventions.

Take Home Menu

1. **Computer-Based Biofeedback Programs to Promote Awareness of Internal Processes**

   a. *Healing Rhythms.* A guided, interactive computer program that provides instruction in mindfulness, breathing for relaxation, and mind–body awareness. It includes beautiful nature-based graphics and soothing music. It comes with a USB-mediated biofeedback monitor that attaches to one's fingers. Website: http://www.wilddivine.com

   b. *Emwave:* Another guided breath-control/meditation program with colorful graphics and computer-assisted biofeedback monitoring. The biofeedback monitor can also be used without the computer. Website: http://www.HearthMath.com/Biofeedback

2. **Developing an Ongoing Mindfulness Practice**

Consider working with one or more classmates to develop a MBSR practice. This might take the form of a group meditation once or twice a week for 30 minutes. You can either meditate silently or use a guided MBSR tape or CD (see resources below) This can be a useful life skill that will serve you well during your education and in your future practice.

3. **Mindfulness-Based Writing**

Use a portion of your field notes to reflect on your self-observations and to practice the elements of acceptance and nonresistance. You can also mindfully reflect on your clinical encounters in the manner suggested in Exercise 3 in Talking Points/Field Notes on page 126.

Further Resources

1. Jon Kabat-Zinn's mindfulness-based stress reduction (MBSR) tapes and CDs can be purchased online: http://www.mindfulnesstapes.com/booktour.html.
2. Open Focus training materials can be obtained at http://www.openfocus.com.
3. Two excellent resources on mindfulness-based cognitive therapy:
   a. Williams M, Teasdale J, Segal Z, Kabat-Zinn G. *The Mindful Way Through Depression: Freeing Yourself From Chronic Unhappiness.* New York: Guilford; 2007. Note: Book contains CD on MBSR.
   b. Brantley J, Kabat-Zinn J. *Calming Your Anxious Mind: How Mindfulness And Compassion Can Free You Anxiety, Fear And Panic,* 2nd ed. Oakland, CA: New Harbinger; 2007.

References

1. Brown KW, Ryan RM. The benefits of being present: Mindfulness and its role in psychological well-being. *J Pers Soc Psychol.* 2003;84(4):822-848.

2. Allan Schwartz, PhD. Adult ADHD: The importance of learning social skills: http://www.mentalhelp.net/poc/view_doc.php?type=weblog&id=220&wlid=5&cn=3. Accessed February 11, 2009.

3. Fehmi L, Robbins J. *The Broad Focus Brain: Harnessing the Power of Attention to Heal the Mind and Body.* Boston: Trumpeter Books; 2007. Note: Book contains CD of Guided Broad Focus Training.

4. Langer E. Matters of mind: Mindfulness/mindlessness in perspective. *Consciousness Cognition* 1992;1(3):239-305.

5. Langer EJ, Imber L. Role of mindlessness in the perception of deviance. *J Pers Soc Psychol.* 1980;39(3): 360-367.

6. Barlow DH, ed. *Clinical Handbook of Psychological Disorders,* 4th ed. New York: Guilford; 2007.

7. Deci EL, Ryan RM. Self-determination theory: When mind mediates behavior. *J Mind Behav.* 1980; 1:33-43.

8. Basmajian JV. *Biofeedback: Principles and Practice for Clinicians,* 3rd ed. Baltimore: William & Wilkins; 1989.

9. Baumeister RF. *Escaping the Self: Alcoholism, Spirituality, Masochism and Other Flights From the Burden of Selfhood.* New York: Basic Books; 1991.

10. Mindfulness.org.au. Mindfulness Related Scales: http://mindfulness.org.au/articles.html#MindfulnessRelatedScales. Accessed February 12, 2009.

11. Bond FW, Bunce D. The role of acceptance and job control in mental health, job satisfaction and work performance. *J Appl Psychol.* 2003;88(6):1057-1067.

12. McCracken LM, Yang SY. A contextual cognitive behavioral analysis of rehabilitation workers' health and wellbeing. Influences of acceptance, mindfulness and values-based action. *Rehabil Psychol.* 2008;53(4): 479-485.

13. Epstein RM. Mindful practice in action: 1. Technical competence, evidence-based medicine, and relationship-centered care. *Families Systems, Health.* 2003;(21):1-9.

14. Shapiro SL, Astin JA, Bishop SR, Cordova M. Mindfulness-based stress reduction for health care professionals: Results from a randomized trial. *Int J Stress Mgt.* 2005;12(2): 164-176.

15. Morales Knight LF. Mindfulness: History, technologies, research, applications. Psy 637: Techniques of psychotherapy. Pepperdine University. Graduate School of Education and Psychology: http://www.knightpsych.com/papers/mindfulness-techniques.pdf. Accessed October 29, 2007.

16. Kabat-Zinn J. *Full Catastrophe Living: Using the Wisdom of Your Body and Mind to Face Stress, Pain and Illness.* New York: Dell Publishing; 1990.

17. Answers.com. Meditation. http://www.answers.com/topic/meditatio. Accessed February 12, 2009.

18. Online Thesaurus: Meditation: http://www. selfknowledge.com/t58666.htm. Accessed February 12, 2009.

19. Tolle E. *A New Earth: Awakening to Your Life's Purpose.* New York: Penguin; 2005.

20. Begley S. Scans of monks' brains show meditation alters structure, functioning. *The Wall Street Journal.* November 5, 2004: http://psyphz.psych.wisc.edu/web/News/Meditation_Alters_Brain_WSJ_11-04.htm. Accessed October 30, 2007.

21. Meditation can boost your gray matter: Buddhist insight practitioners build thicker cortical regions. *Live Science.* November 13, 2005: http://home.att.net/~meditation/monks.brains.html. Accessed October 30, 2007.

22. Davidson RJ, Kabat-Xinn J, Schumacher J, et al. Alterations in brain and immune function produced by mindfulness meditation. *Psychosom Med.* 2003;65:564-570.

23. Grossman P, Tiefenthaler-Gilmer U, Raysz A, Kesper U. Mindfulness training as an intervention for fibromyalgia: Evidence of postintervention and 3-year follow-up benefits in well-being. *Psychother Psychosom*. 2007; 76(4):226-233.

24. Calson LE, Garland SN. Impact of mindfulness based stress reduction (MBSR) on sleep, mood stress and fatigue symptoms in cancer outpatients. *Int J Behav Med*. 2005;12(4):278-285.

25. Gross CR, Kreitzer MJ, Russas V, et al. Mindfulness meditation to reduce symptoms after organ transplant: A pilot study. *Adv Mind Body Med*. 2004;20(2):20-29.

26. UMass Medical School, Center for Mindfulness in Medicine, Healthcare and Society (CFM): http://www.umassmed.edu/cfm/index.aspxis. Accessed November 1, 2007.

27. UMass, School of Medicine, Center for Mindfulness in Medicine, Healthcare and Society (CFM). Professional Education Outline: "The Contemplative Mind in Medicine": http://www.umassmed.edu/cfm/education/contemplative.aspx. Accessed November 1, 2007.

28. Speca M, Carlson LE, Goodey E, Angen M. A randomized, wait-list controlled clinical trial: the effect of a mindfulness meditation-based stress reduction program on mood and symptoms of stress in cancer outpatients. *Psychosom Med*. 2000;62(5):613-622.

29. Sullivan MJ, Wood L, Terry J, et al. The Support, Education, and Research in Chronic Heart Failure Study (SEARCH): a mindfulness-based psychoeducational intervention improves depression and clinical symptoms in patients with chronic heart failure. *Am Heart J*. 2009;157(1): 84-90.

30. Weil A. Breathing: The master key to self healing (audio cassette). Louisville, MO: Sounds True Inc; 2001.

31. American Physical Therapy Association. What Types of Interventions Do Physical Therapists Provide? In *Guide to Physical Therapist Practice*, 2nd ed. *Phys Ther*. 2001;(81):1, Chapter 3, 105-138.

32. Grepmair L, Mitterlehner F, Loew T, et al. Promoting mindfulness in psychotherapists in training influences the treatment results of their patients: A randomized, double-blind, controlled study. *Psychother Psychosom*. 2007;76(6):332-338.

33. Fredrickson BL, Cohn MA, Coffey KA, et al. Open hearts build lives: Positive emotions induced through loving kindness meditation build consequential personal resources. *J Pers Soc Psychol*. 2008;95(5): 1065-1062.

34. Easterlin BL, Cardeña E. Cognitive and emotional differences between short and long term Vipassana meditators. *Imagination Cognition Personality*. 1998;18: 69-81.

35. Fredrickson BL. The role of positive emotions in positive psychology: The broaden and build theory of positive emotions. *Am Psychol.* 2001;56:218-226.

36. Epstein R. Mindful practice. *JAMA.* 1999;282(9): 833-830.

37. Frederickson B. *Positivity: Groundbreaking Research Reveals How to Embrace the Hidden Strength of Positive Emotions, Overcome Negativity and Thrive.* New York: Crown Publishers; 2009.

38. Goleman D. *Social Intelligence: The Revolutionary New Science of Human Relationships.* New York: Bantam; 2007.

39. Demerouti E. Job characteristics, flow and performance: The moderating role of conscientiousness. *J Occup Health Psychol.* 2006;11(3):266-230.

40. Goleman D. Aiming for the brains sweet spot. *The New York Times.* Opinion. Happy Days: At year's end, three writers examine ties to family, friends, and tradition. November 5, 2007: http://happydays.blogs.nytimes. com/2006/12/27/aiming-for-the-brains-sweet-spot/. Accessed November 5, 2007.

41. Weil A. The art and science of breathing: Three breathing techniques: http://www.drweil.com. Accessed February 18, 2009.

42. Yerkes RM, Dodson JD. The relation of strength of stimulus to rapidity of habit-formation. *J Comp Neurol Psychol.* 1908;18:459-482.

43. Jensen G. Mindfulness: Applications for teaching and learning in ethics education. In: Purtillo R, Jensen G, Brasic Royeen C. *Educating for Moral Action: A Sourcebook in Health and Rehabilitation Ethics.* Philadelphia: FA Davis; 2005.

44. Purtillo R, Jensen G, Brasic Royeen C. *Educating for Moral Action: A Sourcebook in Health and Rehabilitation Ethics.* Philadelphia: FA Davis; 2005.

45. Anthropology. *Wikipedia, The Free Encyclopedia*: http://en.wikipedia.org/ wiki/Anthropology. Accessed November 13, 2007.

CHAPTER 6

Emotional Intelligence: Self-Science for Effective Communication

"Knowing others is intelligence;
Knowing yourself is true wisdom."

Lao Tzu (Old Master)
Chinese Taoist Philosopher, c. 600 BCE

Chapter Overview

Recent theoretical advancements related to the intellectual dimensions that drive human potential have resulted in the acknowledgment of those beyond the traditional intelligence quotient (IQ). These dimensions are known as multiple intelligences. This chapter presents a history of multiple intelligence and then moves to an exploration of the interpersonal dimension, now known as emotional intelligence. Emotional intelligence enables the integration of feelings and emotions into our communication, thus setting the stage for authentic relationships. Evidence to support the value of emotional intelligences is provided, along with exercises to enhance its development in the context of engaged professionalism.

Key Terms

Multiple intelligences

Emotional intelligence (EI)

Intelligence quotient (IQ)

The Many Realms of Genius: The Concept of Multiple Intelligences

The music of Beethoven, the art of Picasso, the scientific theories of Einstein—each contribution demonstrates genius in a specific realm of intelligence, and in these examples, each person's contribution changed the world. The unique and profound expression of their individual talents speaks to the existence of specific areas of intelligence. In other words, within each of our brains lies the potential to demonstrate outstanding achievements in a multitude of different ways.

Perhaps you have experienced the joy of excelling in certain areas because of an innate proclivity; you might be a natural athlete, a gifted musician or artist, or you might have the special ability to connect with most of the people you meet. Indeed, many of the attributes that we call "talents" and "strengths" (as discussed in Chapter 3) are simply manifestations of well-developed areas that we now call "multiple intelligences."[1]

As you will learn in the following sections, the concept of multiple intelligence has enhanced our appreciation of the diverse realms of human excellence, one of which is the ability to interact in an authentic and compassionate manner with others.

IQ Alone Does Not Intelligence Make

Until the early 1980s, when Howard Gardner proposed his multiple intelligence theory,[1] and continuing today to a significant extent, standardized intelligence measures such as the Stanford-Binet IQ test have been used to measure human intelligence as a one-dimensional skill set that typically includes logical reasoning, critical thinking, and problem solving.[2,3]

If you have ever questioned the value of using a single standardized intelligence test for the purpose of measuring your academic potential (or perhaps even faced educational consequences because of that score), you might appreciate the need to explore other important aspects of intellectual function. Certainly this was a concern for the families of children whose IQ test scores resulted in their assignment to special education programs or being labeled "mentally retarded" when psychologist Albert Binet first began to administer his standardized tests in the 1920s.[4]

Working in the educational arena, Gardner observed the devastating effects of the inappropriate labeling of children who performed poorly on such measures. Gardner also theorized that a one-dimensional assessment of intelligence could result in the failure to identify and support children with significant potential in other important areas for life success (for example, the child who does poorly in reading but whose creative artwork could lead to a lucrative career as an illustrator). As a response to this one dimensional view, Gardner developed his theory of multiple intelligences, illustrated in **Figure 6-1**.

If you are interested in exploring your own strengths in the multiple intelligences, you will find references for several online tests in the "Take-Home Menu" at the end of the chapter.

As a result of Gardner's work, which eventually included specific pedagogical approaches to develop the multiple intelligences, educators have been encouraged to expand traditional teaching and evaluation methods which focus on a one-dimensional assessment of intelligence. In response to this encouragement, the United States, over the past 20 years, has undergone an explosive growth in the development of "charter schools," federally supported public institutions that offer alternative educational approaches, many of which are specifically designed to engage the multiple intelligences.

For example, one educational approach used in the charter school system is known as the Waldorf method. This approach emphasizes the development of each child's unique intellectual strengths and engages his or her development through a variety of instructional

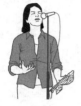

Linguistic Intelligence: A love of words and language in both verbal and written forms. The ability to speak and write in unique, creative, and articulate ways.
Examples: Mark Twain, Toni Morrison

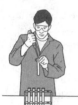

Logical-Mathematical Intelligence: A love of objective, scientific measures represented by facts, numbers, and concrete evidence. The ability to analyze, organize, and manipulate these measurements in valuable ways that increase understanding of the world around us.
Examples: Albert Einstein, Maria Goeppert-Mayer (Nobel Laureate in Physics)

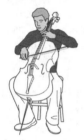

Visual-Spatial Intelligence: A love of the visual world and the relationship of objects within it. The ability to see the world in three dimensions and four directions. The ability to design and construct new objects or to take them apart and put them back together.
Examples: Frank Lloyd Wright, Coco Chanel

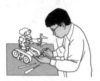

Musical Intelligence: A love of music, song, and rhythm. The ability to easily compose, read, or perform music with an instrument or one's voice.
Examples: Stevie Wonder, Ella Fitzgerald

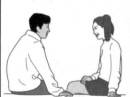

Interpersonal Intelligence: A love of human communication and relationships. The ability to interpret and respond to others in authentic and helpful ways. The ability to build lasting relationships and to promote them in others. Natural compassion and empathy for being human.
Examples: Mother Teresa, The Dalai Lama

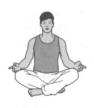

Intrapersonal intelligence: A love of self understanding, wisdom, and insight. The ability to know oneself well and to reflect on the impact of one's interactions and behaviors. The ability to be free of one's ego.
Examples: Thich Nhat Hanh, Anne Frank

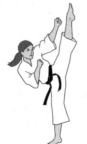

Body-Kinesthetic Intelligence: A love of human form and movement. The ability to effectively engage physical attributes such as strength, balance, coordination, flexibilty, and power. The ability to excel in movement-related pursuits such as dance or athletics.
Examples: Maria Sharapova, Brian Boitano

Figure 6–1. Seven dimensions of genius: the multiple intelligences.

Adapted from: Gardner H. *Frames of Mind: The Theory of Multiple Intelligences.* New York. Basic Books, 1983.

approaches such as music, dance, artwork, and storytelling. The Waldorf method can thus be valuable for children with strengths in the musical, kinesthetic, and interpersonal intelligence dimensions.[5]

The number of charter schools continues to grow in the United States as more communities seek supportive and creative ways to educate their children. As of 2007, over 1 million students were enrolled in 3,500 U.S. charter schools.[6] The success of the charter school movement is a strong testimony to the value of supporting all areas of human potential. Ongoing research in the area of multiple intelligences is currently being directed toward the development and validation of standardized measures for each of the seven dimensions. Such measures might involve creative strategies that have never been used in education. To that end, imagine how effective communication might be assessed as a component of interpersonal intelligence! As this chapter shows, the ability to direct our communication from its internal source is also an intelligence that comprises strengths in specific areas.

The following scenario illustrates how these communication related intelligences may (or may not) exist between individuals.

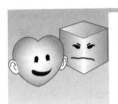

Champ and Blockhead

Champ and Blockhead Assess a Challenging Patient

Blockhead has a straight-A average in PT school and is likely to graduate at the top of his class. He has a photographic memory and hardly spends any time studying (a fact he has shared often with his classmates). Champ, on the other hand, has a B average in his PT classes and is likely to graduate in the middle to bottom third of his class. He must study considerably for these grades and tends to have difficulty doing well on traditional objective exams.

Last week, each of them struggled to complete appropriate tests and measures in a timely manner (45 minutes) on their assigned patients during an early clinical experience.

Blockhead's assignment involved an assessment of Jake, a 7-year-old boy with mild cerebral palsy. As Blockhead began to question Jake on his medical history, Jake became restless and distractible, wanting to play games instead of sitting quietly for the interview, most of which was directed to Jake's mother. Sighing heavily and rolling his eyes, Blockhead ignored his patient's request to play and continued his questioning until Jake finally got up and walked away, looking for a more enjoyable activity. Blockhead tried several times to encourage Jake to return for his questions and became visibly irritated when Jake tried to play a game of hide and seek. Blockhead continued to insist that Jake sit down for the questions. Finally, Jake asked to go home. Upon leaving the clinic, Jake's mother asked that he not be scheduled with Blockhead in the future.

When the experience was over, Blockhead's clinical instructor asked him to self-assess his interaction with Jake. Instead, Blockhead blamed the clinical instructor for providing him with an uncooperative patient who made it impossible to conduct his evaluation, saying, "How could I show you what I really know when all Jake wanted to do was goof around?" When the clinical instructor offered to provide feedback to help Blockhead interact more successfully with pediatric patients, Blockhead replied, "I don't really need to know that, because I'm going into orthopedics when I graduate!"

Champ's clinical experience involved completing an assessment on Felice, a 70-year-old woman with Parkinson's disease. This was Felice's first PT visit, and she was nervous. Although Champ wanted to impress his clinical instructor with his preparation and

Continued

efficiency in performing the appropriate tests and measures, he felt that Felice needed reassurance and decided to direct the assessment according to her comfort level. Thus, the tests and measures were done very slowly, with Champ providing much encouragement and support for Felice. He asked her questions about herself, and as Felice became more relaxed, she began to talk at length about her children and grandchildren, making it difficult for Champ to begin the tests and measures portion of the examination. At the end of the clinic time, Champ realized that he had completed none of these, but Felice stated that she was eager to return for follow-up visits. When Champ was asked to self-assess his interaction with Felice, he was able to clearly identify his challenges and strengths. He was receptive to the feedback given by his supervising faculty member and was able to develop a strategy to improve his efficiency in the future.

Questions

1. Both Champ and Blockhead came to the clinical experience with certain intelligence strengths and challenges. Using the list of multiple intelligences in Figure 6-1, how would you describe these strengths and challenges for Champ? How would you describe these strengths and challenges for Blockhead?
2. If you had been the clinical instructor in this case, how would you address Blockhead's behaviors in terms of the skills needed for effective PT practice? How would you have responded to his comments?
3. What suggestions would you have for both Champ and Blockhead to improve their effectiveness in a clinical setting?
4. Looking at the list of multiple intelligences in Figure 6-1, which do you think are the three most essential for effective clinical performance?
5. How might Blockhead's behaviors affect his overall performance on a clinical rotation? If you were a clinical instructor, would you recommend a passing grade on a rotation where the student had adequate knowledge skills but very poor affective skills? (Hint: you might want to examine the grading instrument that your academic program uses for clinical assignments to determine how this is done.)

If you found yourself struggling with objectively validating and quantifying the interpersonal behaviors shown by Champ and Blockhead in terms of how these affected their overall performance, you can appreciate the challenges of using a single intelligence dimension as a measure of success. You may have also recognized the need for an effective measure of interpersonal intelligence. As a future physical therapist, you probably quickly realized that Blockhead's inabilities to accept responsibility for his actions, to self-assess, and to connect with either his clinical instructor or his patient are not the skills of an engaged professional. However, in the absence of quantifiable ways of measuring these other forms of intelligence (which are related to the intrapersonal and interpersonal domains, as noted in Figure 6-1), a clinical instructor might struggle with failing a student for these behaviors alone. Nevertheless, as our profession directs increasing attention to the importance of such behaviors and quantifying them through several important documents—such as the "Clinical Performance Instrument," "Core Values in Physical Therapy," and the "Generic Abilities Assessment"—current and future practitioners will be expected to demonstrate the full complement of intelligences related to compassionate patient care.

Emotional Intelligence: Self-Science for Success

The challenge of quantifying the interpersonal and intrapersonal elements of multiple intelligence has also garnered significant attention in the scientific community. As a result, research in neurobiology, psychology, and education has resulted in a broadening of Gardner's multiple intelligence theory to include the contributions of feelings and emotions. This integration has resulted in the important concept of *emotional intelligence.*

In 1995, psychologist Daniel Goleman published *Emotional Intelligence.*[7] Building on Gardner's multiple intelligence theory, Goleman further explored elements of the interpersonal and intrapersonal domains. Just as IQ had been previously defined (for the purposes of standardized testing) as critical thinking, problem solving, and logical reasoning, emotional intelligence is now defined as *the element of human intelligence that allows for the successful management of self, relationships and the attainment of meaningful life goals.*[7]

Contained within this definition are four elements that are the key aspects of emotional intelligence. These are listed in **Box 6-1**.

BOX 6-1:   Elements of Emotional Intelligence

1. Self-awareness and self-control*
2. Awareness of the emotions of others (empathy)
3. Motivation of self and others for goal attainment
4. Social expertise

---

*Goleman lists these as two separate elements.
Adapted from Goleman D. *Emotional Intelligence.* New York: Bantam Books; 1995.

Dimensions of Emotional Intelligence

Although theorists who study emotional intelligence may use slight variations in terminology,[7–9] the terms are generally synonymous for the following four components.

Self-Awareness and Self-Control

Self-awareness and self-control are the abilities to identify one's emotions *as they emerge* (which thus includes the prerequisite of mindfulness). If you are aware of your emotions as they happen, you will be more likely to manage them effectively at an appropriate level. Persons who lack self-awareness may not realize the intensity of their feelings until they reach a level that is difficult to control, resulting in emotional reactions that are more likely to be out of proportion to the actual circumstances. Thus, persons who lack self-control are often considered impulsive, moody, or volatile.

As we discussed in Chapter 5, the ability to maintain mindful self-awareness requires ongoing practice and the commitment of attentional resources. We can easily lose sight of our emotional climate and the ability for effective self-control in times of "frazzle," when we are overwhelmed by stress, fatigue, or illness.

Another important aspect of self-awareness and control is the ability to choose appropriate responses or behaviors based on their likely consequences. For example, a person who succumbs to an initial impulse toward rage might inflict considerable harm on others in a variety of ways. Often this harm includes significant damage to relationships or the investment of tremendous emotional energy to repair them.

All of us have had situations that have at first provoked a strong emotional response, as when we are cut off in traffic or a friend makes an innocent remark that we find offensive. Furthermore, minor annoyances and frustrations are a part of everyday life, constantly compelling us to choose appropriate responses to these. Self-awareness and control are critical disciplines enabling us to live with grace and civility in an often chaotic world. Because of this, self-awareness and control are considered the most important aspects of emotional intelligence, affecting each of the other elements.[6]

Implications for Physical Therapy

The Importance of Self-Awareness and Control in Effective Clinical Practice

The current health-care environment is fast-paced, constantly changing, and relentlessly demanding. Self-awareness and control are needed by engaged professionals to assure optimal responses to the many requirements involved in providing effective and compassionate care. In addition to a sensitivity toward the consequences of our actions, another important aspect of self-awareness is a recognition of one's limitations. Practicing beyond the scope of one's competence or licensure or allowing oneself to become burned out and disillusioned are both serious consequences resulting from lack of self-awareness. In these instances, it is important to acknowledge our limitations and the impact of going beyond them. More important is the ability to identify appropriate measures of self-empowerment in such situations. These measures may involve self-care activities such as adequate rest and exercise. They might also include additional education or other strategies to improve competence. Thus, awareness of one's strengths and limitations is an important tool to assure legal and ethical professional practice.

In the final analysis, the effectiveness of our communication is a crucial reflection of our levels of self-awareness and control. If we interact with others in ways that empower, that build alliances and promote positive change in an environment of goodwill, chances are that we are showing a healthy level of competence in this important emotional intelligence skill.

Self-Awareness and Control in Our Patients: An Important Cognitive Skill

The ability to be aware of and to manage our emotional climate is one of the complex, cortically driven cognitive skills known as "executive functions." As you may experience in your interactions with patients recovering from brain injury, such individuals have often lost the ability to interact in socially appropriate ways owing to a lack of self-awareness and control resulting from impaired cortical inhibition to the limbic system. Accordingly, successful rehabilitation of such persons involves teaching either restorative or compensatory strategies for the optimization of self control. For example, Steve, a patient with a brain injury whom I once treated, had the tendency to become rude and aggressive when he had to wait in line. His rehabilitation team thus devised a behavioral modification program to provide rewards for Steve's self-control in such situations, substituting external incentives for the internal awareness that had been impaired by his brain injury. The team worked with Steve to anticipate situations where he might become agitated and helped him to find alternative behaviors. Accordingly, Steve learned to have a book with him for the times when he had to wait in lines. Thus, rather than standing impatiently and letting his frustration grow, he learned to read quietly, distracting himself from a potentially volatile situation.

Talking Points/Field Notes

Observations on Self-Awareness and Control

Discuss the following with classmates and record your observations in your field notes.

1. If you could describe your internal emotional climate as a daytime weather pattern, what would be the generally prevailing conditions? (warm and sunny with a clear sky, rapidly gathering clouds, or a change in temperature, hazy, and overcast). In other words, what is your typical mood? Is it fairly stable, and can you detect changes before a major storm?

2. Do you consider yourself to be a moody person, or have you been told by others that you are moody? If so, why? If not, why? What impact might your moodiness (or lack of it) have on those around you?

3. How easily can your mood change in a given day? What sorts of things tend to affect your mood for better or worse?

4. Describe a time when you had difficulty controlling your emotions (i.e., laughter, anger, sadness, elation). What were the consequences? What did you learn from the experience?

5. What strategies do you use to promote better self-awareness and control for yourself? How have these strategies been helpful?

Your internal communication is a key ally in your quest to develop self-awareness and self-control. As you become more mindful of the continuous narration of your internal voice, you should become more aware of whether it is helpful in maintaining a balanced emotional climate or whether it paints everything with a negative stroke. Recall from Chapter 3 that you can modify your self-talk toward a more optimistic point of view, which you may find to be more empowering in terms of managing your emotions. You are encouraged to continue to monitor your self-talk and to ask yourself, "what am I feeling right now?" on a regular basis.

Awareness of the Emotions of Others (or Empathy)

It certainly follows that if you are able to authentically experience the rich variety of emotions within yourself, that you will be able to detect them in others. While most of us can easily detect the explosive display of emotions of others, many of us may miss the subtle nuances of facial expression and body language that are also used to convey feelings, express needs, and request support. Sadly, in our culture, displays of grief and tearfulness are often discouraged as a sign of weakness to the point where we are uncomfortable in the presence of individuals who express such emotions. We also often struggle with our reactions to emotions related to intimacy, fear, and appropriate anger. Nevertheless, our profession requires that we respond to all patients with unconditional positive regard, compassion, and caring. These virtues require that we be well versed in the healing practice of empathy.

Empathy (derived from the Greek word *empatheia*, meaning "feeling into") has been described by Davis[10] as "merging with another person in a unique moment of shared meaning." Empathy thus means that we first convey our mindful presence to the other individual along with our receptivity to whatever he or she may need to share with us. No doubt you have experienced the richness of a shared empathic moment with another person. Quite likely, you didn't plan for this to happen; however, at some point in your conversation, you could truly feel what the other person was feeling, and this connection resonated between you. After this moment passed, you were probably also able to step back from that shared moment, nonetheless enriched by the experience. The point here is that empathy is a healing connection that empowers and confirms the richness of human experience.

In order to be truly available to the full range of empathic experiences, you must be compassionate with both yourself (allowing and accepting your own feelings) and others (allowing and accepting theirs as well). Empathic persons are generally well adjusted and successful because of this skill, as validated by several research studies. Studies of over 1,000 children showed that those who performed well on a standardized test of empathy, known as the Profile of Nonverbal Sensitivity (which involves having subjects view videotapes to discern the emotions displayed by persons in the absence of verbal communication), were more popular and more emotionally stable than those who did not. Interestingly, these children also did better in school, independent of their IQs.[7] Studies of over 7,000 American adults indicate that high levels of empathy correlate with greater popularity and social adjustment as well as more authentic intimate relationships. As Goleman states, "It is no surprise that empathy helps with romantic life."[7]

Clinical Scenario

Empathy SOS

Angelo is a physical therapist from a large Italian family where pregnancy and birth are frequent events. In fact, his own wife is due to deliver their eagerly awaited first child in just a month. This morning, he is assessing Liz, a 33-year-old athlete who injured her knee in a marathon. When Angelo asks Liz about any recent health changes, Liz becomes tearful and mentions that she had a miscarriage 2 months earlier and just can't seem to get over it. This statement takes Angelo completely by surprise, as this has never happened among his friends or family, and he struggles for an appropriate response.

Questions:

1. What questions might Angelo ask himself in order to better connect with Liz as she shares her feelings?

2. Physical therapists generally want to help their patients get better or to fix things that aren't right in their lives. Is there anything Angelo can say to "fix" this situation?

3. With respect to question #2 above, which responses might be less than helpful?

4. What are helpful things that Angelo could do and/or say to convey empathy for Liz?

Implications for Physical Therapy: Strategies to Increase Therapeutic Empathy

Reflections of Feeling and Content to Convey Empathy

In addition to our mindful presence, we can assure others that we are listening with empathy by using a statement known as a "reflection." Originally developed in the 1960s by psychologist Carl Rogers as part of his therapeutic "client-centered counseling,"[11] reflections are used by listeners to provide support, assure understanding, and promote further disclosure by the speaker. A reflection often involves offering a summary of what has been heard back to the speaker. The summary can involve a direct repetition of the speaker's words, a paraphrase of the same, or an interpretive statement. Depending on the context or purpose of the conversation, we may choose to use reflections that focus on facts and information (content), or emotions (feeling). There is no prescription for an effective reflection of content or feeling; in fact, the best ones arise spontaneously.

Regardless of their form, reflections, particularly those that are feeling-focused, are a useful tool in the demonstration of empathic listening.

Examples of commonly used reflections are shown in **Box 6-2**.

BOX 6-2:   Examples of Reflections That Demonstrate Empathy

FEELING-FOCUSED

You must have felt ... (followed by a feeling and level of intensity such as humiliated, furious, fantastic, ...)

That would be so ... (followed by a feeling such as sad, frustrating, ...)

That must have been ... (followed by feeling and level of intensity such as marvelous, difficult, exciting, ...)

I would have been so ... (followed by an emotion and level of intensity—can be used to show support and agreement with speaker)

CONTENT-FOCUSED

So, what you are saying is ... (followed by a summary)

Are you trying to tell me that ... (followed by summary)

So, let me see if I have this right ... (followed by a summary)

So, what I heard you say is ... (followed by a summary)

When one is using a reflection of feeling with a person, we use our internal communication to identify both the feeling and its intensity that we note during a conversation and our external communication to share this (reflect it) to the person.

For example, in the scenario between Liz and Angelo above, it is fairly obvious that this is an emotional situation for Liz. She has lost something very precious to her. Certainly we can all understand that a loss of this nature is very painful, and comments such as "that must be devastating" or "that must be so difficult for you" indicate that you can enter into this experience for a brief healing moment. On the contrary, failure to recognize the emotional intensity that Liz is feeling, either by an insensitive joke or comment ("my sister has seven kids, I bet she wishes that had happened to her") or a dismissive remark that trivializes the intense emotions ("if you got pregnant once, you can do it again"), will greatly threaten the chances for the development of a therapeutic relationship and can add to her emotional distress.

The Perilous Side of "That Sucks!"

In our fast-paced society with its emphasis on speed and efficiency, there has been an increasing substitution of generic and meaningless slang for thoughtful and accurate reflections of feeling. For example, if we reflexively respond with "that sucks!" to every emotional concern we hear, over time our mindful sensitivity to the feelings of others may lose its acuity. This is because the experience of empathy requires the conscious willingness to enter into a shared emotional experience involving an accurate perception of another person's feelings and the ability to take sufficient pause in order to do so. In contrast, the exclusive use of slang-based reflections enables us to opt out of that perceptive process, keeping us at arm's length from the genuine emotions of ourselves and others. Over time, we may become dulled to these feelings, responding in ways that undermine the authenticity and sincerity of our interactions.

As a physical therapist, you will be called on a regular basis to respond empathetically to persons experiencing a considerable range and depth of emotions. Your effectiveness as a healing clinician will rest in large part on your ability to do this effectively. Needless to say, in addition to your mindful presence, it can be helpful to have a well-developed language related to the description of human emotions that can be used in your expressions of empathy. As you may know, proficiency in any language involves its regular use.

Talking Points/Field Notes

Empathy Language Makeover

The following two exercises can be used to help you sharpen and maintain your emotional language repertoire for effective demonstrations of empathy. You are also encouraged to record your observations about these exercises in your field notes.

Part 1: Expand Your Emotional Language Wardrobe

Work with a small group of classmates. This exercise will be enhanced if at least one member of the group has a strength in the area of linguistic intelligence (such persons are generally quite articulate and should be relatively easy to identify).

Directions: Below are several common human emotions, each followed by a range of intensities. For each emotion, generate a number of descriptors for each intensity. These descriptors should be suitable for use in a clinical practice setting. At the end of the exercise, share your list with other groups to create a larger list. For further additions, you can also consult a thesaurus. (No cheating!)

Joy: Low Moderate High

Fear: Low Moderate High

Anger: Low Moderate High

Disgust: Low Moderate High

Sadness: Low Moderate High

Part 2: Put Your Wardrobe to Use

For the next several days (which could include a weekend or time away from school), resolve to pay closer attention to the nature of feelings shared with you in conversation (be it face to face or technologically mediated). Then, using your internal communication and emotional intelligence to discern the accompanying emotions, generate an appropriate reflection of feeling. Make every effort toward a mindful reflection that includes your identification of this emotion and its intensity. Avoid defaulting to generic responses, particularly those involving slang.

Questions to Consider

1. How easy or difficult was it to refrain from using your usual responses to emotional content? What were the biggest challenges?

2. What effect did more specific reflections of feeling have on your conversations?

3. How did your expanded language assist you in the generation of more specific reflections of feeling?

4. How might you continue to expand your language for the description of emotions? How might this effort affect your personal and professional communication?

5. What impact did this exercise have on your own self-awareness of feelings?

Being Mindful of Your Own Discomfort With Difficult Emotions

Often in situations where another person is sharing emotional content, we may find ourselves becoming uncomfortable. For example, this is a common and well-documented barrier in patient–professional relationships in situations surrounding death.[12] Such studies indicate that discomfort among health professionals in these situations stems from many things, such fear of upsetting the patient, a sense of powerlessness to help the patient, or personal fears or negative death-related experiences on the part of the health-care professional. Thus, rather than being mindful of these feelings and accepting them as a natural response, health practitioners may unintentionally say or do things that rob them of the chance to connect with their patients in an empathic manner.

Bryant cites numerous research examples documenting avoidance tactics used by health-care practitioners with dying patients. These include taking longer to answer their call signals and using technical language to prevent emotional dialogue.[13] Thus, the empathy element of emotional intelligence involves being mindful of your own feelings and reactions to the feelings shared by your patients. Your internal communication can provide helpful cues for you to identify these feelings and to mindfully accept them as they arise.

What If Just I Don't Know What To Say?

Like Angelo, you are likely at some point to interact with patients who share their emotional perceptions about events you have never experienced. Even in the midst of your own feelings of discomfort or helplessness, you can still be empathetic by showing a quiet listening presence. In such an instance, useful self-talk can simply be, "Let me be fully present to this patient." There is also nothing wrong with honestly and sincerely saying, "I can't imagine how you must feel!" This statement lets the speaker know that you can discern a level of emotional intensity and that you are open to continued sharing.

There are two points to made here, the first being that empathy builds relationships, and the second is that empathy can be conveyed without words. Empathy is not about fixing or changing another person's emotional state. It is about meeting people where they are, with full acceptance.

Talking Points/Field Notes

Empathy Builders

The following series of exercises can be helpful in developing your sensitivity to emotions in others. Try at least one of these in the next 48 hours and discuss with a classmate.

Exercise 1. Identifying Emotions in Others

Empathy phone call: Arrange to have a telephone conversation with a classmate where he talks to you about the events in his day. Take turns seeing if each of you can accurately identify the emotions underlying their words and reflect these back to them. Give each other feedback.

Empathy photo review—a group activity that can also be done as a class project: Take pictures of a classmate's face (someone not in your group), having her convey the following emotions: fear, surprise, anger, sadness, happiness, confidence, love, and disgust. (These are the emotions that are often used in tests of emotional sensitivity.) The photo subject should convey these as naturally as possible. Have other classmates try to identify the underlying emotions.

Continued

Talking Points/Field Notes—cont'd ▬▬▬▬▬▬▬

Empathy conversation—a group activity: Each member of the group should have a turn as the speaker and as the listener. The speaker's topic can be anything about which he or she has a level of emotional intensity (either positive or negative) and about which the speaker can talk for 2 to 3 minutes. The listener can then practice using reflections of feeling as appropriate to identify the speaker's underlying feelings. Exchange feedback at the end of the conversation, using the following questions as a guide. Balance check: Please share at your comfort level.

For the Speaker

1. How accurate was the listener in identifying the underlying emotions in your dialogue?

2. How did it feel when the reflections were accurate?

3. How did it feel when the reflections were not accurate?

For the Listener

1. How did it feel to use reflections of feeling?

2. Were your reflections generally accurate? If not, why do you think this was so?

3. What impact did the use of reflections have on the speaker?

Exercise 2. Mindful Awareness of Your Own Empathy Challenges

Examine the following list of patient-related empathy challenges and discuss (and/or record in your field notes) your resulting reactions and self-talk. As you note these reactions, observe them with full acceptance. Then discuss appropriate strategies to demonstrate empathic support with these patients (it might be helpful to ask yourself, "How would I like to be treated if this were me?"). Balance check: Please share at your comfort level.

1. A patient who is tearful

2. A patient in severe pain

3. A patient who is very depressed

4. A patient who doesn't comply with your treatment

5. A patient who is fearful

6. A patient who is demanding

7. A patient who is angry

8. A patient who is impatient

9. A patient who is confused and disoriented

10. A patient who is emotionally needy

Motivation of Self and Others for Goal Attainment

As you well know from your journey thus far toward becoming a physical therapist, you must meet considerable challenges to attain important life goals. As with becoming a physical therapist, many important life goals take several years to be realized, requiring the ability to pull ourselves out of the trenches of discouragement when things don't go as planned and, perhaps most difficult of all, the ability to wait patiently for the sense of self-satisfaction that results from eventual success. Thus the most important aspect of goal attainment is having the motivation to invest significant effort over a period of time, regardless of duration or difficulty. As you probably also know, few goals are successfully achieved without a driving passion and sense of mission to fuel us for the long haul.

To this end, an important benefit of self-motivation is that it allows us to enrich our lives with meaningful goals. More importantly, a strong sense of self-motivation can help us sustain our efforts in the face of discouragement or long stretches of time without reward. Accordingly, the development of meaningful goals and the marshaling of sufficient motivation requires the emotional intelligence skills of self-awareness to determine what is important and personally valuable, self-control for the journey involved, and mindful empathy for self, particularly in times of discouragement.

Inherent in these emotional intelligence skills, effective self-motivation also includes several related attributes that have been shown to positively influence the chance of successful goal attainment.[7] They include an optimistic outlook, impulse control (being willing to delay gratification for a better long-term result), and engagement. Not surprisingly, these are also the key elements of optimal human function described in the discipline of positive psychology and discussed in previous chapters of this text as the foundations of engaged professionalism. Of course it is our internal communication that enables us to develop these skills in service of our life goals.

Talking Points/Field Notes

My Personal Motivation Strategies and Their Results

With a group of classmates, consider the following questions as means of reflecting on the importance of self-motivation in your life thus far. You are also encouraged to record your observations in your field notes.

1. Select a life accomplishment that involved the marshaling of considerable motivation over time and discuss the following. (Balance check: Please share at your comfort level.)

   a. What drove you to work toward this goal? What were the short- and long-term benefits, and how did the goal resonate with your values and mission?

   b. What sort of challenges did you face along the way, and how did you cope with these? How did your self-talk, outlook, and self-control assist you?

   c. What sorts of setbacks or discouragement did you face? How did you recover sufficiently to maintain your focus on the goal?

   d. How did you nurture and energize yourself during the process?

   e. What important things did you learn about yourself in the process of attaining this goal?

Another important aspect of self-motivation and goal attainment is the ability to develop and maintain a supportive network of other persons who assist our process in a variety of ways. No matter how small our goals may seem, the support of others is generally required in some fashion. To that end, one of the most enjoyable responsibilities of my teaching position is that of attending our college graduation ceremonies at the end of each academic term. Over the years, I have observed the practice by many graduates of decorating their mortar board hats with messages of gratitude to parents, spouses, and other key players in their journey through school. Although the decoration of mortarboards is viewed as being somewhat beneath the "pomp and circumstance" of a graduation ceremony, it does provide for a public acknowledgment of the persons behind the scenes.

How do we get people on board to support us in our quest for the realization of our mission and goals, no matter how challenging these may be? This involves the ability to develop authentic relationships based on a level of unconditional positive regard and unselfish caring. For many of us, our parents provided this first glimpse of unwavering support as we grew, unselfishly giving of their time, their love, and their resources to support our goals. Many of us find other allies in extended family members, spouses, partners, friends, and teachers. It can be a gratifying and enriching experience to acknowledge these individuals, perhaps not by putting their names on your mortarboard at graduation, but by writing them a letter, calling or visiting, or extending some unexpected kindness. In the spirit of mindfulness, there is no time like the present.

Talking Points/Field Notes

My Support Network

Again, consider either a past accomplishment or one that you are involved in currently. Discuss the following with classmates and record your observations in your field notes.

1. Whom did you approach for support when you were first deciding to pursue your goal? How did their response affect your decision to move forward on your goal?

2. In what ways did this/these person(s) enable you to pursue your goal? Consider all the many ways they provided assistance (i.e., keeping the house clean, giving you time to work on your goal, etc.).

3. How did you sustain your relationship with this/these person(s) in order to keep your relationship strong while you pursued your goal? What challenges has this involved?

4. How did this/these person(s) help you to cope with any challenges or setbacks that arose in your process? How did they cope?

5. How has/have your relationship(s) been enriched by your shared journey towards your goal?

6. How have you expressed your gratitude to these persons?

In the true spirit of sharing, perhaps one of the most important testimonials of our commitment to the important relationships in our lives is the willingness to support others in the pursuit of their goals. As you complete this discussion, you might consider how you have provided this support.

Implications for Physical Therapy

One of many important roles we play as physical therapists is to optimize our patients' motivation for optimal health and function. This involves having a mindful awareness of their goals, and providing encouragement for them to maintain their efforts. We can be instrumental to this process with a plan of care that challenges without overwhelming, that enables the regular experience of success, and by providing empathy and encouragement when needed. It can be very enjoyable to discover creative ways to help patients stay engaged with their plan of care with exercises and activities that are enjoyable and meaningful as well as devising objective measures of progress that reinforce their efforts. Most importantly, we need to accept where our patients are in their health journey and work with them at their pace. This becomes crucial, particularly when it involves long-term behavior change such as the establishment of a regular exercise program. Specific strategies to optimize patient motivation as they adopt permanent health behavior change will be discussed later in the text.

Helping to Sustain the Patient's Support System

Without a doubt, one of the most challenging life journeys is the adjustment to a significant change in function as the result of an injury or illness. It is not only the life of the patient that is dramatically affected in such an instance but also the lives of his or her friends and family. A patient's recovery and adaptation can be greatly enhanced by a supportive family network, and research indicates that family support is one of the most potent predictors of the discharge destination of patients with stroke (regardless of level of disability).[14] Thus, as physical therapists, it is critical to our patients' overall success to include both them and their families in the "unit of care," meaning that both are considered in the overall plan of intervention. A large number of health-care facilities, particularly those providing inpatient rehabilitation, regularly include both patients and family members in the interdisciplinary team. This practice is extremely valuable in keeping the health-care team's focus directly on the patient and family and can be invaluable in terms of identifying further needs for intervention, support, and education. Accordingly, family members can be encouraged to attend PT sessions for education, information, and support. Working with the patient to educate family members is instrumental in ensuring the patient's success after discharge. In addition, appropriate referrals to other team members such as social workers, psychologists, and spiritual counselors can be invaluable in providing support for the patient and their family in the midst of a health crisis.

Caring for a disabled family member can be emotionally and physically overwhelming. Thus, one of our roles as physical therapists is to identify resources that support both the patient and family. For example, many communities have family respite services that provide assistance to the patient so that family members can go on with important activities that may even include just getting enough rest to maintain their own health. In the next 25 years, the number of adults caring for both elderly parents and their own children (the "sandwich generation") is expected to increase dramatically as the 60 million members of the baby-boom generation reach retirement.[15] Thus, our health-care delivery system will likely include increasing liaisons to community support services that assist these families. As a physical therapist, it is important for you to be aware of the community support services offered in the area of your clinical practice.

A Family Member in Crisis (A True Story)

You have been treating Mr. Al Pinkston, an 82-year-old retired farmer who experienced a right-sided stroke 4 months earlier, for mobility training in your outpatient rehabilitation clinic. His major deficits include significant left-sided weakness, and he now requires moderate assistance to walk indoors with a large-based quad cane and an ankle-foot orthosis (AFO). Al also has moderate expressive aphasia, making it difficult for him to articulate his needs. Al's communication difficulties cause him considerable frustration. He lives with his 80-year-old wife June, who is the primary caretaker in their home. They have two grown daughters who each live 100 miles away and who try to help out with weekend visits at least once a month. Al and June live in a small one-story house about 30 miles out of town. Al has not been able to drive since his stroke. This has been a considerable loss for him, as he has several friends in town whom he used to visit frequently.

June reports that before Al's stroke, he was a gentle, friendly, and soft-spoken man who enjoyed many outdoor hobbies such as hunting, gardening, and woodwork. June reports that in the past month, Al has begun to swear, particularly when she can't understand him, and that he is growing increasingly irritable and withdrawn. June also notes that Al has been eating less and seems to be sleeping much more than usual. June states that Al has also become careless with this personal hygiene, and this has caused several unpleasant interactions between them, as Al is resistant to help.

Continued

Today, before your appointment with Al, June asks to speak to you privately. Once in your office, June begins to cry and tells you that last night while she was trying to take off his AFO, Al began swearing and hit her hard on her back. June is worried about the changes in Al's behavior and is now afraid that he might even hurt her. She asks you for help, saying "I'm really the only person Al has at home, and he's got to let me help him."

Questions to consider:

1. Consider your immediate response to June as she shares this information with you. How do you reflect your concern and empathy (what might you say?)?

2. What additional information might be helpful to obtain from June?

3. Who might you suggest that June contact immediately? What other referrals might be appropriate for ongoing support?

4. What factors might lead you to consider respite care for Al and June?

The rest of the story (no reading ahead!): The physical therapist in this situation was concerned that the progressive increase in Al's irritability, somnolence, and apathy could be related to an organic cause such as depression or might be side effects of his medications. Thus, at the physical therapists suggestion, June contacted Al's physician before leaving the clinic. The physician was able to see Al that day and, after an evaluation, prescribed medication for severe depression. It was also decided that Al should be admitted to a skilled nursing facility for 2 weeks in order to monitor the antidepressant medication and for a course of intensive therapy, including speech and PT for self-care and ambulation training. This course of action was instrumental in enabling Al to return home without further aggressive outbursts, enabling June to care for him until his death from another stroke a year later.

Motivating Each Other: Mentorship

At the professional level, encouraging relationships occur regularly and can contribute significantly to the growth of all persons involved. Engaged professionals make the cultivation and ongoing involvement in such relationships a part of their mission, and it is known as *mentorship.* Hopefully you have already experienced the growth-enhancing support of a mentor, an individual whose ideals, goals, and accomplishments resonate with yours and set an example of what is possible in a profession. Supportive mentors can provide timely opportunities to encourage your professional development; they can encourage your process of self-reflection with insightful feedback and help you maintain a realistic perspective (often based on their own sense of history and experience) when challenges arise. We discuss mentorship in greater depth further on in the text.

Social Finesse: Skillfully Negotiating the Diverse Terrain of Human Relationships

Social finesse is the ability to use empathy to determine appropriate behavioral and communicative interactions in human relationships. Social finesse is predicated on the assumption of unconditional positive regard, which in turn facilitates the authentic expression of feelings, even those of disagreement, in a way that enhances relationships. Persons who excel in the emotional intelligence dimension of social finesse are able to build effective networks in both their personal and professional lives. They are astute in their perceptions of others, they are tactful but assertive, honest, fair, and trustworthy. Often such persons are mentors for others and find themselves functioning as leaders in their organization (either formally or informally).

Social finesse is thus the application of emotional intelligence to the world of relationships. In a nutshell, the person with social finesse uses mindful awareness of self and others to build and sustain authentic and meaningful relationships, using empathy and encouragement to strengthen their authentic connections with others. Failure to use any one of the emotional intelligence skills weakens these connections, making them feel inauthentic and even exploitive.

Implications for Physical Therapy: Social Finesse Applied to Professional Leadership

Social Finesse in the Context of Leadership: Personal Influence [9]

Social finesse is a skill that is readily used in the expert practice of PT for the negotiation of relationships and is critical for effective patient care, health-care-team interaction, and professional growth.

Truly successful organizations involve interactions of committed individuals working in the context of empowering relationships. Thus social finesse is also a prerequisite for effective leadership. Lynn calls the leadership element of social finesse "personal influence."[9] Thus, in the context of leadership, personal influence is used to empower others to anticipate and cope with challenges that often arise in the context of negotiating change. According to Lynn, personal influence is a skill that often distinguishes managers (with their conformity-based emphasis on "doing things right") from leaders (with their empowerment-based emphasis on "doing the right thing"). Personal influence is also helpful in the context of patient care as means of motivation, a critical prerequisite for managing lifestyle changes needed for the achievement of effective outcomes. On a professional level, personal influence is needed on a broad scale, by many individuals, to direct the course of growth for the professional at large.

Aside from the appropriate use of personal influence, effective leaders use social finesse to connect with their colleagues in authentic and personal ways. Effective leaders also truly listen to those with whom they work. They demonstrate genuine caring, and they are approachable and steady in the face of difficulties. The bottom line is simply this: Leaders without emotional intelligence may get things done for a period of time, but the costs of low morale and disengagement eventually undermine the quality of any outcome that should happen to occur.

Clinical Scenario

Finessing a Departmental Change

Peter is the manager of a large inpatient PT department that includes services in orthopedics, burn therapy, oncology, and neurological rehabilitation. Until now, therapists could select the service where they wished to work and remain there as long as they wished. Therapists were also able to rotate to other services as the need arose or if an opening occurred. The majority of experienced staff members in the department had remained on the same service for several years, and a few had become clinical specialists in the related clinical areas.

In looking for ways of strengthening his department, Peter has decided that mandatory rotations between services every 6 months for all therapists would be a useful way of helping the PT staff maintain the broadest scope of clinical skills. He also believes that rotations would discourage boredom and burnout by providing exciting opportunities for the staff to work with a more diverse group of patients, physicians, and other team members. In addition, Peter is also being strongly encouraged by the hospital administration to implement his mandatory rotation plan, as they feel that it would improve options for vacation coverage with hospital staff instead of with expensive outside per diem therapists. The administration also believes that having such

Continued

clinically versatile therapists could improve their market advantage in the community. In order to help generate enthusiasm for his idea, Peter is willing to be a role model. Although he has greatly enjoyed working on the orthopedic service for 2 years, he plans to rotate to another service.

Today, Peter plans to inform his staff about his plan. He knows that he can count on the support of the majority of the newer staff; however, he also knows that the experienced staff members who have remained on the same service will likely oppose the idea. At least one of these experienced staff is very outspoken and has the potential to create discontent among the staff. Thus Peter foresees a dilemma in that he can't afford to lose his experienced therapists, but he also believes that the mandatory rotations could improve the quality of patient care. Therefore he is determined to put his new policy in place as soon as possible.

Discuss the following:

1. Putting yourself in Peter's shoes, consider the emotional intelligence skills presented in this chapter, and discuss how each of these applies to Peter as he orchestrates his mandatory rotation plan.
   a. Self-awareness and control
   b. Empathy
   c. Motivation of self and others
   d. Social finesse

2. What strategies might be helpful to Peter in getting some of the experienced staff "on board" with his idea? How can he empower his experienced staff to help him orchestrate the change?

3. What resources might Peter ask for from administration in order to prepare his department for this change?

4. How do you suggest that Peter respond to therapists who refuse to comply with the mandatory rotations? Should exceptions be made? If so, what does Peter need to consider in terms of:
   a. Morale and productivity of the entire department
   b. The future growth of the department
   c. The relationship between the department and administration
   d. The relationship between the department and other members of the health-care team in the hospital

Beyond IQ: The Importance of Emotional Intelligence in Life Success

While having a high IQ as measured by standardized testing continues to have value in determining academic potential, a larger question is its value in predicting a person's overall life success in terms of overall happiness and satisfaction. In a society that has long emphasized IQ as the consummate measure of intelligence and thus human potential, there has also been the corresponding assumption that a high IQ was the most important element. For many years, the lack of knowledge related to other dimensions of intelligence left this assumption essentially unchallenged.

Then, with the introduction of the concept of multiple intelligences and, in particular, the emphasis on the emotional domain, several studies have recently examined the role of IQ versus emotional intelligence (which the researchers called "EI") in the attainment of a satisfying life.

Goleman[6] provides an extensive overview of IQ versus EI studies in his 1995 book *Emotional Intelligence*. In his summary of these studies, Goleman writes, *"At best, IQ contributes 20% to the factors that determine life success, which leaves 80% to other forces."*

Describing his own observations on the importance of emotional intelligence in the context of a successful existence, Howard Gardner states, *"Many people with IQs of 160 work for people with IQs of 100 if the former has a poor level of interpersonal intelligence and the latter has a high one. In the day-to-day world, no intelligence is more important than the interpersonal. If you don't have it, you will make poor choices about who to marry, what job to take, and so on."*[7]

Evidence for Gardener's observations has been cited in several studies which support the value of EI training in various work settings.[9] For example, in the U.S. Air Force, EI-trained recruiters demonstrated a threefold increase in recruitment success compared to those without such training. The cosmetics company L'Oreal found that sales associates who were selected based on the demonstration of EI competencies outsold colleagues who were not so selected EI by several thousand dollars. Interestingly, the high EI sales associates also demonstrated 63% less turnover than their colleagues with lesser levels of EI skill.

In the health professions, the impact of EI has been studied in nursing,[16] mental health,[17] and medical school applicants.[18] The results of these studies support the value of EI as an important variable for successful practice in each of the respective disciplines.

Studies of Emotional Intelligence in Physical Therapy

Two studies on the impact of EI in PT practice were presented at the 2005 American Physical Therapy Association (APTA) Combined Sections meeting in New Orleans. Boyce, Bell, and Shaughnessy[19] explored the relationship between EI (as measured by the Multifactor Emotional Intelligence Scale), IQ (as measured by the Wonderlic Personnel test), and the academic success of 57 entry-level master's of physical therapy students. A secondary purpose of this study was to determine the efficacy of using EI assessment to predict academic success of physical therapy students. No correlation was found between IQ and academic success; however, the study results also demonstrated a low correlation between EI and academic success and a moderate correlation between IQ and EI. The authors of this study suggested that the measurement of EI might be more useful in the prediction of success in clinical education, "an area that might rely more on practical, motivational and emotional ability than on academic or cognitive ability."

The connection between EI and success in clinical education was explored in another study of physical therapy students. Lewis[20] examined the relationship between EI (as measured by the Mayer-Salovey-Caruso Emotional Intelligence test) and clinical performance (as measured by scores on the APTA Clinical Performance Instrument) among 56 physical therapy students. The study controlled for the variables of cognitive intelligence, age, gender, socioeconomic status, program type, and length of time as a physical therapy student. The results of the study demonstrated that EI was significantly related to two performance measures of the Clinical Performance Instrument (CPI).[21] These performance measures included CPI performance criterion number 14 ("Performs physical therapy interventions in a competent manner") and CPI performance criterion number 11 ("Performs a physical therapy evaluation"). In summarizing the importance of this study, the author stated that because these performance measures are related to EI, and because they are critical to successful clinical practice, "it makes sense to screen for these (EI) abilities prior to admission (to PT programs).[19]

Preaching to the Choir: The Integration of Emotional Intelligence Concepts in Key Physical Therapy Professionalism Documents

Even as we await the results of continued studies that will add to the body of evidence relating the skills of emotional intelligence to the engaged professional practice of PT, many of our key professionalism documents already describe elements of these skills.

Figure 6-2 illustrates the integration of emotional intelligence concepts within three of our key professionalism documents. These documents are the "Clinical Performance Instrument,"[21] "Core Values in Physical Therapy,"[22] and the "Generic Abilities."[23]

Dimensions of Emotional Intelligence
1. Self-Awareness and Control
2. Empathy
3. Motivation of Self and Others
4. Social Expertise

1. <u>The Clinical Performance Instrument for Physical Therapy Student Clinical Education.</u>
   (24 performance criteria. 8 related to professional behaviors). Dimensions of EI can be found in the sample behaviors of each of the 24 criteria, as the following examples illustrate:

   Performance Criterion #2 "Presents self in a professional manner"
   Sample Behaviors:
   "Accepts responsibility for own actions"
   "Demonstrates Initiative"
   "Is punctual and dependable"

   Performance Criterion #3 "Demonstrates professional behavior during interactions with others"
   Sample Behaviors:
   "Treats others with positive regard, dignity and compassion"
   "Accepts criticism without defensiveness"
   "Makes choices after considering the consequences to others"
   "Manages conflict in constructive ways"

   Performance Criterion #6 "Communicates in ways that are congruent with situational needs"
   Sample Behaviors:
   "Communicates verbally and nonverbally in professional and timely manner"
   "Listens actively and attentively to understand others"
   "Initiates communication in difficult situations"
   "Selects the most appropriate persons with whom to communicate"

2. <u>Professionalism in Physical Therapy: Core Values Self Assessment (APTA, 2003).</u> This assessment comprises seven core values related to professionalism, along with indicators of each behavior. The behaviors are:
   Accountability
   Altruism
   Compassion/Caring
   Excellence
   Integrity
   Professional Duty
   Social Responsibility

3. <u>The Generic Abilities Assessment:</u> A set of 10 behaviors required for success in the physical therapy profession (May et al, *Journal of PT Education*, 9:1, 1995). EI dimensions are reflected in all ten behaviors.
   Commitment to Learning
   Interpersonal Skills
   Communication Skills
   Effective Use of Time and Resources
   Use of Constructive Feedback
   Problem-Solving
   Responsibility
   Critical Thinking
   Stress Management

Figure 6–2. Dimensions of emotional intelligence (EI) in key physical therapy professionalism documents.

Implications for Physical Therapy Practice

The ability to exert the dimensions of emotional intelligence described in this chapter are key elements of both effective personal and professional behaviors. Because the delivery of physical therapy interventions takes place in the context of personal interactions, the skills of self awareness, empathy, and motivation are critical for success in this endeavor. Of equal importance is the ability to navigate the social environment in which our treatment is delivered. Thus the development of emotional intelligence skills will enhance both internal and external communication. The next chapter further explores the role of emotional intelligence in our interactions with others.

Chapter Summary

1. The areas of excellence in human performance relate to seven intelligences (proposed by Howard Gardner), which include linguistic, logical-mathematical, visual-spatial, musical, interpersonal, intrapersonal, and body kinesthetic types. Emotional intelligence contains elements of the interpersonal and intrapersonal domains.

2. Emotional intelligence involves self-awareness and control, empathy, motivating self and others, and social finesse. These skills are each important in effective communication with self and others in the context of engaged professionalism.

3. Empathy involves the conscious willingness to share the feelings of another person. Empathy can be demonstrated through reflections of feeling, which involve the accurate interpretation of another person's emotions and their intensity, which is then conveyed to them as a measure of support. The habitual use of generic or slang responses to the emotional concerns of others may impair authentic and appropriate demonstrations of empathy.

4. Motivation of self and others is an important skill in PT practice and involves the ability to develop effective therapeutic communication, demonstrate empathy, and provide meaningful activities that support patient goals.

5. Social finesse is a prerequisite of effective leadership and engaged professionalism.

Take Home Menu

1. Online tests of multiple intelligence. There are several online sites that provide free tests of multiple intelligence. You may enjoy visiting one of these sites and learning more about your particular strengths. These sites include:
   a. Multiple intelligences: http://www.bgfl.org/bgfl/custom/resources_ftp/client_ftp/ks3/ict/multiple_int/index.htm. Accessed December 31, 2007.
   b. Seven intelligences; Adult Version: http://www.mitest.com/o7inte~1.htm. Accessed December 31, 2007.
   c. Learning Disability Resource Community. Multiple intelligence test: http://www.ldrc.ca/projects/miinventory/miinventory.php. Accessed December 31, 2007.
   d. Businessballs.com. Howard Gardner's multiple intelligences: http://www.businessballs.com/howardgardnermultipleintelligences.htm#multiple%20intelligences%20tests. Accessed December 31, 2007.

Continued

█ **Take Home Menu—cont'd**

2. Online emotional intelligence tests. The following sites offer free, no-registration-required tests of emotional intelligence. They are meant to provide general information. Standardized and validated emotional intelligence tests are administered by persons who are trained in their administration and usually involve a fee.
   a. Emotional Intelligence Test R-2: http://www.psychtests.com/cgi-bin/tests/transfer.cgi. Accessed December 31, 2007.
   b. E-IQ test: http://www.helpself.com/iq-test.htm. Accessed December 31, 2007.

References

1. Gardner H. *Frames of Mind: The Theory of Multiple Intelligences.* New York: Basic Books; 1983.

2. Strydom J, Du Plessis S. IQ test: Where does it come from and what does it measure? Audiblox: http://www.audiblox2000.com/dyslexia_dyslexic/dyslexia014.htm. Accessed November 26, 2007.

3. Project Zero at the Harvard Graduate School of Education. Multiple Intelligence Schools: http://www.pz. harvard.edu/Research/MISchool.htm. Accessed November 26, 2007

4. I.Q. test: Where does it come from? Audiblox: http://iq-test.learninginfo.org/iq01.htm. Accessed December 30, 2007.

5. Waldorf learning methods and theories: http://www.educationatlas.com/learning-theories-waldorf.html. Accessed November 28, 2007.

6. US charter schools: http://www.uscharteshool.org/pub/uscs_docs/o/history.htm. Accessed November 27, 2007.

7. Goleman D. *Emotional Intelligence.* New York: Bantam Books; 1995.

8. Weisinger H. *Emotional Intelligence at Work.* San Francisco: Jossey Bass; 1998.

9. Lynn AB. *The Emotional Intelligence Activity Book: 50 Activities for Promoting EI at Work.* New York: AMACOM, Division of American Management Association; 2002.

10. Davis CM. *Patient Practitioner Interaction: An Experimental Manual for Developing the Art of Health Care.* Thorofare, NJ: Slackk; 1994.

11. Rogers C. *On Becoming a Person: A Therapist's View of Psychotherapy.* New York: Houghton Mifflin; 1961.

12. Cooper J, Barnett M. Aspects of caring for dying patients which cause anxiety to first year student nurses. *Int J Palliat Nurs.* 2005;11(8):423-430.

13. Bryant C. *Handbook of Death and Dying.* Newbury Park, CA: Sage Publications; 2003.

14. Wee JY, Hopman WM. Stroke impairment predictors of discharge function, length of stay and discharge destination in stroke rehabilitation. *Am J Phys Med Rehabil.* 2005;84(8):604-612.

15. The Sandwich generation. Many Americans are taking care of their parents as well as their own children. CBS Evening News, May 8, 2006: http://www.cbsnews.com/stories/2006/05/08/eveningnews/main1600179.shtml

16. Cadman C, Brewer J. Emotional intelligence: a vital prerequisite for recruitment in nursing. *J Nurs Mgt.* 2001;9:321-324.

17. Freshwater D. Emotional intelligence: Developing emotionally literate training in mental health. *Mental Health Practice.* 2004; 8(4):12-16.

18. Carrothers RM, Gregory SW, Gallagher TW. Measuring the emotional intelligence of medical school applicants. *Acad Med.* 2000;75:456-463.

19. Boyce DA, Bell DP, Shaughnessy J. The correlation of emotional intelligence, academic success, and cognitive ability in master's level physical therapy students. Poster presentation, American Physical Therapy Association, Combined Sections Meeting; New Orleans, LA, February, 2005.

20. Lewis ES. A study of emotional intelligence, cognitive intelligence, and clinical performance of physical therapy students. Poster presentation, American Physical Therapy Association, Combined Sections Meeting; New Orleans, LA, February 2005.

21. American Physical Therapy Association. *Clinical Performance Instrument.* Alexandria, VA: American Physical Therapy Association; 1997

22. American Physical Therapy Association. *Professionalism in Physical Therapy: Core Values.* Alexandria, VA: American Physical Therapy Association; 2003.

23. May WW, Morgan BJ, Lemke JC, et al. Model for ability based assessment in physical therapy education. *J Phys Ther Educ.* 1995;9(1):3-6.

Part 3

External Communication

This section addresses *external communication*, which is used to form authentic and meaningful connections in both personal and professional contexts. Persons with high levels of external communication skills are generally able to develop satisfying interpersonal relationships, which empower all areas of their lives.

External communication is grounded within the broad realm of *social intelligence.* In turn, social intelligence involves two major constructs, *social awareness,* the ability to perceive and adapt to the parameters of the prevailing social culture, and *social skills,* specific communication strategies that promote effective connections. These constructs are respectively explored in Chapters 7 and 8.

Chapters 9 and 10 address external communication in the context of developing an empowering therapeutic alliance with the patients we are called to serve. This partnership can be greatly enhanced through an appreciation of generational differences (as discussed in Chapter 9) and the challenges of the of illness experience (which is explored in Chapter 10).

CHAPTER 7

External Communication and Social Awareness

"Only Connect."

E. M. Forster
English novelist and essayist, 1879–1970

Chapter Overview

External communication is the means by which we share our thoughts, feelings, and ideas with others. This chapter first explores the importance of external communication in the development and maintenance of authentic connections with others. The ability to communicate with others in a way that promotes mutual empowerment and affirmation is known as *social intelligence.* Social intelligence first involves social awareness, the ability to understand and adapt to the often unspoken norms and behavioral expectations of differing groups. These elements are described and explored in this chapter.

Key Terms

Social intelligence	Culture
Social awareness	Professional socialization
Social skills	

External Communication Connects Us With Others

The Importance of Connection

The quotation at the beginning of this chapter, "only connect," is an elegantly simple testimony to the fundamental and biologically driven human need for meaningful relationships. From the moment of birth and throughout our lives, we are nurtured, encouraged, and challenged by our relationships with others. Supportive human connections are essential for optimal health, happiness, and quality of life.[1]

Positive connections with others can enhance cognitive skills such as learning, creativity, and memory. Supportive relationships enhance our work productivity, academic performance, and potential for achievement.[2-4]

In the health-care setting, patients who experience a compassionate connection with their health-care providers are more likely to adhere to prescribed treatment regimens and to have better functional health outcomes than those without such relationships. They are also less likely to require placement in extended care facilities, even in the presence of significant disability.[5-9] Having supportive connections with patients is also good malpractice insurance. Clinicians who develop positive relationships with their patients are less likely to have legal action taken against them.[10]

The benefits of positive relationships have far-reaching effects at the organizational level of health care, contributing to improved productivity and quality of service. For example, nurses with supportive managers have better patient safety outcomes than those without.[11] The ability to develop supportive relationships is an essential trait for effective leadership. The efforts of many persons are required for significant organizational change. Thus leaders who can motivate their colleagues towards their goals and vision will be much more successful in their roles. In contrast, leaders who rely largely on impersonal policies or mandates (such as financial gain) will seldom achieve long-term success.[12]

Finally, research in positive psychology has clearly demonstrated the link between happiness and the presence of a strong social support network. In her 2007 book *The How of Happiness: A Scientific Approach to Getting the Life You Want*, Sonja Lyubomirsky, a research professor in the area of positive psychology, provides an extensive evidence-based review of the elements of human happiness and well-being. The findings on social connections all point to a strong positive relationship between happiness and high levels of satisfaction with one's family life, social activities, romantic partner, and colleagues.[13]

Thus positive human relationships are an invaluable resource that afford each of us the opportunity for a rich and fulfilling life. As with the cultivation of any resource, the investment of dedicated time, effort, and skills is paramount for success. In our current society, with its immensely diverse array of human interests, experiences, and world views, how does one effectively build meaningful and lasting alliances? These are key questions in the emerging field of social intelligence. No doubt you have already experienced the life-enhancing benefits of strong relationships.

Sociograms are drawings of social networks. This concept was developed by psychiatrist Jacob Moreno to assist psychologists, teachers, and organizational leaders in identifying and facilitating the productive social alliances within their institutions.[14]

Let us begin our investigation of social intelligence by identifying and affirming these individuals through the construction of a modified sociogram.

Talking Points/Field Notes

My Social Network

Identifying one's social network can be a reassuring exercise, particularly in life situations where you can benefit from support. **Figure 7-1** shows a modified sociogram depicting a typical social network. For this person, the sociogram consists of family and friends (the large circle), followed by one family member and two groups of "buddies" with whom the relationships are less intimate. The arrows going both ways in the inner circle signify a mutually supportive relationship between this person and the members of her network. One-way arrows can also be used to depict the major direction of support if it is not mutual.

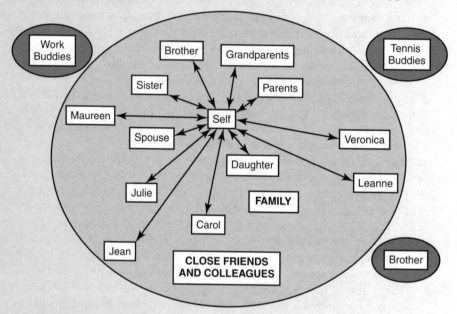

Figure 7–1. Representation of a close social network (a modified sociogram).

Directions

1. Make a chart or drawing representing your social network, beginning with those closest to you (these persons can be family, friends, colleagues, or whomever you choose).

2. If you like, you can also represent relationships that are less intimate but still enjoyable and beneficial in your life. Often these are persons who share a specific interest or purpose, such as a classmate or member of your church, sports team, or club.

3. You can also add the year when your friendship or relationship began. This will give you a perspective of the longevity of your relationships.

4. If you choose, you can use arrows to depict the directions of support from each of these individuals. For example, a relationship where both individuals give each other support would be depicted by two-way arrows. Less reciprocal relationships might be depicted by one-way arrows, pointing towards the receiver of the support.

Reflect on the Following in Your Field Notes and, if Comfortable, Share With a Group of Classmates

1. Explain your diagram and your reasons for the various placements of individuals. How have they enriched your life? How have you enriched their lives?

2. Are there similar characteristics among these persons? How might they be different?

Talking Points/Field Notes—cont'd ■━━━━━━━━━━━━━━━━━━

3. How do you nurture the important connections in your life? What do you think are the most important considerations for maintaining strong connections with your "inner circle," particularly during the busier times in your life?

4. How has your sociogram changed in the past 2 years? It might be interesting to repeat this exercise at the end of your PT education. Becoming part of a dynamic profession such as physical therapy will provide numerous opportunities to develop close friendships with colleagues in the coming years.

External Communication as the Currency of Connection

Given the importance of positive human connections, why aren't all of us as successful as we would like in our ability to achieve and sustain them? It might be useful to consider that our external communication is a form of currency, a medium of exchange, through which we offer the "commodity" of our friendship, knowledge, or services. Therefore how do we strengthen the value of our communication currency in the relationship market?

In the world of finance, currency is used to obtain goods and services. Certain forms of currency (the American dollar and the European euro) are considered "legal tender" for these transactions. In contrast, other mediums of exchange (such as drugs or counterfeit money) are not considered appropriate for settling accounts in most financial relationships.

The appropriate use of communication for interpersonal exchanges has similar results as the use of appropriate currency for financial transactions. Unfortunately, people sometimes select inappropriate forms of currency to settle their interpersonal accounts (which could involve managing conflict, solving problems, or expressing emotions).

For example, the use of impersonal technological methods for emotionally potent communication (such as delivering a terminal diagnosis on an answering machine) would likely result in a "debt" of relationship damage on the part of the offender. Consider the real-life example presented below.

Clinical Scenario

Canned by Computer

Jess is a physical therapist who has provided weekend and vacation relief in her town's community hospital for the past 15 years. She is well respected in the 20-member PT department and has received outstanding annual performance evaluations from Samantha, the PT department director. Jess and Samantha have also enjoyed a long-standing social relationship outside of work.

There is significant paperwork involved in the annual performance evaluation process, including a lengthy hospital-mandated written assessment of all employees that must be completed by the director. In addition to the annual reviews, the hospital also requires the department director to maintain several other records for each employee, such as documentation of TB tests, CPR certification, and completion of continuing education courses.

Unbeknownst to Jess, Samantha is experiencing significant job stress because of increasing productivity demands. Thus, Samantha decides that maintaining the required employee paperwork for the three relief staff is no longer a good use of her time. However, this decision also means that Samantha will need to terminate the employment of Jess and the other two relief staff.

In order to carry out this termination, Samantha sends Jess and the other two employees a brief e-mail stating that their services are no longer needed at the hospital owing to increasing paperwork demands. When Jess receives this e-mail on her home account, she is offended by this method of communication and too upset to reply.

Continued

One week later, Samantha resigns from her hospital position. Shortly afterward, Jess receives a telephone call asking her to be a character reference for Samantha, who is applying for a supervisory position at another facility.

Questions for Consideration

1. Discuss Samantha's use of e-mail to terminate Jess's employment. Do you consider this an appropriate method of communication in this situation? Under what circumstances, if any, might e-mail be justified as a means of terminating an employee?

2. What other communication methods would be appropriate for terminating an employee in Jess's situation?

3. How might you respond to Samantha if you were Jess? What form of communication would you use?

4. E-mail can be a useful form of communication if used appropriately. What considerations might you use in determining whether or not to use this method for various types of communication?

5. Should Jess consider Samantha's actions in deciding how to respond to the request for character reference for another supervisory position?

External Communication in Practice: Building Connections for Professional Empowerment

As the previous example demonstrates, the appropriate use of words, their methods of delivery, and awareness of their likely impact are important considerations in the use of external communication to ensure the health of our relationships. When used thoughtfully with positive mutual intent, external communication can promote collegiality and empowerment among groups or individuals, much in the way the use of legal tender can facilitate economic growth. A 2002 study of 164 PTs provides interesting insight into the use of external communication as an effective medium of exchange for reducing a debt of frustrations in clinical practice.[15]

These therapists were surveyed to determine:

1. Their satisfaction with PT as a career choice. ("If you had to do it all over again, would you choose PT as a career?")

2. Whether or not they were frustrated with clinical practice. ("Do you find the practice of PT frustrating?")

3. The primary sources of their frustrations. (Respondents could select from a list and add their own as well.)

4. Their strategies for addressing these sources. (Respondents were asked to explain methods for reducing them.)

The results of the survey indicate that 89% of the subjects were satisfied with PT as a career choice. Interestingly, 67% of the respondents also indicated that they viewed the practice of PT to be frustrating. **Table 7-1** illustrates the five top frustrations identified by the respondents.

Table 7–1. Top Sources of Frustration in Physical Therapy Practice

Source	Number and Percentage of Respondents	
1. Inability to help patients enough	n = 62/83	75%
2. Not enough time to achieve goals	n = 55/82	67%
3. Lack of respect from other professionals	n = 41/63	65%
4. Too large of a patient load	n = 48/77	62%
5. Lack of teamwork	n = 44/72	61%

From Mueller K. Take this job and love it: Factors related to job satisfaction and career commitment among physical therapists. Platform presentation. 14th Congress, World Confederation for Physical Therapy. Barcelona, Spain; 2003.

Other frustrations included lack of autonomy, excessive paperwork and documentation requirements, and restrictions imposed by managed care.

Interestingly, the respondents who were satisfied with their career choice but frustrated with some elements of practice viewed these challenges as an opportunity to develop new approaches involving several different strategies. Thus most of these respondents developed methods that were positive and empowering.

Eighteen different approaches were identified, which were divided into two major categories. Eight of the strategies related to improving efficiency, either by streamlining procedures (such as the use of standardized documentation) or by improving professional competency in areas related to managed care and clinical practice.

The remaining 10 strategies involved the use of external communication strategies to:

1. *Build collaborative relationships* with interdisciplinary colleagues in order to improve the sharing of information related to their work responsibilities.

2. *Improve their level of influence* in their various work settings through involvement on task forces and committees. This involvement allowed them to influence decisions that positively affected their work, thus empowering them toward greater autonomy and efficiency.

3. *Educate others about the role of physical therapists in the health care system.*
   The respondents provided in-service education to colleagues, nurses, and physicians. They also engaged in marketing efforts within their workplace, their communities, and in conjunction with national initiatives of the American Physical Therapy Association (APTA). These efforts also resulted in greater autonomy and respect.

Box 7-1 summarizes the communication strategies used by the respondents.

This study supports the use of effective communication as a powerful tool for positive organizational change. In order to be successful in their efforts, the therapists in this study employed several important skills. First, they had a solid understanding of the culture of health care, which directed their external communication in effective ways. Second, they developed a network of collegial support in order to both strengthen and broaden their level of influence. Next, they understood and harnessed the sources of formal and informal power within the workplace. In addition, they sought appropriate contexts for instituting change, such as involvement in committees and task forces. Finally, they recognized the importance of educating consumers about their professional role, seeking involvement in their communities and in their profession at large.

BOX 7-1:   Communication Strategies Used by 164 Physical Therapists to Address Frustrations of Clinical Practice

1. Network with colleagues to improve bargaining power.
2. Enhance team cooperation through formal and informal communication.
3. Increase communication with team members through committees and task force involvement.
4. Pursue self-education about the intricacies of managed care to better advocate for patients.
5. Expand patient education efforts.
6. Educate physicians about role and benefits of PT.
7. Market the profession through exemplary professional behaviors, education, and communication to consumers and team members.
8. Enhance professional competence through continuing education and graduate work, then sharing this expertise.
9. Be politically active; contact and educate legislators about initiatives that affect clinical practice.
10. Actively support APTA initiatives affecting practice.

From Mueller K. Take this job and love it: Factors related to job satisfaction and career commitment among physical therapists. Platform presentation. 14th Congress, World Confederation for Physical Therapy. Barcelona, Spain; 2003.

Talking Points/Field Notes

My Satisfactions, Frustrations, and Strategies

Every decision has its frustrations or challenges. Reflect on the following questions and record your observations in your field notes.

1. What major frustrations are you experiencing in your role as a physical therapy student?

2. Choose the top two frustrations and identify approaches that would effectively address these. How do these strategies involve communication? Consider internal as well as external forms.

3. Can you be satisfied with a decision (presumably, in this case, to become a physical therapist) and frustrated with certain aspects at the same time? What effect does this generally have for you personally?

4. How can you go about making frustrations an engaging challenge? What examples might you have to show this? How is communication (internal and/or external) involved?

As you will discover in the coming sections, the ability to understand the prevailing social culture is an essential requirement for the determination of appropriate communication skills. This skill, known as *social awareness*, is the major focus of the remainder of this chapter. First, however, we explore its relationship to the larger context of social intelligence.

Elements of Social Intelligence: Setting the Stage for Effective External Communication

Evolving from the original concepts of Gardner's multiple intelligence theory, explored in Chapter 6, social intelligence pertains to the ability to develop and sustain healthy, caring relationships that *benefit each party involved*. Thus social intelligence involves the ability to evoke positive change in self and others.

The components of social intelligence have been explored by several researchers over the years. Ongoing studies are in progress to define these in a universal manner, which can then be evaluated through standardized assessments.

Daniel Goleman has proposed two dimensions (or specific skill sets) related to social intelligence: *social awareness* and *social skills*.[16] Other researchers have also identified specific behaviors relating to both social awareness and social skills. These studies involved having subjects identify attributes that they felt were important measures of both of these areas.[17–19]

Box 7-2 illustrates the two dimensions of social intelligence proposed by Goleman.

BOX 7-2:   Two Components of Social Intelligence

1. SOCIAL AWARENESS: INTERPRETING THE SOCIAL WORLD
   - The ability to empathically interpret other people's feelings, thoughts, and emotions
   - Knowing the unspoken expectations, rules, and behavioral norms of different social contexts

2. SOCIAL FACILITY: COMMUNICATING EFFECTIVELY IN THE SOCIAL WORLD
   - Using social awareness to facilitate effective interactions with others
   - The ability to synchronize nonverbal communication to promote harmonious connections (nodding or smiling at the right time, appropriate use of body language)
   - Presenting oneself positively in all situations (making a good first impression and sustaining it in future interactions)

Adapted from Goleman D. *Social Intelligence*. New York: Bantam; 2006.

Table 7-2 illustrates behaviors related to the two domains of social intelligence identified by other researchers.[16–18]

As you review this table, consider whether or not you agree with its components. In addition, reflect upon whether you consider these appropriate in our current society. As you might be aware, social norms and expectations can change considerably over time. Many of these norms fall under the guise of "etiquette," which pertains to socially acceptable standards for behavior. For example, in my childhood, breast-feeding in public was rarely seen and considered shocking. Today, many persons have no objection to this behavior, and it has thus become more prevalent.[20]

Table 7–2. Specific Behaviors Related to Emotional Intelligence

Sternberg, Conway, Ketron, and Bernstein (1981)[17]	Kosmitski and John (1993)[19]
Accepting others for what they are	Understanding people's thoughts, feelings, and intentions
Admitting mistakes	
Displaying interest in the world at large	Dealing effectively with others
Being on time for appointments	Knowing the rules and norms of human relationships
Having a social conscience	
Thinking before speaking or acting	Learning and accepting other people's perspectives
Having curiosity	
Avoiding snap judgments	Adapting well to all social situations
Making fair assessments	
Assessing the relevance of information to a problem at hand	Showing warmth and caring
Showing sensitivity to other people's needs and desires	Being open to new ideas, experiences, and values
Being frank and honest with self and others	
Showing interest in the immediate environment	

Talking Points/Field Notes

Attributes of Socially Skilled Communicators

1. In a small group, discuss, list, and rank the top ten social skills of the best communicators you know. Feel free to add your own ideas as well. Compare your list to the behaviors listed previously in Tables 7-1 and 7-2. How are they different?

2. Consider the relevance of these skills to your future work as a PT. Would your list change?

3. The lists in Table 7-2 were developed at a time when the use of technological communication was less prevalent than it is today. What rules of etiquette (social norms) have arisen as a result of our increased reliance on technology? Are there any rules you would add?

4. If you could select one social skill from your list to work on, what would this be? Why did you choose this? How would you go about working on this?

Goleman describes social awareness and social skills as the predominant elements of social intelligence.[16] The next section describes social awareness as a primary determinant for appropriate external communication. In other words, we will be operating under the premise that the context of your communication is as important as its content.

The "context" aspect pertains to the environmental and cultural elements that guide appropriate communication behaviors. Social awareness is the skill that contributes sensitivity and responsiveness to these.

Social Awareness: Playing by the Rules of the Prevailing Social Culture

Our external communication involves considerably more than the delivery of words. In the broad context of social interaction, there are many explicit (clearly stated) and implicit (tacitly understood) guidelines that govern the dynamics of our interpersonal exchanges.

If you have ever traveled out of the country, you have perhaps had the embarrassing experience of violating one of these guidelines. Perhaps you used a word or gesture that is considered part of everyday discourse in the United States but offensive in another culture. For example, in Australia, the "thumbs-up sign" means something along the lines of "up yours." In Turkey, pointing the sole of your shoe at another person is considered an insult.[21,22]

As these examples show, sensitivity to the prevailing social culture is paramount for successful communication in that other environment.

The term *culture* pertains to a shared set of values and behaviors that is passed on from one generation to the next. The set of behaviors in any given culture can be vast and include language, forms of dress, etiquette, and sources of authority. Some of our strongest and most pervasive cultural rituals may derive from our ethnic or religious heritage (such as being Asian or Jewish). Cultural differences are a key contributing factor to the rich diversity that is a part of our society. Sadly, a lack of appreciation, understanding, and tolerance of these differences is also a contributing factor to much of the conflict that sometimes occurs in the world.

Each one of us brings a set of cultural experiences to our interactions. Whether or not we are aware of it, these experiences have profound influence on our perceptions and expectations about communication. The topic of cultural diversity is immensely broad and has important implications for effective communication in our current global economy. Hopefully, you will have numerous opportunities to explore this topic in the course of your professional education. In the context of external communication and social awareness, culture is an important consideration in the determination of appropriate communication strategies. A brief exploration of this topic follows.

Talking Points/Field Notes

My Cultures and Their Influence

In your field notes, construct a drawing illustrating the various cultural influences that have affected your life thus far. Considerations can include your ethnic and racial heritage, your gender, and your socioeconomic background, education, religion, and primary language. As you consider these, reflect on the rituals, traditions, behaviors, and expectations of each of these.

Figure 7-2 illustrates the elements contained within the Italian ethnic heritage.

Continued

Talking Points/Field Notes—cont'd

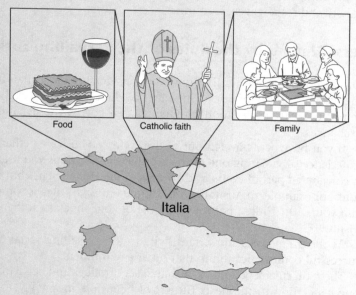

Figure 7–2. A culture drawing: elements of Italian heritage.

When you have completed the representation of your cultures, reflect on the following and share with a small group if desired.

1. Looking back to your earliest memories, what rituals stand out and why? How have you preserved these rituals as you have reached adulthood?

2. Recall the first time that you became aware of cultural differences in your life. What element was the source of the difference? What impact did this have? How did you respond?

3. Recall a time when cultural differences affected your communication. What was the challenge and how did you respond?

4. What are ways that we can communicate caring and compassion in the midst of cultural differences?

In addition to our family culture, most of us function in several other cultures as well. For example, the profession of PT, with its own set of values, language, and role expectations, is a culture, as is your academic program, or any campus organizations to which you belong. Each of these cultures has its own set of behavioral rules and expectations, which you must follow in order to be an accepted member. In each of these cultures, the more experienced members educate you about these traditions, either formally or informally, so that you develop awareness of the group's behavioral norms. For example, as a physical therapy student, you are undergoing a professional socialization process whereby you are learning the rules of our professional culture from your academic and clinical instructors. These rules include those for appropriate language, behavior, and demeanor. **Figure 7-3** illustrates elements of the culture of PT.

On a more general scale, social awareness involves the ability to identify and respond to the expectations of any social culture in which you find yourself. For the purposes of this discussion, we will consider a social culture as any group of individuals who are brought together for a common purpose. Thus, a professional meeting, your classroom environment, or a community organization would be considered a social culture.

Reflect on the following example.

Figure 7–3. Elements of the culture of PT.

Values:	The Code of Ethics, Standards of Practice for Physical Therapists
Language:	Models of Disablement, The International Classification of Function (ICF), Practice Patterns, Medical Terminology
Role Identity:	Health professionals recognized as "practitioners of choice" for the diagnosis of, interventions for, and prevention of impairments, functional limitations, and disabilities related to movement, function, and health. (APTA 2020 Vision Statement)
Societal Status:	A recognized position in the health-care delivery system conferred by a professional socialization process involving education at the post-baccalaureate level. A growing level of prestige related to increasing autonomy and the move towards doctoral education.
Social Control:	Internal regulation of the profession by educational programs, a professional organization (the APTA). External regulation by licensing boards, accrediting bodies, and other stakeholders in the health-care industry (other professionals, insurance payors, etc.).

Clinical Scenario

Assessing a Social Culture

Noah has been out of PT school for 5 years. During that time, he has built a successful PT practice that operates a pro bono clinic for uninsured patients once a month. Noah has also been very involved in supporting the growth of his small community, sponsoring several successful fund-raisers for various improvements. Thus, Noah is quickly gaining respect as an emerging civic leader and has been invited by the mayor to participate in a local advisory council for his city government. The members of this advisory council will include respected leaders in commerce, law, and medicine, most of whom are older and more traditional than Noah. To kick off the advisory council, Noah has been invited to dinner at the nicest restaurant in town.

Key elements of the invitation read as follows:

> *You and your guest are invited to dinner*
> *At the Historic Oak Leaf Restaurant*
> *Cocktails will be served at 7:00 pm*
> *Dinner to follow at 8:00 pm*
> *Dinner Forum: The most pressing issues*
> *facing our community (Bring your ideas!)*
> *Dress is business casual*

Discuss the Following in a Small Group

1. Noah has recently come out as gay. He has just started dating Mitch, a physical therapist who works at the local hospital. Attending this dinner with Mitch would be the first public indication of Noah's sexual orientation. While both Noah and Mitch are comfortable about this, they have concerns about the potential impact of Noah's being openly gay on his aspirations to be a community leader. How might these two go about making their final decision?

2. Noah does not drink and does not really enjoy cocktail parties. Would there be any compelling reason to consider attending the cocktail portion of the evening in this case?

Continued

3. Noah's most pressing community issue is the growing number of persons without health insurance who are attending his pro bono clinics. It is common practice in Noah's community for small business owners to hire only part-time help in order to avoid paying for medical benefits. Although Noah would like to speak out against this practice, some of these individuals are prominent civic leaders who will be attending this dinner. In addition, the physicians who will also be attending regularly refuse services to uninsured patients.

4. How might Noah interpret "business casual" dress with a group of older, more traditional individuals?

5. Noah will be meeting several of the other attendees for the first time. What strategies might he use for small talk with these persons?

As this example shows, even a simple invitation may involve the need for thoughtfully assessing the spoken and unspoken norms for a given social culture. Noah will need to demonstrate a level of social awareness that will influence the decisions he makes with regard to the upcoming evening and the persons involved. He will also have to consider the consequences of his decisions on many levels, including his personal integrity and sense of self, his desire to be recognized as a community leader, and his need to maintain a viable business. In other social contexts (such as a group of supportive friends getting together for a weekend barbecue), these decisions and consequences might be quite different. There are several elements within each social culture that should be considered in terms of their potential impact on communication. **Figure 7-4** illustrates elements of a social culture that require awareness.

Let us now consider each of the elements of a given social culture in further detail.

Individual Agendas

Whether or not we are aware of it, we approach every social interaction with an "agenda" involving the realization of personal needs, desires, or goals. These needs can include a desire for acceptance and friendship or the goal of obtaining a valued service (as in the

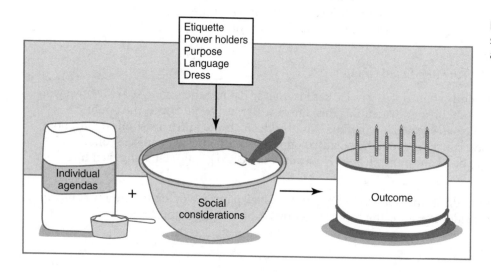

Figure 7–4. Elements of a social culture that require awareness.

Etiquette
Power holders
Purpose
Language
Dress

Individual agendas

+

Social considerations

Outcome

case of our patients). In Noah's situation, attending the community advisory council dinner could provide a valuable opportunity for him to expand the scope of his leadership abilities. Operating from this agenda, Noah would probably assess the social culture in a way that would direct his communication towards success in this domain. Assuming that Noah's primary goal was to be recognized as a community leader, how would your answers to any of the previous questions be different?

What if, on the other hand, Noah's primary agenda was to promote greater acceptance of all individuals in his community, regardless of their sexual orientation? How then might Noah's assessment of the social culture surrounding the community advisory council dinner drive his communication? How might your answers to the previous questions change?

Just as each of us approach our interactions with an agenda, so does everyone with whom we interact. It is thus helpful to be sensitive to this pervasive element of social interaction, because it can have a tremendous impact on the outcome of a situation. For example, when the agendas of an individual or group conflict, a process of negotiation is often necessary in order to resolve this and maintain the relationship. Negotiation and conflict resolution are addressed further on in this text.

Talking Points/Field Notes

Agendas in My Communication

Discuss the following and record your observations in your field notes.

1. Recall a time when you approached a specific interaction with a clear agenda. (If you cannot readily think of an example, consider an interview for employment or acceptance into a PT educational program.)

2. In what ways did you assess the social culture of the interaction beforehand? What considerations arose as a result of your assessment?

3. How did you direct your communication in order to be successful in meeting your agenda? (Refer to Figure 7-3.)

4. How might the outcome have been different if you had communicated in your most typical manner (i.e., as you would in relaxed circumstances with close friends)?

Purpose

Just as we may not always be consciously aware of the individual agendas that we bring to the various social cultures in which we interact, the true purpose of most of these is usually not explicitly stated. For example, although Noah was invited to a restaurant for the first meeting of his community advisor council, the dinner itself was meant to provide more of a pleasant backdrop to the real purpose of business networking. For another group of individuals (such as those in the restaurant business), the meal itself could well be the central focus of the evening.

Thus, lack of awareness of the underlying purpose of our social gatherings might result in failed agendas and possible misunderstandings. Persons who consistently misjudge or ignore the implicit or explicit purposes within their various social cultures often appear awkward, ignorant, or rude. Consider, for example, the following.

Pizza Meeting Mishap

Kevin is the owner/manager of an outpatient orthopedic PT clinic. He is interested in developing a new marketing approach to be directed at consumers and referral sources in his community. Kevin and the four experienced members of his PT staff often have productive and enjoyable "pizza meetings" at their favorite Italian restaurant. The staff enjoy these events, which are a pleasant mix of work and fun. Therefore, Kevin offers to take his staff out for a pizza meeting one evening after work to share marketing ideas. Paul, the newest member of the staff, agrees eagerly to the invitation without question, as do the rest of the group.

On the appointed evening, everyone except Paul shows up on time. Kevin orders everyone's favorites pizzas and they order pitchers of soda to share. While they wait for the pizza (and for Paul), they all enjoy friendly conversation and also begin identifying ways to market the practice. Everyone is enjoying this time together when Paul arrives, his arm around a young woman. He introduces her as his girlfriend Kay and explains that she has moved from another state, declaring, "She just got here, so we're celebrating!" Then he says, "I see you all have your drinks" and orders a pitcher of beer for himself and Kay. The pizzas arrive and everyone enjoys the dinner. Kay seems very shy and listens quietly as the group talks. Paul offers his thoughts about marketing ideas, but because he keeps turning his attention to Kay, he is not able to participate fully in the group conversation. When the check arrives, Paul doesn't offer to pay for the beer. Although everyone graciously thanks Kevin for dinner, he goes home without the usual personal and professional satisfaction that comes from the pizza meetings.

Questions

1. In which ways did Paul demonstrate a lack of awareness regarding the purpose of the pizza meeting? In what ways could Paul have better prepared for the evening in order to communicate more appropriately?

2. How might you react to a colleague who behaved as Paul did during the meeting?

3. How might Paul have assessed the social culture of the pizza meeting before attending?

4. If you were Kevin, how might you follow up with Paul about the evening?

In your future professional life, it is likely that you will also attend many gatherings in which work and fun are combined. The "fun" element is essential for building the alliances and support that enhance long-term professional engagement. However, given the overall professional context of such events, it is wise to assume—unless you can be certain otherwise—that the old adage "business before pleasure" applies.

Language

The selection of appropriate language often depends on the specific culture. In your professional socialization process of becoming a physical therapist, you are learning the language of clinical practice, which contains terminology related to patient examination, diagnosis, and intervention. While these terms will serve you well in talking with colleagues and other team members, you are likely to confuse a patient if you ask him to "horizontally adduct your glenohumeral joint." For many patients, you will need to use lay terms (e.g., "bring your arm across your chest") to assure understanding. Moving back and forth between clinical and lay terms will become easier for you with practice; it is a skill that will enhance your professional confidence.

On the other hand, professionalism also means that you refrain from using casual language or lay terms inappropriately. For example, forms of address that we might use in our intimate relationships ("honey" or "sweetie") or vernacular anatomic terms ("move your butt") are likely to be considered offensive or patronizing when used with patients.

Although the use of slang and profanity appear to be gaining increasing use in the public arena, such language is still not appropriate in professional settings. In a recent business-related article, "casual" speech was likened to casual clothing: "Both can be useful in the right environment," the article states. "But when employed inappropriately, they mark a person as unprofessional, as someone who doesn't understand that business is serious."[23]

Power Holders

In all social cultures, individuals vary in terms of their ability to influence others and direct outcomes. Rosabeth Moss Kanter has studied characteristics of empowering work environments. Her research has led to development and validation of a theory of structural power.[24] According to Kanter, power is defined as the ability to accomplish tasks through access to four specific domains: information, support, resources, and opportunity. Sources of power can be either *formal* or *informal*.

Formal power is generally conveyed by a specific title (such as president or chief executive officer), which gives its holder access to all four power domains. Access to these domains then enables those with formal power to direct the work of the organization and the persons involved. Formal power can be described as "top down" (coming from the top and moving to lower levels).

Informal power is equally strong but derived from alliances with formal power holders as well as with peers and subordinates. Persons with informal power are also able to affect outcomes within the organization through their ability to secure the support and cooperation of others at all levels. For example, the boss who asks her administrative assistant for input on hiring decisions is conveying informal power to her subordinate. In cases where formal power is abused, the holders of informal power may able to use their influence to remove such a person from her position. Informal power thus moves in all directions within an organization.

Support for Kanter's theory has been found in studies involving nurses[25] and physical therapists[26] who were working in a hospital environment. In these studies, the two groups of clinicians were asked to rate their perceptions of work empowerment. The results of these studies indicated a moderate level of empowerment in both groups. Most interestingly, those with the highest levels of empowerment were able to effectively engage informal and formal power sources for access to the domains of support, information, opportunity, and resources. This engagement involved effective communication skills.

Social intelligence is a critical prerequisite for the ongoing success of all power holders. Formal power is sometimes bestowed upon individuals who lack sufficient social intelligence to motivate others towards the goals of an organization (i.e., the tyrannical CEO who is appointed by investors because of his or her financial knowledge). Informal power, however, is generally earned through strong social intelligence skills, and in many cases, eventually leads to the attainment of formal power. As Kanter's research with nurses and physical therapists has demonstrated, individuals with access to both formal and informal sources of power have the greatest opportunities and thus the greatest success in an organization.

While formal power sources are usually easier to identify, persons with informal power are often less obvious, even holding lower positions in the organization. An important aspect of social intelligence is the ability to identify and interact effectively with both sources.

PTA Power Put-Down

Arlene is a physical therapist assistant (PTA) at large acute-care hospital. With over 20 years of experience at this facility, she enjoys strong collegial relationships with the PT staff and goes out of her way to help them when needed. In turn, the PT staff view Arlene as one of the most valued members of the department. In fact, Arlene recently won the hospital's "Ray of Light" outstanding employee award.

With her easygoing personality and dedicated approach, Arlene has gained the respect of persons at all levels in the hospital. To that end, Paul, the department director, often finds that Arlene's insights about staff concerns and morale are helpful to him in optimizing staff engagement.

Arlene and the other PTAs rotate among the PT staff, sharing assigned patients as schedules and patient complexity dictate. Arlene has just been assigned to work with Claire, a Doctor of Physical Therapy graduate and recent hire. Like many new graduates, Claire is working hard to demonstrate that she is fully competent and independent in her work, seldom seeking out the other staff for any form of support or collegial interaction. When Arlene offers helpful and well-intended suggestions from her many years of experience, Claire brushes her off.

One day, while Arlene is in a stall in the women's restroom, a colleague enters, apparently talking on her cell phone. Arlene quickly recognizes the woman's voice as Claire's. Arlene is shocked to hear her say, "Arlene thinks she can tell me how to do my job and that's just (expletive) because I have worked years for my doctoral degree and she's just a (expletive) PTA!"

Questions

1. In what ways is Claire ignoring important elements of her work-related social culture? (Consider the elements described thus far.)

2. How might Claire's failure to acknowledge these elements affect her professional effectiveness?

3. If you were Arlene, how might you respond to Claire's behavior in the restroom? What sort of specific concerns might Arlene have regarding this?

4. Should Arlene address her concerns directly to Claire, or this is an issue for the department's director?

5. Despite her position, Arlene appears to hold significant informal power in her workplace. How do you think one acquires this?

6. How does a newcomer to a specific social culture identify and interact with the informal power holders? Why might this be helpful?

The example of Claire speaks to the wisdom of using extreme care with our language in all situations. Even when we are "off duty," we are still visible in our communities as representatives of our profession. To that end, one faculty colleague recalls sitting behind some students at a movie theater where he could plainly (and painfully) overhear their disparaging remarks about his class.

Etiquette

Its definition is as follows: "etiquette pertains to practices of behavior dictated by social convention or authority."[27]

Most social cultures contain both explicit (clearly stated) and implicit (tacitly understood) rules of conduct, which are intended to promote order and goodwill among persons. Explicit rules such as, "All pets must be on a leash" or "No trespassing" are usually obviously stated (often by signs or documents), enforced by legal sanctions, and thus hard to ignore.

Most forms of etiquette, particularly those that pertain to this discussion, are implicit, meaning that they are verbally shared by the culture's "teachers" and internalized by the "learners." For example, as a child, your parents most likely taught you how to eat politely, meet new people, and show respect to others. Implicit rules thus involve knowledge of the internalized norms of a given culture. For example, tipping your hair stylist for good service, entering a line at the end, and using a tissue or handkerchief to blow your nose are all internalized norms for etiquette in our society. No fine awaits those who fail to observe these norms, although our personal ethics (our standards of right and wrong) may be called into question. Persons who have a strong sense of implicit etiquette generally adhere to these norms because it is the right and ethical thing to do for the good of society. This sentiment is eloquently described by author Rushworth Kidder in his definition of ethics as "obedience to the unenforceable."[28]

In some cases, the lines between etiquette, laws, and ethics are difficult to distinguish, leaving the individual to decide the best course of action. For example, a patient might feel that it would be good manners to give his physical therapist a check for $100 in simple gratitude. However, it is unethical (and, in states where the PT Practice Act is aligned with the APTA Code of Ethics, illegal) for PTs to accept such gifts. The topic of ethics is beyond the scope of this book, but because of its potential intersection with law and etiquette, you should be certain that you are familiar with both your state practice act and the PT code of ethics by the time you graduate from your academic program.

Good etiquette involves mindful consideration of others, a commodity that may escape us when we are overwhelmed by the demands of our lives. As we rush through our days, we may sometimes unwittingly overlook the little courtesies that promote kindness in our connections with others. Thus, as I observed during a recent visit to a fast-food restaurant, we might see people rudely barking orders to the servers at the counter ("gimme a burger"), leaving their trash on the tables for others to clean, and talking loudly into their cell phones while their mouths were stuffed with food. Each time we interact with another person, even a total stranger whom we will probably never see again, mindfulness suggests that we treat him or her with the graciousness and respect conveyed by basic etiquette. In the context of our profession, our code of ethics demands this of each of us.

Despite what may appear to be an increasing laxity of implicit manners, these rules are still extremely important in professional settings. Accordingly, numerous universities—such as Ball State University, Southwestern University, Louisiana State University, and the University of Missouri—are now offering courses in basic etiquette for students as a way of enhancing their employment options after graduation. In promoting the need for such courses, one administrator stated, "Good manners and etiquette at formal dinners is a deal-breaker in the business world...and knowing which fork to use and what to do with your elbows is as important as exam grades or degrees."[29] Even the American Bar Association, the national professional organization for lawyers, has posted information for acceptable manners among its members.[30] According to these sources, the most common assaults on poor manners are related to a simple lack of consideration for others. Frequent examples include ordering the most expensive item at a business dinner, taking too large of a serving at a buffet and thus leaving others without food, drinking inappropriately, or having loud cell phone conversations that disturb others. Other concerns focus around poor communication skills, including constant interrupting of others, treating subordinates rudely, and asking intrusive questions.

As mentioned previously, many work-related functions occur in the context of social gatherings. Unfortunately, a poor impression related to lack of manners is likely to undermine professional success, regardless of the level of work-related skills. If you are ever in doubt about the appropriate etiquette for a situation, it may be wise to ask a trusted colleague or observe carefully before acting on incorrect assumptions that could have a negative effect on your professional and personal success.

Finally, the rules of implicit and explicit etiquette continue to evolve to meet the changes in society. For example, as technological forms of diversion and communication become more common, there are evolving rules for the appropriate use of iPods, cell phones, and computers. In fact, the use of these devices has spawned an entirely new form of manners training known as "netiquette" (a blend of the terms *network* and *etiquette*). For example, the use of all capital letters in e-mails is considered "shouting" and thus is discouraged by netiquette experts.[31] To that end, international business companies such as IBM and Intel have developed guidelines for appropriate ways to conduct electronic communication.

Talking Points/Field Notes

Mindful Manners

For the next 48 hours, resolve to be as polite as you can in all your interactions with service professionals, friends, and family. Refrain from using your cell phone in any situation where it could be disruptive. See how often you can sincerely use the basic terms of "please," "thank you," and so on. You can even try to be a more courteous driver. As you go about this exercise, observe the use of manners by those around you. Then reflect on the following and record your observations in your field notes:

1. In which ways did you change your customary use of etiquette in your everyday interactions? How challenging was it to remain mindful about this for 48 hours?

2. What kind of responses did you notice? How did these responses make you feel?

3. Describe the results of your observations regarding the use of manners by those around you. Were there any differences in the use of etiquette among different groups of people (i.e., with respect to age or gender)?

4. Were there any situational elements that corresponded to either more or less use of etiquette (i.e., at the grocery store versus in church)?

5. What insights did you gain with this exercise? How would things be different in society if everyone were mindful about their etiquette?

Dress

Of all the elements of social culture, the idea of appropriate dress might well be the most controversial. Because our manner of dress is in some ways an expression of our individuality, it can be difficult to have this dictated for us by others. Nevertheless, whether we like it or not, our clothing invites all sorts of judgments about our socioeconomic status, ethnicity, and personality. These judgments, which can sometimes provoke negative interpersonal behaviors, are the rationale for the increasing prevalence of uniforms in both private and public schools in the United States. Accordingly, in the year 2000, the National Association of Elementary School Principals (NAESP) conducted a phone survey of 755 principals, which revealed that 21% of all U.S. public schools had a uniform policy (up from just 3% in 1996). Most interestingly, a California-based study on the social effects of school uniforms reported a 90% drop in disciplinary suspensions and an 85%

decrease in assaults among students in kindergarten through grade 8. Thus, in the words of one principal, "school uniforms level the playing field, keeping the focus on the educational process rather than on who has the coolest designer jeans."[32]

Selective choices in clothing can also be useful to individuals or groups. For example, in the health-care industry, specific garments (such as lab coats and hospital scrubs) are still used to convey authority and professionalism to patients and others. Experienced physical therapists might still remember the professions' early uniform, consisting of white shoes, blue pants, and a white top with the triangular shoulder patch designating membership in APTA. In its early years, the patch was probably helpful in providing a sense of professional identity to early practitioners. However, the patch was retired from the APTA membership in 1988. At that point, the APTA house of delegates decided that it was no longer appropriate, especially given our profession's move to greater autonomy and postgraduate education (for example, there are no patches for physicians, lawyers, or other doctoral-level practitioners).

Even though our profession no longer claims a specific uniform (the white shoes proving to be highly impractical), many practice facilities still have dress codes, and some use standard articles of clothing (such as polo shirts with facility logos) to convey a level of professionalism that can be reassuring to patients.

Given the impact of clothing on the perceptions of others, it is wise to consider the statement we wish to make through our choices. Again, sensitivity to the dictates of the social culture will be instrumental in your ability to make thoughtful selections. As you continue your professional education, you might begin to observe the general modes of dress seen at professional conferences and clinical settings. You may also note differences in clothing trends among persons of different ages, and these differences might affect your choices, depending on the generational composition of the various social cultures you encounter. For example, in a clinic staffed mostly by practitioners over the age of 40, the clothing standards might be more formal (with "casual Fridays" meaning khaki pants and polo tops) than in one with younger staff (where "casual Fridays" could mean denim). Again, if in doubt, it is best to inquire. Many academic programs suggest that students contact their internship sites prior to arrival in order to determine the appropriate dress for that facility.

Clinical Scenario

Interview Impressions (Yet Another True Tale)

Joe is the director of a skilled nursing facility. Today he is interviewing Jeremy, who has been practicing for 2 years in another city. Joe finds Jeremy in the waiting room of the PT department. Jeremy is wearing a leather jacket, corduroy jeans, and tennis shoes. As Joe approaches, Jeremy sits engrossed in a magazine while listening to music on his iPod and drinking a cup of coffee. As Joe greets Jeremy with a handshake, Jeremy smiles, pulls off his iPod ear buds and stuffs them into his pocket. Jeremy and Joe proceed into Joe's office (where Jeremy sets his coffee cup on Joe's desk), and the interview begins. At one point in the discussion (in which Jeremy asks good questions, offers insightful opinions, and conveys genuine interest in the staff position), Jeremy's cell phone vibrates in his pocket and he turns it off without comment. At this point, Joe decides to ask Jeremy his typical final interview question: "Give me one great reason why I should hire you." Jeremy leans forward and looks Joe in the eye. He replies with a laugh, "Dude! You need to hire me because I am simply the best man for this job!" The interview ends, and 2 hours later, Joe receives an e-mail from Jeremy, thanking him for the interview and restating his interest in the position.

Continued

Questions to Consider

1. If you were Joe, how might you evaluate Jeremy's display of social awareness related to an interview situation (i.e., his dress, manners, language)? Which of these, if any, might be cause for concern?

2. Would any of these behaviors have a negative impact on your decision to hire him, even in spite of a good interview?

3. Would your assessment of Jeremy's behavior be different if he were applying for an administrative position in the skilled nursing facility instead of a staff one?

4. Comment on the value of interview thank-you notes in Jeremy's case and in general. If you were Joe and had initially decided against hiring Jeremy, would his thank-you note cause you to reconsider?

5. If you did not hire Jeremy and he called asking for feedback to improve future job interviews, what specific advice would you have for him?

Implications for Physical Therapy Practice

The foregoing elements of social culture, when observed and effectively considered, can greatly enhance your external communication and your ability to make meaningful connections with others. The social culture of PT is played out in many different environments related to patient care, professional activities, as well as educational and community settings. Because of the diversity of these environments, ongoing development of our social awareness can optimize our communication effectiveness, particularly when combined with strong social skills.

Chapter Summary

1. Supportive human connections promote overall function and well-being in all areas of our lives. The ability to forge and sustain these connections involves context-appropriate external communication.

2. External communication is used to build alliances, optimize our level of influence, and educate others. Physical Therapists must be skillful in each of these areas.

3. Social intelligence is the study of the attitudes, behaviors, and skills that promote meaningful connections with others. The two major elements of social intelligence are social awareness and social skills.

4. Sensitivity to the environmental context of our communication involves social awareness.

5. Persons with shared traditions, values, and norms for behavior form a social culture. Most of us function within many social cultures.

6. The elements of social awareness include personal agendas, purpose of interactions, power sources, language, etiquette, and dress.

Take-Home Menu

1. Free online etiquette quiz. How do your business manners rate? About.Com. Small Business: Canada: http://sbinfocanada.about.com/library/nosearch/bletiquettecorrect1.htm. Accessed December 11, 2007.

2. Your Turn at Champ and Blockhead: Because the many aspects of social culture are subtle and highly individual, it can be very interesting to discuss these differences in the context of a case study. Working in pairs or a small group, construct your own Champ and Blockhead scenario based on an aspect of this chapter, perhaps building on an actual experience. When you are done, you can either present your scenario to the class for a large discussion or swap scenarios with another group for a smaller dialogue.

3. Development of physical therapy student code of classroom conduct: Many physical therapy student programs provide incoming students with guidelines for expected professional behaviors in the classroom. In the program in which I teach, students asked for an opportunity to write their own guidelines. The resultant document was very thorough, addressing areas such as text messaging in class, coming to school when sick, and eating in lectures. Working in a group, construct a code of conduct for your classroom culture. When all groups have completed this, share with the class at large and discuss. Do you think it would be helpful to have classroom code of conduct. Why or why not?

References

1. Baumeister RF, Leary MR. The need to belong: Desire for interpersonal attachments as a fundamental human motivation. *Psychol Bull.* 1995;117(3):497-529.

2. Baumeister RF, Twenge JM, Nuss CK. Effects of social exclusion on cognitive processes: Anticipated aloneness reduces intellectual thought. *J Pers Soc Psychol.* 2002;83:817-827.

3. Furrer C, Skinner E. Sense of relatedness as a factor in children's academic engagement and performance. *J Educ Psychol.* 2003;95:148-162.

4. Thau S, Auquino K, Poortvliet PM. Self-defeating behaviors in organizations: The relationship between thwarted belonging and interpersonal work behaviors. *J Appl Psychol.* 2007;92(3):840-847.

5. Masters KS, Stillman AM, Spielman GI. Specificity of social support for back pain patients: Do patients care who provides what? *J Behav Med.* 2007;30(1):11-20.

6. Penttinen J, Nevala-Puranen N, Airaksinen O, et al. Randomized controlled trial of back school with and without peer support. *J Occup Rehabil.* 2002;12(1):21-29.

7. Tyre P. Poker buddies for life: In sickness and in health, many boomers turn to their close friends, not family, to get the support they need. *Newsweek.* February 20, 2006, page 61.

8. Worthington K. Customer satisfaction in the emergency department. *Emerg Med Clin North Am.* 2004;22(1):87-102.

9. Neumann M, Wirtz M, Bollschweiler E, et al. Determinants and patient-reported long-term outcomes of physician empathy in oncology: a structural equation modeling approach. *Patient Educ Counsel.* 2007;69(1-3):63-75.

10. Blackman C, Luyet R. Who gets sued? Business Consultants Network Connect. September 26, 2006: http://www.bconnetwork.com/connect/WhoGetsSued.html. Accessed January 15, 2008.

11. Laschinger HKS, Leiter MP. The impact of nursing work environments on patient safety outcomes. *J Nurs Admin.* 2006;36(5):259-267.

12. Stichler JF. Social intelligence: An essential trait of effective leaders. *Nurs Women's Health.* April/May 2007:189-193.

13. Lyubomirsky S. *The How of Happiness: A Scientific Approach to Getting the Life You Want.* New York: Penguin Press; 2007.

14. Scott J. *Social Network Analysis: A Handbook,* 2nd ed. Newberry Park, CA: Sage; 2000.

15. Mueller K. Take this job and love it: Factors related to job satisfaction and career commitment among physical therapists. Platform presentation. 14th Congress, World Confederation for Physical Therapy. Barcelona, Spain; 2003.

16. Goleman D. *Social Intelligence.* New York: Bantam; 2006.

17. Sternberg RU, Conway BE, Ketron JL, Bernstein M. People's conceptions of intelligence. *J Pers Soc Psychol.* 1981;41:37-55.

18. Kihlstrom JF, Cantor N. Social Intelligence. In Sternberg RJ, ed. *Handbook of Intelligence.* Cambridge, UK: Cambridge University Press, 2000:359-379.

19. Kosmitzki C, John OP. The implicit use of explicit conceptions of social intelligence. *Pers Indiv Diff.* 1993;15:11-23.

20. Berkeley Parents Network. Breast feeding in public: http://parents.berkeley.edu/advice/nursing/public.html. Accessed January 17, 2008.

21. Axtell RE. *Gestures: The DO's and TABOOS of Body Language Around the World.* Hoboken, NJ: John Wiley & Sons; 1998.

22. Harrison G. Motivational training: The awesome power of body language: http://www.motivationaltraining.com/articles/body-language/bl6%20.htm. Accessed February 12, 2008.

23. Sinclair M. Keep slang and profanity out of business. *Bus J Milwaukee.* February 7, 2003: http://www.bizjournals.com/milwaukee/stories/2003/02/10/smallb6.html. Accessed February 18, 2008.

24. Kanter RM. *Men and Women of the Corporation,* 2nd ed. New York: Basic Books; 1993.

25. Laschinger HKS. A theoretical approach to studying work empowerment in nursing: A review of studies testing Kanter's theory of structural power in organizations. *Nurs Admin Q.* 1996;20(2):25-41.

26. Miller PA, Goddard P, Laschinger HKS. Evaluating physical therapists' perception of empowerment using Kanter's theory of structural power in organizations. *Phys Ther.* 2001;81(12):1880-1888.

27. *The American Heritage Dictionary of the American Language,* 4th ed. New York: Houghton Mifflin; 2000.

28. Kidder R. *How Good People Make Tough Choices: Resolving the Dilemmas of Ethical Living.* New York: HarperCollins; 2003.

29. Faragher J. Manners maketh the man. *The Work Clinic: Your Counsel and Career Advice.* January 14, 2008. Available on line: http://www.personneltoday.com/blogs/workplace-advice/2008/01/manners-maketh-the-man-workpla.html. Accessed February 19, 2008.

30. Schneider D. Office etiquette essentials: American Bar Association. *Your ABA: E-News for Members.* April, 2007: http://www.abanet.org/media/youraba/200704/article12.html. Accessed February 19, 2008.

31. Hambridge S. *RFC 1855: Netiquette.* Intel Corporation: http://www.dtcc.edu/cs/rfc1855.html. Accessed February 20, 2008.

32. Public School Uniform Statistics. *The Education Bug,* Available online: http://www.educationbug.org/a/public-school-uniform-statistics.html. Accessed February 18, 2008.

CHAPTER 8

The Application of Socially Skilled External Communication: Building Effective Alliances

"What is beauty? Beauty is something that can be appreciated by others. A beautiful mind is one that can be appreciated by others—usually through conversation."

Edward de Bono, MD, PhD, (1933–),
World renowned authority on creative thinking and author of
How to Have a Beautiful Mind

Chapter Overview

Persons with a high level of social intelligence use their keenly tuned awareness to determine the spoken and unspoken behavioral requirements of the prevailing culture. Next, they use specific skills to engage others in an authentic way to develop and sustain meaningful relationships. These skills involve effective self-presentation, synchronizing content and emotions, and the use of engaging conversation. This chapter explores each of these elements in the context of building effective alliances for successful professional endeavors.

Key Terms

Impression formation

Active listening

Synchrony

Nonviolent communication

Neurolinguistic programming

Social Skills for Alliance Building: The Stages of Relationship Development

This section explores the stages of alliance building and discusses effective external communication skills to enhance each of these. Relationships progress through a series of related stages involving *impression formation*, *building rapport*, and *attachment*.

Impression Formation

In your classes on patient assessment, perhaps you have been told, "Your evaluation begins the moment you lay eyes on the patient." The point of this adage is that your patients will present many important cues about themselves before even saying a word. Your awareness of these cues can be instrumental in facilitating your establishment of an authentic therapeutic connection. Regardless of the setting, whenever we meet someone for the first time, we are also engaged in the mutual process of self-presentation and the resultant formation of a first impression. This first impression influences the perceptions that guide our subsequent interactions with the person involved. Obviously, favorable first impressions are more likely to result in positive future interactions. In our fast-paced world, first impressions are used to determine suitability for employment, acceptance to educational programs, and even the potential for romance. The current concept of "speed dating," where participants engage in a series of brief conversations (lasting as little as 3 minutes) with potential romantic partners, is based largely on how quickly people form first impressions. Interestingly, a 2005 study at the University of Pennsylvania found that participants in speed dating sessions had made their decisions in the first three seconds.[1]

First impressions are the result of subconscious multisensory neurological processing, known as "rapid cognition."[2] As soon as a person with whom we are about to interact enters our field of vision, our brains rapidly process visual input about their general appearance, including their posture, body language, and facial expression. Before a single word is exchanged, we have already made a subconscious assessment about their openness to interaction. For example, in most social circumstances, you are more likely to approach a person who regards you with a smile and a relaxed, open posture as opposed to one who presents an expressionless gaze and rigid cross-armed posture. The formation of a first impression is thus well under way, and our very first assessments of this person are either confirmed or altered as we enter into dialogue.

Talking Points/Field Notes

My Personal Dynamics of First Impressions

Discuss the following and reflect on your observations in your field notes:

1. What are specific attributes that I convey in making a good first impression?

2. How do I use my communication skills in order to be successful?

3. What attributes lead me to form a good first impression of others?

4. How often do I find that my first impression does not change over time?

5. Describe a situation where my first impression of another person changed. What generally causes this to happen? What can I learn from this?

First impressions are considered by social scientists to be the first step in both relationship development and human survival (i.e., knowing instinctively to avoid a person with a menacing look). Accordingly, the process of *impression formation* has been a topic of research for over 40 years.[3] Human subjects have demonstrated high levels of reliability in their ability to interpret the emotional components of facial expressions, and it has been shown that this process occurs in approximately 39 milliseconds.[4] Because facial expressions are universal, we can thus convey warm approachability in any culture with a sincere smile. If you have ever been in a gathering of strangers and approached a person because of his welcoming facial expression, you have experienced the power of this universal human signal.

The next step in the process of impression formation involves the interpretation of sensory cues related to verbal and nonverbal communication. During this time, each person continues their mutual process of assessment related to verbal and nonverbal communication.[5] **Figure 8-1** illustrates the evidence-supported components of the impression formation process.[5]

As Figure 8-1 illustrates, we determine a person's approachability primarily by his or her facial expression. As we begin to interact with that individual, our impression-formation

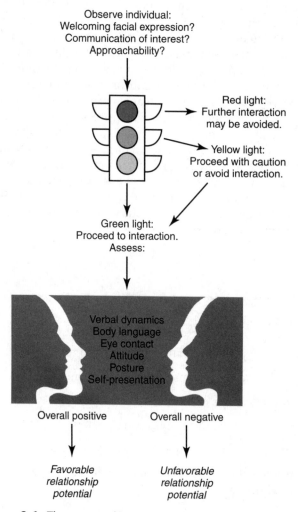

Figure 8–1. The process of impression formation.

process continues as we interpret body language, demeanor, gestures, eye contact, and finally, verbal cues. Once this process is complete (again, all of this being accomplished subconsciously and almost instantly), we will either feel inclined or disinclined toward further interactions. Before turning our discussion toward communication skills that enhance positive impressions, let us consider the Champ and Blockhead scenario.

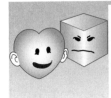

Champ and Blockhead

Champ and Blockhead Present Themselves at a Professional Gathering

It is the opening night reception of the American Physical Therapy Association Combined Sections Meeting. Over 6,000 physical therapists from across the United States have gathered for an exhilarating week of education, professional business, and social networking. The opening night reception is a great place to meet current and potential professional colleagues.

Champ and Blockhead are attending this reception for the first time, having just graduated the previous spring. *You, too, are attending this meeting, and are about to meet each of these colleagues.*

Blockhead does not want to be at this gathering but came with a group of colleagues with whom she was having dinner after the reception. Because Blockhead considers these networking events to be stressful, she has had a couple of drinks to relax. Arriving at the reception, she stays close to Champ and a few colleagues from work, hoping to avoid the task of making small talk with anyone new.

At this point you have just entered the room, and you recognize one of the persons in Champ and Blockhead's group as an old classmate. You approach the group and notice Blockhead standing quietly, so you introduce yourself to her. As you offer Blockhead a handshake, you ask her if she is enjoying the reception. Blockhead returns your handshake with a clammy, limp grasp and replies offhandedly that she really hates these gatherings and is hoping to leave as soon as possible. Indeed, with her slumped posture and lack of affect, she looks utterly miserable. Trying to further engage her in conversation, you express empathy by saying "Yeah, these things can be a little awkward, but at least it's a great way to see old friends." Blockhead then complains about the food, the music, the hotel setting. As she continues her litany, you note that your mood is starting to drop, and you make a mental note to avoid her for the rest of the evening.

At this point, Champ approaches you and introduces herself with a warm smile. She looks you in the eye, smiles warmly, and shakes your hand with a comfortable grasp. She tells you that this is her first time at this conference and that she has long been looking forward to coming. When you ask her about the courses she plans to attend, she answers with enthusiasm, explaining that she is hoping to build her expertise in a certain area and that there happens to be three talks that will help her. This leads you to share that you have the same interest, and you begin an enjoyable conversation.

Discuss the following in a small group:

1. Describe the elements of your first impression of Blockhead. Which elements of her self-presentation had the greatest impact on your assessment?
2. Describe the elements of your first impression of Champ. Which elements of her presentation had the greatest impact on your assessment?
3. Individually, list the top five elements that you believe are the most important aspects of self-presentation for a positive first impression. Compare answers as a group and see if you can agree on a single list.

Social Skills to Enhance Positive Impressions: Elements of Self-Presentation

Not surprisingly, interpersonal communication makes a significant contribution to our first impression. As we continue our discussion of social intelligence, we will explore important social skills which promote successful first interactions and the formation of positive impressions. A long history of research in the area of impression formation has provided useful insights about the elements of effective self-presentation.[3,6]

These elements include *congruency in verbal and nonverbal communication*, and *choosing an attitude for engagement*.

Congruency Between Verbal and Nonverbal Communication

Self-presentation involves sensitivity to the messages we convey through both verbal and nonverbal sensory modalities. In face-to-face situations, the content of our words is strongly overshadowed by the embellishment and emphasis provided by our body language, facial expressions, gestures, and tone of voice. In sincere and authentic communication, these cues all complement each other to produce a genuine message that inspires trust. In this regard, perhaps the highest compliment is found in the saying, "What you see is what you get," which speaks to a person who displays consistency in both verbal and nonverbal communication. In the rapid process of impression formation, we interpret the "take-home message" of an individual's combined verbal and nonverbal communication to determine his or her sincerity, likeability, and trustworthiness. Not surprisingly, social science research has shown that consistency between verbal and nonverbal communication is likely to facilitate a good impression and engender trust.[2,6]

Positive first impressions are enhanced when a person's verbal and nonverbal cues are congruous, meaning that their body language conveys the same thing as their tone of voice, words, and gestures. For example, if a person exclaims, "Delighted to meet you!" while smiling with raised eyebrows and facing squarely toward you in a relaxed, open posture, you are likely to form a first impression of this individual as sincere and trustworthy. If, on the other hand, this same exclamation is accompanied by a backward lean, hunched shoulders, and narrowed eyes, your first impression might lead you to question this person's intent.

As mentioned previously, research on the impact of communication indicates that language itself contributes only 7% of the meaning of a conversation, while body language and tone of voice contribute 55% and 38%, respectively. Thus, whenever we are presented with inconsistencies between verbal and nonverbal communication, we will most naturally respond primarily to the message conveyed through the latter.[7] This finding has important implications for the value of attitude, as our carefully chosen words can easily be contradicted by our subconscious (and often faultlessly honest) body language. The study of body language involves the understanding of over 120 human gestures and symbols, making this topic too broad for full exploration here.[8] However, for the purposes of effective self-presentation, especially in the first crucial seconds of impression formation, it is worthwhile to consider the type of body language that is most likely to be successful. This is known as "open" body language—postures, gestures, and facial expressions that convey readiness to engage, interest in others, and genuine warmth. **Table 8-1** depicts common symbols associated with open body language.

Table 8–1. Open and Closed Body Language	
Open Body Language: Conveys Interest, Liking, Readiness to Engage	**Closed Body Language: Conveys Dislike, Tension, Avoidance**
Facing other person squarely (ventral to ventral)	Turning head and/or body away from other person
Being at same level and position as other person (both standing, sitting, etc.)	Placement of objects between the two other persons (e.g., large desk)
Forward trunk lean	Backward trunk lean
Hands visible and open	Hands clasped together or fisted
Arms relaxed at sides	Arms crossed in front
Eye contact	Looking away
Head nod	Shaking head
Relaxed but erect posture	Stiff posture
Smile	Eyes narrowed or squinting, unsmiling
Legs stretched, open (if crossed, pointed toward other person)	Legs tightly crossed, pointed away from person
Touching person's arm, shoulder Offer of handshake Comfortable distance (12–36 inches) moving toward person	Increasing the distance from other person
Jacket unbuttoned	Jacket buttoned

Choosing an Attitude for Engagement

As discussed in the last chapter, all human interactions involve individual agendas. Even more importantly, we also bring a level of personal energy to each interaction, and this is largely determined by our attitude, which we can consciously change in our internal communication.

You have undoubtedly noticed that you are more likely to be successful in your interactions (and in the accomplishment of your agenda) if you demonstrate the mindfully present attitude of full engagement. In contrast, consider how it feels to interact with a person who is disengaged and sporting an attitude which clearly conveys that he or she would rather be somewhere else. Such negative attitudes are almost palpable and can have a significant impact on your own mood. As it turns out, such a cause–effect relationship has significant implications for our interactions. There is considerable evidence supporting the presence of a *negativity bias* among adults, which involves a greater sensitivity to negative information.[9] Negativity bias is thought to be related to neurological mechanisms involving the fight-or-flight response, which are mediated through the brain's amygdala. Thus, negative input is processed more rapidly and provokes a stronger emotional response than positive input.[10] With respect to impression formation, negative perceptions of others are more powerful and exert more bias than positive ones.[11]

In other words, among all the elements involved in impression behavior, most people will remember the negative elements, which will have the greatest overall influence of the final "verdict." Thus, the communication of a negative attitude is likely to leave a powerful and lasting impression. **Figure 8-2** illustrates elements of negative attitude and the negativity bias.

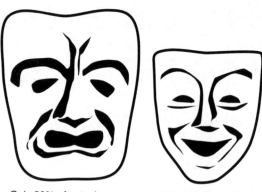

Only 30% of actual events   70% of actual events

Figure 8–2. The negativity bias: Our brains tend to amplify negative events, even when their frequency of actual occurrence is low. In turn, our responses are often disproportionately negative.

We cannot always choose our agendas or our social interactions. In the course of any given day, we will interact with other persons in a variety of contexts in order to carry out our activities of daily living. Nevertheless, whether we are giving a talk in class or relaxing with friends after a long week, we can choose the attitude that we bring to these situations. In turn, an engaging attitude will have tremendous impact on our enjoyment and sense of accomplishment in all that we do. The consistent bearing of a positive attitude is grounded in mindfulness. Thus, if we choose to live mindfully, we will be continually aware of the prerogative that each of us has to be joyfully present to everyone we meet. The bottom line is this: if our life circumstances dictate that certain interactions are inevitable, why not make them as enjoyable and rewarding as possible?

As we have already discussed, positivity can be consciously developed and has been demonstrated to have a mediating effect on the number and effect of what psychiatrist Daniel Amen calls automated negative thoughts (ANTS). For some persons, ANTS can comprise up to 80% of their internal dialogue.[12,13]

Two prominent theories of communication, neurolinguistic programming (NLP)[14] and nonviolent communication (NCV),[15] address the importance of a positive attitude for effective interactions with others. Both approaches suggest communicating from the heart in order to reflect an attitude of caring and compassion for others. To that end, one NLP practitioner suggests pointing your heart in the direction of anyone that you talk to, all the while projecting a "beam" of joy and openness. Although this advice might seem simplistic, it is actually a powerful way of connecting positively with others and making a good impression.[16] You might recall from our earlier discussions of NLP that each of us has tremendous potential to achieve whatever we desire. Accordingly, one of our most important tools toward that end is our attitude.

Talking Points/Field Notes

Creating Positive Expectations for Our Interactions

Directions: This exercise involves two dimensions: optimizing your attitude before interactions and conveying this attitude during interactions.

Optimizing Your Attitude

As much as possible in the next week, generate a positive attitude toward each of your interactions before they begin. Hold this positive attitude in mind, particularly in instances where you engage with others in a situation or task that you don't normally enjoy. It might be helpful to preprogram your internal communication with a

Talking Points/Field Notes—cont'd ■

statement such as "I greatly enjoy being with. . . ." It can also be helpful to visualize yourself enjoying the interaction as much as possible. If you tend be shy in new social situations, your suggestion can include a confidence-building statement such as "I am completely relaxed and joyful in all my interactions." In difficult situations, it can be enormously helpful to affirm "I will be fully present to this person and helpful in all that I do and say."

Conveying Your Attitude

As you engage in your interaction, use words, body language, and other self-presentation skills to convey an attitude of mindful enthusiasm and interest. Make every effort to maintain your full attention on the person you are talking to.

Observation and Discussion

Record the effects of your change in attitude on the resulting interactions. In a group, share your experiences as you discuss the following:

1. As you review the week, did you notice a similarity in the types of interactions that you tend not to enjoy? In which ways did you "reprogram" your attitude toward a more positive approach?

2. How did the change in attitude affect the quality of these interactions?

3. How did you modify your verbal and nonverbal communication to convey an optimal attitude for interaction? What results did this have on the quality of your interaction?

4. How challenging was it to maintain your full attention on the other person during your interaction?

5. How do you think the quality of your interpersonal interactions might change if you consistently adopted a positive, mindful approach to each one?

Building Rapport: The Bridge to Acceptance

Rapport is defined as a "relationship based on mutual trust, understanding, and emotional affinity."[17] In its earliest stages, rapport is the natural consequence of effective self-presentation and positive impression formation. It involves a subconscious but felt sense of being in harmony with another person's feelings, thoughts, and perceptions. Interactions where rapport is present are exhilarating in many ways, because it is an indicator of mutual acceptance. It is no mistake that we tend to build rapport most quickly with those whom we genuinely like or respect (in other words, those whom we accept on some level) as well as with those who convey these sentiments to us. A level of acceptance is thus an essential requirement for the formation of genuine human relationships as well as a necessity for the delivery of compassionate health care. The professional concept of "unconditional positive regard" for all patients is built on the premise that every human being possesses some quality worthy of our respect. Thus, in interactions where no rapport is present, it may simply be that we have not yet identified that resonating trait upon which we can build a genuine relationship.

Studies on the nature of rapport suggest that there is one underlying element that can be expressed on many different levels. It is simply this: we build rapport with persons who are like us in some way. In our elective relationships (those we freely choose), there is generally a shared interest, personality quality, or even physical characteristic with which we can identify. This identification is fertile ground for the sharing of communication, which eventually leads to some level of relationship.

Although we probably cross paths with numerous interesting persons with whom we could become great friends in the right circumstances, this is most likely to occur in the context of a shared interest such as exercising at the same gym or attending the same professional meeting. Accordingly, it is not unusual for persons in the same profession to marry, as this provides many opportunities for shared interest. "Like marries like," with similarities in educational level being one of the most common elements.[18]

For example, a recent study showed that almost 50% of women physicians marry other physicians.[19] However, many of our interactions may be with persons where no shared interest is apparent. Nevertheless, studies on rapport demonstrate that there are powerful ways to enhance possibilities for mutual understanding. These approaches involve the specific social skills that are explored in the next section.

Social Skills for Building Rapport

In order to build rapport, we must first put others at ease in order to facilitate comfortable and authentic dialogue. Because we are most comfortable (and most likely to be at our best) in the presence of persons who we perceive to be like us in some way, the skills of rapport building involve strategies which foster a common ground. Consider, for example, how you feel in the presence of a person who intimidates you. Intimidating persons often create the perception of a divisive power differential that keeps us at bay. In such situations, we are likely to feel emotionally stressed and even physically uncomfortable. We may notice that our tongues are tied and our thoughts are frazzled as we wrack our brains for things to say in order to bridge the gap. This absence of emotional resonance is often depersonalizing, and it is never comfortable to feel less than human.

Thus, the strategies for building rapport involve forging bonds that foster similarities in our many modes of communication. Our conversational skills are of critical importance of course, but so are the ways in which we use our nonverbal communication to develop and reinforce commonalities. Thus we can develop rapport through nonverbal as well as verbal means, and the skills involved include *synchrony, engaging conversation*, and *active listening*.

Synchrony

As we have discussed thus far, one of the most important predictors of rapport is the shared perception of similarities. Although this perception is subconscious on many levels, it is undeniable and immensely powerful. Consider any situations where you have met another person and felt an instant liking. Given the speed at which humans make such judgments, this liking has to do with many factors beyond the exchange of words. Specifically, we tend to feel instant liking of persons whom we perceive as being like us. In turn, this perception of similarity tends to facilitate comfort and ease. Conversations where synchrony exists are enjoyable, spontaneous, and energizing. We feel a connection to the other individual that engenders feelings of goodwill and warmth. Synchrony is so important, in fact, that no genuinely comfortable social interaction can occur without it.

In the realm of social intelligence, synchrony refers to the ability to interpret and respond to the full complement of verbal and nonverbal behaviors. This complement of behaviors is known as "microlevel" actions. When we are in rapport with another person, a natural display of synchrony involves the subconscious matching of that person's gestures, body language, facial expression, and vocal intonations.

Feldman[19] describes synchrony as a process where persons engaged in interpersonal communication perceive and respond to each other's microbehaviors (tone of voice, direction of gaze, facial expressions, level of arousal, muscle tone, body orientation, and even breathing patterns) so that they coalesce into a shared emotional tone. Furthermore, the ability for each individual to respond to second-to-second changes in these behaviors is an essential element for effective participation in any positive emotional interaction.[20,21]

According to Goleman,[22] synchrony is one of three elements necessary for rapport. The second is full attention (which we have discussed in terms of a mindfully present attitude). The third is the generation of positive feelings (which arise from our enthusiasm for being with the other person). These three elements build upon each other. Not surprisingly, in order to be effective in the social skill of synchrony, you must first devote your full attention to the other person and you must care enough about him or her to seek the establishment of rapport.

In seeking to establish rapport with another person, we can either enjoy the presence of spontaneous synchrony (if it occurs) or we can facilitate rapport through consciously synchronizing our verbal and nonverbal cues to those of the person with whom we are interacting.[22]

Although the idea of deliberate synchrony might seem contrived, it is a skill intended not for the manipulation or coercion of others but rather as a measure of putting them at ease to facilitate their best expression of self. Boothman[15] likens the practice of deliberate synchrony to the use of a specialized electrical adaptor in a foreign country. According to this analogy, the adaptor serves as a connecting device through which electrical power is accessed. In the same manner, consciously synchronizing our communication allows us to connect to another person, accessing an optimal interaction.

The human ability for synchrony is an important developmental skill, which is supported by specialized neurons in the central nervous system.[23] These "mirror neurons" are located in the motor system, producing a specialized response after observation of the same action. Thus, a smile in one person evokes a smile in another.

At the developmental level, synchrony is a critical element for healthy attachment and emotional connections between mother and infant. Synchrony is readily observable between mothers and their infants as this emotional connection proceeds. An infant will synchronize movements of the limbs, jaw, and tongue to the rhythm of the mother's voice and movements.[24] Thus, by the time we reach adulthood, we have hopefully become well versed in the use of synchrony to create and sustain rapport in our relationships. However, as with any subconscious behavior, we are probably relatively unaware of our ability to use this important social skill. Just as you have likely begun to engage in analysis of human gait in a variety of situations, you can also develop your observational skills in the area of synchrony. As you sharpen your skills, you will quickly be able to assess the effect of synchrony on the level of rapport, as the following examples illustrates.

Searching for Synchrony

In an intimate and elegant restaurant, Susan and John are having their first date over dinner. Despite the sumptuous visual stimuli created by glowing candles, sparkling crystal, and masterful table-side food preparation, Susan and John appear oblivious to these potent distractions. Instead, they give their full undivided attention to each other as they converse in warm, quiet tones. While John talks, Susan leans inward toward him, eyes sparkling, nodding agreement. When Susan talks, John regards her with a warm smile that radiates from his entire face. As their conversation proceeds, Susan and John begin to mirror each other's facial expressions, voice quality, and gestures. They frequently laugh at the same time, use similar facial expressions, and even eat in unison. Their communication flows with a relaxed and spontaneous back-and-forth exchange that enhances the cozy intimacy of the room.

Mike and Claudia are also having their first date at a nearby table. Claudia seems to be doing most of the talking, and her high-pitched tone can be heard at nearby tables. As she holds court, Mike leans back in his chair, listening with a tight smile as his eyes occasionally dart around the room. Underneath the elegant tablecloth, Mike's foot taps impatiently. Claudia continues to gush, interrupting Mike on several occasions. Then, as Claudia tells Mike what appears to be a wildly humorous story, he leans forward and responds quietly, the rigid smile replaced by a somber, narrow-eyed expression. At this point, Claudia looks away and picks up her cell phone from the table, nervously looking at the screen. Mike glances at his watch.

If you were asked to predict the likelihood of future dates between each of these couples based on this description of their initial attempts to connect with each other, chances are that you would quickly be able to do so. Although both couples engaged in the exchange of words to a degree, their impact varied considerably. John and Susan displayed synchrony in its many forms, sharing tones of voice, body movements, and gestures. This "dance" of synchrony creates a positive energy that could readily be observed by those around them.

In contrast, the lack of synchrony between Mike and Claudia could be likened to a visibly awkward dance where neither partner knows who is leading, so that they keep stepping on each other's toes. Rather than the comfortable flow of conversation that occurs when synchrony is present, Claudia appeared to "hold court" during her interaction with Mike, depriving him of any opportunity to respond. Thus, instead of a dance, Mike and Claudia's interaction could be described as the conversational equivalent of "parallel play," a developmental phenomenon in which young toddlers play beside each other in a self-absorbed manner without interacting.[25] The potential for synchronizing with another person is optimal in face-to-face interactions and moderately limited in telephone conversations, where the only input is aural. As we become increasingly reliant on cyber communications, where there is little or no need for synchrony, it is possible that our opportunities to develop the perceptual abilities required for synchrony may atrophy over time.

Interestingly, the term *parallel play* was recently used to describe the pitfalls of a form of online communication known as a weblog ("blog"), where writers divulge thoughts, opinions, and sometimes highly personal information to an audience whose replies are seldom invited or acknowledged.[26,27]

This observation, made by a director of a large online education company,[27] begs the question of how reliance on cyber communications such as blogs might affect the dynamics of face-to-face conversation and the formation of genuine relationships.

Talking Points/Field Notes

Developing Awareness of Synchrony

Directions: This exercise has two major components, in-class and out-of-class practice and observation. The in-class exercises should be done in groups of four persons.

In-Class Practice/Observation

These exercises are done in random order, so that the observers are unaware of whether the interaction is in synchrony or out of synchrony. In practicing synchrony, the point is not to directly mimic every aspect of the other person's behavior so that it feels contrived or uncomfortable but to complement one or more elements in a comfortable, complementary fashion. Synchronizing voice volume, speed of talking, open versus closed posture, and general level of emotional intensity are helpful ways to put the other person at ease, which is again the point of synchrony.

Talking Points/Field Notes—cont'd ▪

1. In synchrony: Two classmates will have a 1- to 2-minute conversation on a current event or other topic of mutual interest. Between them, they should decide which one will attempt to synchronize with the other. It may help to consider your verbal and nonverbal communication dynamics when you are enjoying an interaction with another person.

2. Out of synchrony: Two classmates will have a 1- to 2-minute conversation as above, but one of them will move out of synchrony with the other. It may help to consider your verbal and nonverbal communication dynamics when you are not enjoying an interaction with another person.

The other classmates will observe the interaction and comment on the level of rapport in each condition. They should not know whether or not the interactions are portraying synchrony. Everyone should have the opportunity to observe, practice synchronizing, and feel the effects of having a person be in and out of synchrony with them.

Questions for Discussion and Reflection

1. Discuss how it felt to have someone be in synchrony versus out of synchrony with you in terms of your own sense of comfort and rapport.

2. Discuss how it felt to practice synchronizing with another person. Which elements did you choose to synchronize and why?

3. When you were observing, how accurately were you able to identify the condition of your classmates being in or out of synchrony? What did you notice in terms of their rapport and communication dynamics in each situation?

4. How might awareness of synchrony be helpful in enhancing your communication with patients in order to establish rapport?

Out-of-Class Practice/Observation

1. For the next few days, observe the presence or absence of synchrony in conversations around you (without staring or being obtrusive of course). Note the level of comfort and apparent rapport between the persons involved.

2. Practice synchronizing in a few conversations, ideally with persons you do not know well (this can even be among classmates).

Reflect on the impact this had on your conversation dynamics in your field notes.

Implications for Physical Therapy

In establishing a therapeutic alliance with our patients, we must first develop rapport. This in turn promotes the building of genuine trust, compassion, and unconditional positive regard. If we are successful in forging this connection, we will also optimize our chances for successful patient management. From your own experiences, you can perhaps recall a situation where you wanted to change health-care providers owing to the lack of therapeutic rapport.[28]

Patients who lack rapport with their health-care providers will have greater difficulty following through with their treatment regimens and have poorer outcomes than those who do.[29,30] Lack of rapport and poor communication have also been linked to medical error, a factor contributing to the deaths of 44,000 persons each year in the United States.[31,32] Thus, regardless of the context, relationships that involve caring for another person do contain a level of emotional connection.

Synchrony SOS (Another True-Life Tale)

Ian is a physical therapy student on his first day of a clinical rotation in a skilled nursing facility, where many of his patients are considered "frail elderly." In contrast, Ian is 6½ feet tall and a competitive body builder who weighs 260 pounds. Having grown up in New York City, he tends to talk quickly, loudly, and directly. Ian greatly enjoys conversation and is good at small talk. He is energetic and loves to encourage his patients to reach their functional potential. This is Ian's first time working with this patient population.

Ian is about to begin an assessment of Ruth, who is 82 years old and has severe arthritis and osteoporosis. She is ready to begin gait training after a recent fall, in which she sustained a hairline acetabular fracture. Ruth is 5 feet tall and weights 100 pounds. She has just been transported to the PT department in her wheelchair. Ian walks up with a smile and greets Ruth in his booming voice. Ruth sees Ian looming over her and responds, wide-eyed, in a slow, quiet voice. After a couple of questions, Ruth asks for a blanket, saying that she is cold, and Ian quickly realizes that perhaps Ruth is not comfortable with him.

Questions

1. Consider the elements of verbal and nonverbal communication discussed in this chapter thus far. Which of these might Ian modify/synchronize in order to put Ruth at ease?

2. How can Ian's conversational skills be helpful in establishing rapport? Specifically, what questions might Ian ask Ruth in order to put her at ease and facilitate rapport between them?

3. How can Ian demonstrate unconditional positive regard and compassion for Ruth?

In the situation described above, Ian learned to speak more slowly and quietly as well as to position himself at Ruth's level whenever possible (and especially to avoid standing over her). He also learned that Ruth needed encouragement to build her confidence after her fall and that he needed to proceed slowly with her exercises in order to avoid pain. After asking Ruth about the things she enjoyed most, Ian found out that they both loved old-time jazz, swimming, and chocolate. Ian then decided to work with Ruth in the facility's therapeutic pool, where they exercised to music; after that, they shared hot chocolate. The pool exercises were helpful in decreasing Ruth's joint pain and she made significant progress in her gait training. After one month, Ruth was able to return home to live with her daughter.

Engaging Conversation: The Importance of Small Talk

Our ability to engage others in conversation is the ultimate expression of our social intelligence. Through conversation, we convey our interest and readiness to be in relationship with others. Strong relationships are built on the mutual acceptance and understanding that ensues from the disclosure of personal thoughts and feelings. However, most of us have internal boundaries that dictate the appropriate timing and depth of these revelations.[33]

Everyone's boundaries are different and are a complex composition of numerous elements, including levels of extraversion (attention focused on the outside world of people and events) or introversion (attention focused on the internal world of thoughts, feelings, and perceptions). In addition, each of us varies in our approach to personal disclosure. For example, you may know people who are quite forthcoming in sharing information about themselves, as well as others who guard themselves carefully. Each of us also has a level of comfort in terms of receiving the disclosure of others, a threshold that separates comfortable sharing from "too much information." Thus, the dance of conversation is a careful exploration of mutual boundaries, interests, and emotional availability for the purpose at hand (whether this is a therapeutic relationship between patient and therapist, a collegial relationship with other physical therapists in the workplace, or the expression of romantic interest).

Thus, regardless of individual differences in emotional boundaries between persons, most conversations generally involve a necessary exchange of casual and friendly information where persons in dialogue put each other at ease, show interest, and convey their agendas. The type of conversation in this initial exchange is known as *social talk* (or what many of us know as small talk) and far from being a waste of valuable time (e.g., in a busy clinic with a new patient), research suggests that it is a prerequisite for the future strengthening of the relationship.[34] This is because even when we are discussing seemingly banal topics like the weather or the latest sports scores, we are conveying a level of emotional arousal. When two persons in social conversation detect the sharing of emotions related to nonpersonal topics, the stage is set for personal levels of disclosure. Furthermore, those who share similar responses to events are likely to have more cohesive and longer-lasting relationships.[35] Finally, while we tend to relate better with those who display similar levels of emotional positivity or negativity,[36] there is evidence to suggest that we are more likely to form a positive first impression if our small talk reflects positive emotions (such as admiration, warmth, and optimism).[33,37]

Although the term *social lubricant* has often been cynically applied to the use of alcohol to promote relaxation and enjoyment in social situations, in reality, the ultimate social lubricant is conversation. In developing conversational skills, you may find the guidelines illustrated in **Box 8-1** helpful.

Another interesting approach to conversation is to examine the issue at hand from many different perspectives. DeBono represents these perspectives as "thinking hats,"

BOX 8-1:   Suggestions for Social Conversation

1. Adjust your attitude
   Approach conversations with optimism. Expect rapport and enjoyment, just as you do when you are attending a gathering of good friends.
2. Show interest
   Interesting people are interested in others. Ask open-ended questions to generate deeper levels of discussion. Consider the power of "Why do you think so?"
3. Listen
   The best conversationalists actively listen to others. Don't pretend to listen when you're not, or mentally argue, or rehearse your next statement or question. By listening actively, you can spontaneously generate relevant questions or reflective responses.
4. Turn the spotlight on the other person
   Everyone's most expert topic is themselves. One of the best ways to get to know someone is to ask them about their background, interests, or opinions.
5. Look for possibilities
   The use of imagination can create fascinating conversation. Look at topics from many different perspectives and bring these into your dialogue.
6. Remember your social skills
   This is about manners, not interrupting and watching for body language, which signals engagement. Try synchronizing a few elements to enhance rapport.
7. Share the floor
   A conversation is reciprocal. Don't dominate or sermonize. After answering a question from the other person, it is helpful to ask "and what about you?"

Continued

BOX 8-1:   Suggestions for Social Conversation—cont'd

8. Keep learning

Be a lifelong learner. Developing your own interests can provide interesting fodder for conversation. Keep up on the news. Even knowing a little bit about a lot can be useful. Conversations are a great way to learn the world around you.

9. Stay present to the other person

Beginning each interaction with the affirmation "I am fully present to this person" can often lead to authentic and meaningful conversation. It is particularly helpful in challenging situations.

10. Graceful exits

When mingling, recognizing other persons' schedules can be a graceful way to end a conversation. Such exits can include, "I know you have lots of people to talk to, so I'll let you go," or "It's been great talking to you." On the other hand, using food or the restroom as a diversion (e.g., "Well, I think I'll go check out the food table") might provoke the response, "I'll go with you!"

which relate to emotions, facts, possibilities, positive outcomes, judgments, and the "big picture."[38] According to DeBono, many of our conversations focus on facts and judgments and could be greatly enhanced by a simple shift in perspective. **Figure 8-3** illustrates the six different perspectives and how they might apply to the topic of health-care costs.

TOPIC: THE HIGH COST OF HEALTHCARE

THE BIG PICTURE:	What are the overall social implications of high healthcare costs? What is our goal in addressing this problem?
FACTS:	How many Americans have no health insurance? How much have insurance premiums risen over the past 5 years?
FEELINGS:	What would it feel like to be refused medical care because of insurance restrictions? How would you feel if your insurance claim was denied?
JUDGMENTS:	What is wrong with the current system? Who is to blame?
POSITIVE VALUES:	How might an insurance-based emphasis on evidence-based practice make us a stronger profession? How has our profession become more accountable in the face of managed care?
POSSIBILITIES:	What if every work site allowed time for meditation? What if insurance covered health club fees?

Figure 8–3. Six conversational perspectives. *(Adapted from DeBono E. Six Thinking Hats. Toronto, Canada: MICA Management Resources; 1999.)*

Talking Points/Field Notes

Exercises to Develop Engaging Conversation

Each of these exercises can be completed and discussed in a small group. You can do all of these or select specific ones, depending on time and interest.

1. Develop an interest in *anything*. Good conversationalists have a broad range of interest on all levels. With an inquisitive mind, it is possible to generate questions and comments that can provide for stimulating conversation.

Talking Points/Field Notes—cont'd ■━━━━━━━━━━━━━━

Directions: Each member of the group is asked to write two nouns (which can represent a person, place, or thing). For example: *goniometer, Las Vegas, Mary McMillan*. Each person should share his or her list and, as a group, use each list to generate up to 20 open-ended questions that would make for interesting conversation. If you are having difficulty generating questions, refer to the perspectives listed in Figure 8-3. Once you have completed this exercise, discuss your experiences with classmates and record your observations in your field notes.

2. Hosting a dinner party (includes role play): As a group, you are hosting a dinner party to which you can each invite one person you have always wanted to meet, either living or dead. Once each of you has identified this person, consider at least three questions you would want to ask him or her. Share your person and your questions with the group, so that you now have the full "guest list." Then take turns being the dinner party host with everyone else in the group playing the roles of the guests (the persons you have all identified). As the host, consider how you would use conversation to make introductions and put each of your guests at ease. Note: Role plays can be both enjoyable and educational if you take them seriously enough. Once you have completed this exercise, discuss your experiences with classmates and record your observations in your field notes.

3. Field notes exercise—my open-ended world: One of the ways to expand the creative side of your communication is to consider the topic from an open-ended perspective (who, what, when, where, why, is, does, etc.).

Directions: Generate a list of *at least* 100 open-ended questions. They can pertain to any subject. This exercise will be more mentally challenging and interesting if you write all the questions in one session. Here are a few examples generated from PT students:

  a. What would the United States be like today if the southern states had won the Civil War?

  b. What would happen if there were a safe, noninvasive, and effective way to prevent and reverse obesity?

  c. Where does the spirit go after death?

After you are done with this exercise, you might want to examine your list for any prevailing themes. What does this say about your interests? Discuss your experiences with classmates and record your observations in your field notes.

Implications for Physical Therapy

The ability to engage your patients in conversation, particularly in the early stages of rapport building, is an essential skill. Although a diagnosis or concern brings patients to our door, they also bring along their stories, interests, and relationships as part of their life picture. As you will learn in Chapter 10, the experience of being a patient can be depersonalizing. In turn, depersonalization can have a host of negative emotional consequences (such as frustration, powerlessness, and fear), which can interfere with the healing process. Our engaging conversation can remind both ourselves and our patients that they are far more than a diagnosis. Furthermore, through making an effort to understand patients in the full context of their lives, we can often help them identify meaningful goals that will motivate them to succeed. The following case scenario provides an opportunity to consider the use of conversational skills for rapport and the establishment of therapeutic goals.

Use of Small Talk in the Initial Patient Interview

You are on your final internship in a community hospital near an Amish community. Sarah Fisher, a member of this group, is 35 years old; she has been referred for inpatient PT following the sudden onset of lower extremity weakness and optic neuritis. She has just been diagnosed with multiple sclerosis. Upon reading her chart, you learn that Sarah is married and has six children between the ages of 5 and 15. Sarah has been very active in her community, enjoying gardening, quilting, and baking.

You meet Sarah for the first time in the PT department, where she arrives in a wheelchair, accompanied by her husband Jacob and three of her younger children. Her demeanor is reserved, and as you introduce yourself, Jacob says gently, "This is our first time in a hospital, so excuse us if we are a little nervous."

Consider the following questions:

1. How can the information in Sarah's chart be helpful for social talk that will put her at ease and also assist you in determining her PT needs?

2. How would you begin your interaction with Sarah? How would you explain your role as a physical therapist in a way that she and her family could understand?

3. What specific things might you say to Sarah's husband and children to engage them?

4. If you had just received a diagnosis of multiple sclerosis, what questions might you have? What might you say to Sarah to support and encourage her as she learns about her disease process?

5. What specific questions might you ask Sarah regarding her daily activities in order to formulate a functional and meaningful plan of care?

Active Listening: "We Have Two Ears and One Mouth for a Reason"

What is the most important skill for being a good conversationalist? In answering this question, many of us might focus on "output" features such as wit, humor, and eloquence. These skills are inarguably important, but mostly in structured communication contexts such as lecturing to a large audience or delivering a stand-up comedy routine.

When we speak of interactive forms of dialogue, the most important skill is active listening, which means focusing our full, undistracted attention on the speaker in the present moment. Only in this manner can we accurately perceive and authentically respond to the full complement of the speaker's verbal and nonverbal signals. Thus it cannot be emphasized enough that *active listening is the foundation of effective communication.*

Sadly, active listening is a skill that most of us do not practice enough. *Practice* is an operative term here, because active listening takes mindful, concentrated *effort.* Mindfulness is needed to direct our attention to the present moment and to narrow the focus of our attention to the speaker. Concentrated effort is required to filter out distractions, whether they occur in the environment (a ringing telephone) or within our own minds (daydreaming or planning our dinner menu). Active listening is thus a skill that requires continual commitment and recommitment. For example, many of us might find ourselves falling out of practice in times of stress and will need to consciously redirect our focus. Nevertheless, active listening is a highly worthwhile endeavor, as your communication will become more authentic and meaningful as a result. In your role as a physical therapist, active listening can dramatically improve the quality of your patient care. In your everyday life, active listening can enrich your relationships at all levels. The following exercises can be useful in assessing and developing your active listening.

Talking Points/Field Notes

Exercises for Active Listening

Each of these can be done in small groups in the manner of talking points and can also be reflected upon in your field notes.

1. Active listening quiz: It has been said that each of us were given two ears and one mouth in order to do twice as much listening as talking. How well do we do this? **Table 8-2** contains a listening quiz. Take this assessment, giving your honest answers. Then discuss your answers in a small group and reflect on these in your field notes.

Table 8–2. Active Listening Quiz

Select the answer that best describes your general listening habits. Use the following key:

A = Always

O = Often

E = Every now and then

S = Seldom

Questions	Responses
1. I daydream while listening.	
2. I fidget while listening.	
3. I have to ask the speaker to repeat what he or she has said.	
4. I interrupt the speaker.	
5. I finish the speaker's sentence.	
6. I "steal the floor" or "one-up" the speaker ("that's nothing, let me tell you...")	
7. I hear, "You're not listening!"	
8. I rush the speaker.	
9. I get distracted by things around me.	
10. I tune out the speaker.	
11. I rehearse what I am going to say next.	
12. I mentally argue with the speaker.	
13. I feel bored.	

Continued

Talking Points/Field Notes—cont'd ▬▬▬▬▬▬▬▬▬▬▬▬

2. My listening saboteurs: We all have various "listening saboteurs," which prevent us from listening with our full mindful attention. Do any of these creatures live in your brain? See **Box 8-2**.

BOX 8–2:   Listening Saboteurs

Read the following descriptions of negative listening habits that can sabotage authentic dialogue. Can you relate to any of these characters?

Pretender:	Pretends to listen and even acts like he's listening but his thoughts are somewhere else.
Big But:	Has to argue every point as soon as possible ("but..."). Wants to be right and have you see things her way.
Captain Hook:	Uses your stories as a hook for his own better version. Favorite sayings include: "You think that's bad? Let me tell you about..." or "That reminds me of...."
Convo Klepto:	The master of interruption: Breaks into your conversation and steals the floor.
Wizard:	Has a solution or advice to all your problems and wants you to know as soon as possible ("If I were you...").
Wannabe:	Knows exactly how you feel about everything.

Adapted from Lynn B. *The Emotional Intelligence Activity Book: 50 Activities for Promoting EQ at Work*. New York: AMACOM: American Management Company; 2002.

If you are like most of my students (and me as well), you have probably noted that your active listening skills could be enhanced with a little more practice. There is no magic spell that will make you a better listener and no specific way to go about this except for the consistently mindful investment of effort.

If you are still wondering whether active listening is a worthy use of your attention, given all the other demands you face, consider this: *If you are not actively listening to the persons in your life, what makes you think they are actively listening to you?* From our discussion on synchrony, it should be obvious that active listening is an essential element for accurate, empathic attunement. Thus, if you are not actively listening to another person, you prevent the mutual achievement of synchrony between you in a true reflection of "what goes around comes around."

There is an important adage from neurolinguistic programming (NLP) that states, "The meaning of your communication is the response you get."[39] Thus, when you actively listen to others and empathetically connect in the process, the dynamics of your interaction will deepen as understanding evolves between you.

It is both empowering and healing to feel understood. This has been demonstrated in the psychotherapeutic process, beginning in the late 1950s with the work of Carl Rogers, whose "client-centered therapy" approach was grounded in the use of active listening. Rogers noted that active listening improved his clients' self esteem, awareness, and problem-solving skills. Most importantly, his clients, having experienced the benefits of being listened to, began to actively listen more to others and thus reported that their relationships improved. Since the time of Rogers' initial research, these findings have been supported in other psychotherapeutic studies.[40] The rhythm of our lives is often one of frantic, technologically expedited urgency. Many of us may go through entire days without actively listening to (or being listened to) the persons around us. Thus, when an opportunity for active listening presents itself, it may feel awkward and contrived. Nevertheless, you are encouraged to persist, keeping in mind that this form of communication is the central ingredient for lasting authentic relationships. With this in mind, you are invited to try the following activities.

Talking Points/Field Notes

Practice in Active Listening

The following activities will assist your practice in active listening. As you complete these, you can discuss their results in a small group and in your field notes.

In-Class Activity: Listening Dyads (This Exercise Is Done In Pairs)

In this exercise, each of you will take turns practicing active listening and being actively listened to. You will each have a 2-minute opportunity to speak on any topic about which you can speak personally and comfortably (e.g., your overall experience as a PT student, a favorite hobby, what you did over a recent holiday). Your instructor will keep time.

Speaker: Share your thoughts with the listener as freely and comfortably as you can. This activity is not about talking fast to fill up the 2 minutes but rather about sharing comfortably whatever comes to mind.

Listener: Your role is to actively listen with your full attention on the speaker. You may not interrupt, interject, or say anything except one- or two-word encouragers such as "yes, go on," "uh huh," and so on. Do not fidget and try not to take your focus off the speaker for the entire 2 minutes. When the first 2-minute session is over, change roles and repeat this activity, using the same or different question as desired.

Questions About Your Role as a Listener

Each person should use this scale to assess his or her listening skills during this activity:

1 = **very difficult**, 2 = **difficult**, 3 = **somewhat difficult**, 4 = **easy**, 5 = **very easy**

While listening to your classmate, how difficult was it for you to:

1. Keep your mental focus entirely on the speaker without being mentally distracted?
2. Avoid mentally rehearsing your responses or what you might say if you were talking?
3. Avoid mentally arguing with the speaker if you disagreed?
4. Avoid feeling like you wanted to interrupt the speaker with a wisecrack or comment?
5. Refrain from fidgeting or playing with an object such as a pen?
6. Maintain eye contact with the speaker (what percentage of the time do you think you kept eye contact)?
7. Use body language (posture, position, movement) to show interest in the speaker? Consider specific ways in which you did this.
8. Discern the speaker's emotional content?
9. Encourage the speaker to continue?
10. Use your face to listen? Consider the impact of facial expressions and nonverbal gestures such as smiling, nodding, etc.

Share your self-assessment with your partner. Does he or she agree? What suggestions does your partner have? What challenges did you identify during this exercise? How might you address these in your future listening efforts?

Continued

Talking Points/Field Notes—cont'd ■ ▬

Questions About Your Role as Speaker

1. What impact did being listened to have on the quality of your conversation?

2. How did it feel to speak without interruption, knowing you had the full attention of the listener?

3. How might you feel about a person who actively listens to you versus one who does not? How likely are you to share future concerns with a person who actively listens versus one who does not?

Out of Class Activity: Active Listening in Real Life

For the next 24 hours, consciously make the attempt to actively listen in all face-to-face and telephone conversations. You might wish to contact a friend or family member that you haven't spoken to in a while and catch up in person or on the phone.

The following suggestions apply: Do not fidget or do anything else except sit and listen. Limit environmental distractions (TV, computer, driving, etc.). This exercise is about the quality versus the quantity of your exchanges, so don't feel compelled to make your conversations longer than appropriate. Rather, simply affirm being in the moment for the duration of each interaction, however long or short it may be.

At the end of 24 hours, reflect on your experience using the following questions:

1. How was the quality of your interactions affected by your use of active listening? Does any specific situation come to mind?

2. How did your active listening affect the quality of your comments and responses?

3. How did your active listening affect the speaker's interactions with you? (Did you feel more "listened to"?)

4. How difficult was it to actively listen? What specific challenges did you face?

5. What value do you think active listening has in your dialogues?

Implications for Physical Therapy

Engaging your patients through active listening may well be one of the most important things you can do to assure the quality of their care. Several studies support the relationship between the active listening of health-care providers and high levels of patient satisfaction, compliance, and positive outcomes.[41,42]

However, in the busy health-care environment, you may sometimes feel conflicted between the desire to take the time to connect with your patients and the need to meet documentation and productivity requirements (e.g., how do you document or bill for a conversation with a patient?). However, you may quickly discover that time spent in actively listening to patients actually saves time in the long run, as you will be able to more effectively meet their needs, engage their cooperation, and empower them toward successful outcomes.

Clinical Scenario

Active Listening in Action

Jared is a physical therapist at an urban inpatient rehabilitation center and is completing a PT examination on Augusto Sanchez. Augusto is an athletic 19-year-old with T-12 complete paraplegia resulting from a fall from a ladder that occurred during his work as a construction laborer. As Jared explains the general program of spinal cord rehabilitation (including bed mobility, transfers, and wheelchair skills), Augusto becomes upset, interrupts Jared, and says, "You haven't said a thing about walking! I don't care about the other garbage you are talking about! I want to walk out of here! How can you help me with that?"

Questions

1. What underlying emotions might Jared need to attend to as he listens to Augusto?

2. How can Jared respond to Augusto in a way that lets him know that he has been heard?

3. Patients with T-12 paraplegia can learn to ambulate with long leg braces and crutches, but this is so strenuous that many such patients eventually abandon the activity. Knowing this, how can Jared support Augusto toward this goal while instructing him in the other important mobility skills he will need to function independently?

4. How can Jared engage Augusto in a dialogue exploring his athletic interests in the context of goal setting?

The rest of the story: Jared acknowledged Augusto's desire to ambulate and told him that he would definitely be able to work toward this. Jared also was very honest with Augusto with respect to the energy demands and strength requirements of ambulation with braces and crutches. He told Augusto that training in balance, transfers, and wheelchair skills would help build the necessary upper body strength required for ambulation. This motivated Augusto to work hard in rehabilitation, where he progressed rapidly. Upon attempting gait with braces and crutches, Augusto decided that he would likely stand mostly to maintain bone strength in his lower extremities. Augusto's story has a happy ending. As Augusto completed his rehabilitation, Jared encouraged Augusto to try out for the local wheelchair basketball team. Over the course of time, Augusto proved to be an outstanding wheelchair athlete and decided to train for the Paralympic Games. Jared's ability to listen to Augusto's desires and interests helped him to support Augusto toward a successful outcome.

As this example illustrates, active listening sets the stage for successful patient interactions. The topic of building effective patient–therapist interactions is covered in more detail in Chapter 10.

Attachment: Sustaining Authentic Relationships Through Effective Communication

Besides being among the most important human needs, healthy interpersonal attachments are important for optimal physical, emotional, and cognitive function.[43]

In a relationship predicated on mutual acceptance, there is generally an emotional bond of goodwill and affection known as attachment. Originally proposed by psychologist John Bowlby[44] to describe the intense emotional bond between mothers and their infants, attachment theory has been expanded to include the dynamics of any interpersonal relationships based on mutual goodwill, including those between peers, coworkers, and caregivers.

In most deep friendships, both attachment and acceptance coexist and build upon each other. The communication progression that we have discussed thus far—impression formation, rapport building, and the related skills of synchrony, engaging conversation, and active listening—are all critical skills for sustaining meaningful relationships. Thus a degree of attachment exists whenever there is a mutual feeling of goodwill, interest in each other's well-being, and commitment to a relationship. The many attachments in our lives will therefore have a multitude of contexts (those with classmates, work friends, romantic partners) and will also have a corresponding level of goodwill, interest, and commitment. As these virtues are conveyed through our communication, it is fair to say that the more important our attachments, the greater the investment of our authentic communication (in terms of its depth and consistency over time). But just what is meant by authenticity and how does this affect our relationships?

Authenticity: What I Say Is Who I Am

Authenticity has been defined as communication that reflects one's true self[43]; it pertains to the ease with which we communicate our honest values, feelings, and needs. The depth and range of this comfort will likely vary in our relationships, depending on their context. Nevertheless, most of us are likely to avoid relationships that require us to deny our values or to act disingenuously. If you have ever felt pressure to behave in a way that makes you uncomfortable, no doubt you were facing a threat to your personal authenticity.

Not surprisingly, a recent study demonstrated that the depth of attachment between persons is related to the level of their shared authenticity.[45]

In other words, our deepest attachments will be persons who allow us to express ourselves in the most genuine ways. As we have discussed previously, the benefits of authentic attachments are numerous in terms of physical and emotional health. In addition, there is evidence to suggest that the ability to engage in authentic attachments is related to success in goal achievement.[46] No doubt success in goal achievement is facilitated when we can be honest about what we need. Moreover, if we can share this honesty in the context of meaningful relationships, we will likely experience greater support and empowerment toward success.

Authenticity can be viewed as a continuum of progressively deeper layers of self-disclosure. Even though we will likely choose not to reveal the intimate aspects of our lives to everyone we meet, we can nevertheless convey an important measure of authenticity in our desire to be mindfully present, to engage and to listen to the persons in our lives to the best of our abilities. The skills of social intelligence can help us interpret cues that guide our communication and our expression of self, and the awareness of the importance of authentic communication can be helpful in guiding us toward its expression. Thus, in addition to the deeper levels that contain our innermost thoughts and feelings, authenticity also speaks to our core values, our beliefs about what is important in terms of our interactions with others. Although our inner boundaries may rightfully preclude the disclosure of deep emotional content in everyday situations, our core values should be evident in all our interactions, regardless of context.

The consistency with which we convey our authentic values builds trust in relationships. For example, you might be more likely to rely on a friend who is consistently thoughtful and caring as opposed to one who is kind only when they want something from you. Thus, it is important to reflect on the elements of our authentic self that we wish to present everyday to those around us. **Figure 8-4** represents these layers of authenticity, beginning with the core values which we convey in all relationships and our inner thoughts and feelings, which we reserve for intimate relationships.

Figure 8–4. Levels of authenticity: A set of core values and virtues to consistently convey in all communication, and our innermost thoughts and feelings, which we reserve for intimate relationships.

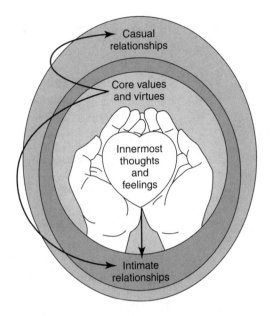

This is not to suggest that we have two different selves but rather that we have a continuum of depth that unfolds in our relationships as we develop stronger levels of attachment.

Implications for Physical Therapy

In our practice as physical therapists, the development of trust between us and our patients is essential to an effective therapeutic partnership. Accordingly, in 2003, APTA adopted a set of seven core values intended to guide the authentic expression of professional interaction. These values are *accountability* (accepting responsibility for our actions), *altruism* (putting the patient's needs before our own), *compassion and caring* (the consistent display of unconditional positive regard), *excellence* (providing the best possible care), *integrity* (consistency between our thoughts, words, and actions), *professional duty* (practicing legally, ethically, and competently), and *social responsibility* (acting for the greater public good).

Our profession has thus embraced these core values as essential elements that we must consistently convey through our communication. In other words, they are "nonnegotiable" elements of authentic PT practice.[47]

Talking Points/Field Notes

The Nonnegotiable Elements of My Authentic Self

Consider the core elements of your authentic self (what you hope to convey as a reflection of self in all of your interactions). These elements can include desirable attributes or virtues such as intelligence, compassion, or enthusiasm. Then complete the following, discussing your results in a small group and reflecting in your field notes.

    a. Which four core elements (or more, if you desire) do you seek to convey in all of your everyday interactions (with colleagues, supervisors, friends)?

    b. How do these change when you are with people who are the closest to you? What other attributes may emerge?

Continued

Talking Points/Field Notes—cont'd

   c. How easy is it for you to be your authentic self in most situations?

   d. In which circumstances might you not be authentic and why? How does this make you feel?

   e. What do you think are the most important elements to sustain a strong attachment?

As these two chapters on social intelligence and external communication have suggested, there are many considerations in the pursuit of effective communication. No one is effective all the time; that is not even a realistic goal. Instead, as you reflect on these elements, consider them in terms of a lifelong journey in the same way that you will hopefully pursue learning and development in other areas. As your future unfolds, you will likely confront circumstances that cause you to take stock of your communication skills and to make appropriate adjustments therein. It is this ongoing self-awareness and commitment to optimal communication that will serve you well as an engaged person and professional.

Implications for Physical Therapy

Each of the external communication skills discussed in this chapter (making a good first impression, building rapport, active listening, and engaging conversation) has profound implications for successful PT practice. All patient care is completed in the context of a caring and respectful relationship, which requires the same external communication skills as in any other. Thus, you are encouraged to develop these skills for the benefit of successful relationships in all of your work-life roles. You will find that multiple arenas of practice will reinforce each other, so that increased comfort in one area will facilitate ease in the others.

Chapter Summary

1. This chapter explored the use of social skills and external communication in the process of relationship development, which consists of *impression formation, rapport building,* and *attachment.*

2. Impression formation is the process by which we present ourselves to others and convey our interest and desire to engage. Open body language, an optimistic attitude, and a welcoming facial expression are all ways in which we can create a favorable first impression.

3. Rapport building is the process where we engage emotionally, creating alliances and finding areas of shared experience. Positive regard, synchrony, and engaging conversational skills are helpful in promoting rapport.

4. Attachment pertains to a sustained emotional connection between individuals. The level of attachment can vary greatly depending on the level of trust and self-disclosure. We all have inner boundaries that guide our choices in terms of appropriate levels of sharing.

5. Authenticity pertains to the consistency with which we convey the core elements of ourselves in our communication. These core elements pertain to our core values and virtues as well as our innermost thoughts and feelings. Authenticity involves staying true to ones core values in all situations while sharing innermost aspects of self in ones closer relationships.

Take-Home Menu

1. Analyzing Synchrony. Watch a conversation on a movie or television show with the sound off. See if you can detect body language related to engagement and synchrony (or lack of it). See if you can predict the quality of the relationship depicted before turning the sound back on.
2. Take the APTA Core Values Self-Assessment. If you have not already done so in class, do so now. Which areas were the most challenging? How might you address these in your future practice? You will find this on the APTA website, http://www.apta.org under "core documents."
3. Acquire a Listening Partner. In the practice of active listening, it is very helpful to have a partner with whom you can practice (and who will do this for you). After sharing a dialogue, give each other feedback.

References

1. *Falling in Love in Three Seconds or Less.* February 11, 2005. University of Pennsylvania, Office of University Communications: http://www.upenn.edu/pennnews/article.php?id=747. Accessed March 7, 2008.

2. Gladwell M. *Blink: The Power of Thinking Without Thinking.* New York: Little, Brown; 2005.

3. Hamilton DL, Driscoll DM, Worth LT. Cognitive organization of impressions: effects of incongruency in complex representations *J Pers Soc Psychol.* 1989;57(6):925-929.

4. Bar M, Neta M, Linz H. Very first impressions. *Emotion.* 2006;6(2):269-278.

5. Hamilton DL, Katz LB, Leirer VO. Organizational process in impression formation. In Hastie R, Ostrom TM, Ebbesen EB, et al, eds. *Person, Memory: The Cognitive Basis of Social Perception.* Hillsdale, NJ: Erlbaum; 1980:121-153.

6. Mehrabian A. *Silent Messages: Implicit Communication of Emotions and Attitudes.* Belmont, CA: Wadsworth; 1981.

7. Mehrabian A, Wiener M. Decoding of inconsistent communication. *J Pers Soc Psychol.* 1967;6(1):109-114.

8. Brenner RC. *Body Language in Business.* Brenner Books: http://www.brennerbooks.com/bodylang.html. Accessed March 6, 2008.

9. Ito TA, Larsen JT, Smith NK, Caioppo JT. Negative information weighs more heavily on the brain: The negativity bias in evaluative categorizations. *J Pers Soc Psychol.* 1998;75(4):887-900.

10. Verplankten B, Friborg O, Trafimow D, Woolf K. Mental habits: metacognitive reflection on negative self thinking. *J Pers Soc Psychol.* 2007;92(3):526-541.

11. Denrell J. Why most people disapprove of me: Experience sampling in impression formation. *Psychol Rev.* 2005; 112(4):951-978.

12. Amen D. *Change Your Brain, Change Your Life.* New York: Three Rivers Press; 1998.

13. Shimoff M. *Happy for No Reason: 7 Steps for Being Happy from the Inside Out.* New York: Free Press; 2008.

14. Bandler R. *Using Your Brain for a Change. Neuro-Linguistic Programming.* Moab, UT: Real People Press; 1985.

15. Rosenberg M. *Nonviolent Communication: A Language of Compassion.* Del Mar, CA: PuddleDancer Press; 1999.

16. Boothman N. *How to Make People Like You in 90 Seconds or Less.* New York: Workman; 2000.

17. *The American Heritage Dictionary of the English Language,* 4th ed. Boston: Houghton Mifflin; 2000.

18. Zernike K. Why are there so many single Americans? *New York Times, Week in Review: Ideas and Trends,* January 11, 2007: http://www.nytimes.com/2007/01/21/weekinreview/21zernike.html?pagewanted=2&_r=2. Accessed March 10, 2008.

19. Sobecks NW, Justice AC, Hinze S, et al. When doctors marry doctors: a survey exploring the professional and family lives of young physicians. *Ann Intern Med.* 1999;130:312-319.

20. Feldman R. On the origins of background emotions: From affect synchrony to symbolic expression. *Emotion.* 2007;7(3):601-611.

21. McFarland D. Respiratory Markers of Conversational Interaction. *J Speech Hearing Lang Res.* 2001;44:128-145.

22. Goleman D. *Social Intelligence.* New York: Bantam Books; 2006.

23. Bates AT, Patel TP, Liddle PF. External behavior monitoring mirrors internal behavior monitoring. *J Psychophysiol.* 2005;19(4):281-288.

24. Beebe B, Lachman FM. Representation and internalization in infancy: Three principles of saliency. *Psychoanal Psychol.* 1994;11:127-166.

25. Parten MB. Social participation among preschool children. *J Abnorm Soc Psychol.* 1932;27:243-269.

26. Oracle website: http://www.oracle.com/corporate/press/2007_dec/embedded-vendorshare-idc.html. Accessed January 11, 2008.

27. Feldsteinn M. Blogging as parallel play. *E-literate.* July 5, 2004: http://www.mfeldstein.com/blogging_as_parallel_play/. Accessed January 11, 2008.

28. Boudreax ED, Ary RD, Mandry CV, McCabe B. Determinants of patient satisfaction in a large municipal ED: The role of demographic variables, visit

characteristics and patient perceptions. *Am J Emerg Med.* 2000;18(4):394-400.

29. Carter W, Inui T, Kukull W, Haigh V. Outcome-based doctor-patient interaction analysis: II. Identifying effective provider and patient behavior. *Med Care.* 1982;20:55.

30. Richards T. Who is at the helm on patient journey? *BMJ.* 2007;335(7610):76.

31. Kohn LT, Corrigan JM, Donaldson MS, eds. *To Err is Human: Building a Safer Health System.* Committee on Quality of Health Care in America, Institute of Medicine. Washington, DC: National Academies Press; 1999.

32. Reader TW, Flin R, Cuthbertson BH. Communication skills and error in the intensive care unit. *Curr Opin Crit Care.* 2007;13(6):732-736.

33. Adams J. *Boundary Issues: Using Boundary Intelligence to Get the Intimacy You Want and the Independence You Need in Life, Love, and Work.* Hoboken, NJ: John Wiley & Sons; 2005.

34. Peters K, Kashima Y. From social talk to social action: Shaping the social triad with emotion sharing. *J Pers Soc Psychol.* 2007;93(5):780-797.

35. Anderson C, Keltner D, John OP. Emotional convergence between people over time. *J Pers Soc Psychol.* 2003;84:1054-1068.

36. Gump FF, Kulik JA. Stress, affiliation and emotional contagion. *J Pers Soc Psychol.* 1997;72:305-319.

37. Wyer RS, Budesheim TL, Lambert AJ, Swan S. Person memory and judgment: Pragmatic influences on impressions formed in a social context. *J Pers Soc Psychol.* 1994;66:254-267.

38. DeBono E. *Six Thinking Hats.* Toronto, Canada: MICA Management Resources; 1999.

39. Andreas S, Faulkner C. NLP: *The New Technology of Achievement.* New York: William Morrow; 1994.

40. Angus L, Kagan F. Empathic relational bonds and personal agency in psychotherapy: Implications for psychotherapy supervision, practice and research. *Psychother Theory Res Pract Training.* 2007;44(4):371-377.

41. Lanson SD. Compliance, satisfaction and physician-patient communication. In Bostrom R, ed. *Communication Yearbook 7.* Beverly Hills, CA: Sage; 1983.

42. Wanzer ME, Booth-Butterfield M, Gruber MK. Perceptions of health care providers' communication: Relationships between patient-centered communication and satisfaction. *Health Commun.* 2004;16(3):363-384.

43. Baumeister RF, Leary MR. The need to belong: Desire for interpersonal attachments as a fundamental human motivation. *Psychol Bull.* 1995;117(3):497-529. Accessed March 10, 2008.

44. Bowlby J. *A Secure Base: Parent-Child Attachment and Healthy Human Development.* New York: Basic Books; 1988.

45. Lopez FG, Rice KG. Preliminary development and validation of a measure of relationship authenticity. *J Counsel Psychol.* 2006;53(3):262-371.

46. Elliot AJ, Reis HT. Attachment and exploration in adulthood. *J Pers Soc Psychol.* 2003;85(2):317-331.

47. American Physical Therapy Association. Professionalism in Physical Therapy: Core Values Self Assessment: http://www.apta.org/AM/Template.cfm?Section=Search&section=Leadership&template=/CM/ContentDisplay.cfm&ContentFileID=287. Accessed April 1, 2008.

CHAPTER 9

Effective Communication Through the Generations

"Each new generation is a fresh invasion of savages."

William Hervey Allen (1889–1849),
American author

Chapter Overview

For the first time in history, the workplace includes members of four different generations. The world view of each group is shaped by the unique social events and trends of their early lives, which change through the years. As a result of these differing perspectives, generational differences can arise, potentially resulting in misunderstandings that impair effective communication. This chapter describes the defining characteristics of each generation and their impact on attitudes and expectations related to engaged professionalism. Strategies to promote effective intergenerational communication in the context of PT practice are described and explored.

Disclaimer: The generational characteristics described in this chapter are not intended to stereotype or to suggest that each group will behave in predictable ways. Rather, the collective attributes described reflect behavioral trends, the awareness of which can enhance communication.

Key Terms

Generations

Professionalism

Communication

Introduction: The Relationship of Generational Studies to External Communication

Our study of external communication has been grounded in the context of social intelligence and its components of awareness and skills. As you will discover in this chapter, each generation creates its own social culture. Today's society now features the unique world views of four distinct generations spanning a 100-year age range. As a physical therapist you will interact with each group in several contexts: as a patient, colleague, and teacher. The ability to apply effective communication skills to your interactions with each generational group can be enhanced by awareness of their prominent behaviors and expectations. The following are examples of how generational differences can affect communication:

1. A 60-year-old insurance case manager notes that the quality of written communication from one PT facility has deteriorated in the past month. Several notes have been submitted with spelling errors, poor grammar, and incomplete sentences. This facility has just hired several young new graduates who rely on computer-based documentation.

2. Following complaints from several middle-aged patients, a clinical site feels compelled to rewrite its student intern professional dress code to include "no visible tattoos or facial piercings."

3. A new PT department manager, 35 years old, finds himself in conflict with his 50-year-old supervisor over the latter's elaborate procedures for budget requests. The supervisor feels that these have always worked in the past and is reluctant to make any changes.

In each of these examples, differences in generational norms may contribute to the potential for negative judgments, leading to conflict. Having an understanding of these differences can shift the focus away from subjective evaluations and toward the objective identification of solutions.

"When I Was Your Age..." The Nature of Generational Differences

When it comes to the acknowledgment of intergenerational differences, probably no saying is more exasperating than "When I was your age. . . ." No doubt you have already been on the receiving end of this reproach, usually delivered by someone over the age of 30 and related to some perceived transgression in work ethic, form of dress, or social behavior. Nevertheless, despite the high irritation factor of this admonition, the irony is that in all probability, you too will inflict it upon a young adult at some future point. Such is the nature of generational differences, a timeless societal reality that was described by ancient Greek philosophers such as Plato, Socrates, and Aristotle. One of these (allegedly Aristotle) wrote[1]:

> The children now love luxury. They have bad manners, contempt for
> authority, they show disrespect to their elders. . . . They no longer
> rise when elders enter the room. They contradict their parents,
> chatter before company, gobble up dainties at the table, cross their
> legs, and are tyrants over their teachers.

The term *generation* speaks to a group of individuals who are born at a similar point in history and move through time as a cohort. As each group progresses through its lifespan (particularly the first 15 years), it tends to acquire a shared set of values and attitudes pertaining to the surrounding world. According to Strauss,[2] a new generation arises approximately every 22 years, and each shares elements of a distinct "group personality." Thus far, 18 generations have come and gone through the course of American history, and at any point in time, society is represented by members of as many as six (ranging up to 108 years in age).[2]

Interestingly, Strauss believes that there are four generational types: idealist, reactive, civic, and adaptive, which repeatedly emerge in succession as time evolves. According to Strauss, history is shaped largely by the generation in middle age. This is illustrated by the fact that the average age of all U.S. presidents, during their tenure, is 55.[3] Members of the middle-aged group have typically been in the workforce long enough to assume prominent levels of power in their respective occupational spheres. This prominence then allows them to exert considerable influence in the key societal institutions of government, education, religion, and the military.

The unfolding of historic events also has a profound influence on the cohorts in early adolescence (which Strauss identifies as "coming of age") or young adulthood (which Strauss calls the "rising generation"). The shared attitudes and world view of these younger generations are profoundly shaped by the societal impact of strategies employed by the generation in middle age.

For example, in 2008, the generation in middle age are members of the cohort known as baby boomers (born between 1943 and 1960). During the boomers' tenure as the principal power brokers of our society, members of this "idealist" generation have had a pivotal role in responding to societal events such as terrorism, climate change, and the pressures of a competitive global economy.

In the meantime, members of two younger generations, "reactive" generation X (born between 1961 and 1982) and "civic" millennials (born between 1983 and 2000), are observing the impact of boomer initiatives from different points in their lives. Each of these younger groups will collectively evaluate the boomers' effectiveness in addressing these societal issues. Their resulting perceptions and attitudes will then affect the way they address such challenges when they reach middle age and assume higher levels of power.

Presumably, each generation exercises its influence in ways that are well intended but also a reflection of their collective values and ideals. The rising generation will observe its elders through the lens of its own collective world view and may thus arrive at a different assessment of the boomers' accomplishments.

As an illustration of generationally different attitudes, the boomers tend to be competitive and ambitious, with many placing their careers above other commitments.[2] Observing the impact of such prioritization on health and relationships, many members of generation X have rejected the boomers' single-minded work ethic in favor of a greater life balance.[4] Consequently, a significant difference has evolved between boomers and "Gen Xers" with respect to a desirable level of work investment. The resultant lack of understanding between these two cohorts has led to the boomers' unfortunate characterization of generation X as "slackers," while members of generation X sometimes disdain their elders as "workaholics."

This intergenerational disconnect doesn't stop there. As a rising generation X grapples with the societal effects of middle-age boomer management, the youngest generation, the millennials, are coming of age and forming their own peer personality. Possibly in response to generation X's independent self-reliance, the millennials appear to be among the most socially connected and altruistic generations ever (hence Strauss's "civic" label). As a result, the millennials are also one of the busiest cohorts, with 20% being involved in volunteer work.[5] Furthermore, a 2006 national survey indicated that 61% of this generation feels "personally responsible" for making a difference in the world.[5]

Time will tell how the millennial generation makes its mark on society, but the early indications are promising. However, as history has repeatedly shown, it is likely that our nation's very youngest children, members of the latest generation to emerge, will deconstruct the millennials' approach in favor of their own.

Interestingly, our nation's youngest cohort, which began in 2001, is being called the "homeland generation" (possibly because of the current concerns about national security).[6] Members of this generation will face its own set of societal challenges as their lives progress. According to Strauss's model of repeating generational types (shown in Fig. 9-1), the "homelands" will be an "adaptive" group whose characteristics will be similar to those of the current oldest generation, the veterans.[6]

Generational differences typically emerge as the adolescent generation begins to seek freedom and independence at the same time that their parents grapple with increasing structure and responsibility. Accordingly, we can probably all remember the emerging perceptual shift of our teen years, during which our parents were demoted from "all knowing" to "clueless."

According to Strauss, this evaluative shift in perception is known as "de-authentication,"[2] which contributes to generational conflict. Not surprisingly, the de-authentication process is reciprocal, as evidenced by a reactive adult perceptual shift where the children in their lives change from "perfect darlings" to "selfish teenagers." Needless to say, when de-authentication occurs between generations, communication breaks down and misunderstandings ensue.

Fortunately, this generational divide may resolve to some degree as members of the younger generation assume increasing responsibility in their own lives. As young adults confront the relentless and simultaneous challenges of maintaining satisfying employment, managing long-term relationships, paying bills, and raising children, they may once again rekindle a strong appreciation for their parents. Nevertheless, differences in generational attitudes often persist in other ways, often manifesting themselves in the domains of work and career.

The resolution of generational differences is more likely in the face of understanding and acceptance. Each generation leaves a mixed legacy of both negative and positive societal contributions. Recognizing that all of us are similar, the development of generational differences should foster a greater sense of community among all groups. It is hoped that the information in this chapter will help you to communicate in a way that brings out the best in persons of all age groups.

Implications for Physical Therapy

As physical therapists, one of our major privileges is the ability to work with individuals representing every age group. Each patient brings a marvelous historical and personal perspective to the therapeutic interaction. As you will also learn, each generation shares similar age-related health concerns, which are greatly affected by the prevailing health-care climate. Our sensitivity to each of these factors can help us foster an effective partnership with patients of all ages.

As you will also discover, generational differences are having an unprecedented impact on the professional and workplace spheres of our lives. Each generation has a unique perspective on the appropriate demonstration of professional behaviors.[4] Understanding the nature of these differences can help us adapt in ways that promote collegiality and productive working relationships.

In the following sections, the origin and nature of differences affecting the current generations are discussed. Even more importantly, communication strategies that transcend these differences and promote optimal relationships with members of all generations are explored.

Talking Points/Field Notes

Generational Differences in My Life

These exercises are designed to promote awareness and empathy for the impact of generational differences in your own life. It is hoped that this will motivate you to develop communication strategies that will promote understanding and cooperation with persons of all ages. You are encouraged to reflect on these exercises in your field notes.

1. When did you first become aware of a generational difference between your age group and members of your parent's generation? What were the circumstances? What was the impact?

2. What do you think are some major attitudinal differences between your age group and that of your parents? Which of these do you think has caused the greatest misunderstanding? Which of these do you feel has been helpful?

3. What do you think are the most common criticisms of your generation? What is your response to these?

4. What are your most common criticisms of older generations? If there is a representative of this generation in your class (an older student or faculty member), it would be interesting to have a class discussion about his or her response.

5. What do you admire the most about the older generations? What do you think they admire the most about your generation? (Suggestion: Have this conversation with a member of the older generation!)

6. In which ways does your communication change depending on the generation of the person? How do these changes affect your interaction?

Four Generations of Colleagues and Patients

For the first time in history, the workplace is made up of members of four generations. This is because longer life spans and socioeconomic incentives have compelled increasing numbers of older individuals to remain actively involved in their professions, often well into their seventies. Thus, the composition of today's workplace may include persons who differ in age by as much as 50 years. As we have already noted, each generation has a unique perspective that dictates their attitudes and values related to work, relationships, and, more importantly, their communication. **Table 9-1** illustrates the major elements of each generation.

The Veterans, 1925–1942 (Also Known as Silents or Traditionals): Institutional Architects

Historical Perspective

Members of this generation, known as the veterans, were born during a tumultuous time: the period of the Great Depression, the polio epidemic, and World War II. Facing the hardships related to war, disease, and poverty, veterans were forced to adapt and make do. Many of the men in this generation, along with their fathers, were military veterans who served in World War II and the Korean War.

Thus, steeped in the military culture, members of the veterans' generation learned to follow the chain of command and to respect those in authority. The veterans are a

Table 9–1.	**Characteristics of the Four Predominant Generations (in 2008):**			
Generation	**Years of Birth**	**Representatives**	**Key Societal Events**	**Percent in Workforce**
Veterans	1925–1942	Martin Luther King, Jr Elvis Presley	Great Depression World War II Cold War	6
Boomers	1943–1960	Oprah Winfrey Bill Gates	Vietnam War Civil Rights Era First Man on Moon	40
Gen X	1961–1981	Barack Obama Jodie Foster	AIDS Crisis Corporate Downsizing Computer Age	33
Millennial	1982–2000	Prince William Sasha Cohen	September 11, 2001 Iraq War Hurricane Katrina	21

hard-working generation who built many of our country's leading corporations and institutions. As a result, members of this generation currently control 75% of U.S. financial interests.[7]

The concept of "give and take" is a central tenet of this generation, whose members played a crucial role in the support of our government during the challenges of World War II. In return, the government rewarded their efforts through the GI bill, which gave many returning veterans the opportunity for a college education. Taking advantage of the postwar housing boom of the late 1940s and 1950s, the veterans settled into the nation's first suburbs and forged a standard of living that was substantially higher than that of their parents.[2]

Because of these generous initiatives, the veterans viewed their government as a kindly benefactor who would take care of them. Indeed, federally subsidized education, housing, and hospitals[8,9] created a specialized welfare system that benefited white males in particular.[8] Thus, not only did the government provide members of this generation with homes and education, the Social Security Act of 1935 promised ongoing financial support upon retirement. Having paid into the social security system throughout their lives, the veterans expect to collect on this investment.

The veterans had an instrumental role in the development of major institutions that serve us today, including the PT profession. Under their guidance, our profession began to emerge from its technical underpinnings to a full-fledged health-care discipline with its own body of knowledge. **Figure 9-1** illustrates the growth of the PT profession during the time of the veterans' generation.

Finally, this generation has a strong work ethic, along with a belief in the importance of "paying your dues." They tend to be more on the formal side, and they value loyalty, tradition, and respect. This generation grew up with few technological devices with which to enhance their communication (their primary devices being telephone and typewriter). As a result, they are often extremely articulate with both the spoken and written word, and many were thoroughly schooled in spelling, grammar, and punctuation.

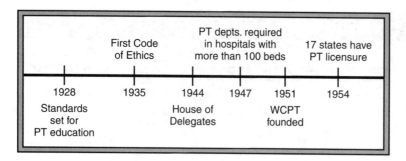

Figure 9–1. The growth of the PT profession during the time of the veterans' generation.

Veterans as Patients

Many members of the veterans' generation are now in their seventies and eighties, reaping the benefits of a sophisticated health-care system that has increased their life span. While many enjoy robust health, research also indicates that the overall quality of life and general health of the 1.4 million surviving veterans who served in the military is lower than that of their nonmilitary peers.[10]

As a whole, adults over the age of 60 also face a higher burden of disease, especially chronic conditions such as arthritis, diabetes, heart disease, and cancer. In 2008, some 70% of adults over the age of 60 had two or more of these chronic conditions.[11] In addition, the National Institute on Aging reported in 2007 that one in seven American adults over age 71 had some type of dementia.[12]

Medicare is the primary health insurance carrier for most Americans over the age of 65. In recent years, however, rising costs have resulted in significant reductions in Medicare spending, shifting the financial burden from government to patient. As a result of these cutbacks, along with the ongoing expenses related to chronic health conditions, many members of the veterans' generation are finding themselves paying increasingly more "out of pocket" for their care. Even those with supplemental insurance may be financially challenged by numerous copays for office visits, medical procedures, and medication. Sadly, this is not what the veterans expected. Because this generation helped to create a health-care system that promoted reasonably priced, widespread access to services, many veterans consider the current managed-care system an affront to their dreams of a benevolent health-care system that would take care of them.

Accordingly, it is important that these patients clearly understand their rights and benefits with respect to their health care. Without such knowledge, they may challenge billing practices and become frustrated with what they consider to be unreasonably high charges. They need clear explanations of what they are being charged for. Furthermore, many veterans are living on limited incomes and thus have to be frugal when it comes to out-of-pocket expenses. It is therefore helpful for them to know what other resources exist—for example, community sources of reduced-cost equipment or assistive devices.

Since many of these patients grew up during the Depression, they learned to do without or did it themselves. They may need encouragement to actively participate in their plan of care, especially if they have never exercised before.

The veterans were the last generation to grow up without computer-based technology, and many of them lack the knowledge and skills to access Internet-based health-care information. A 2005 study by the Pew Internet & American Life Project indicated that only 26% of persons over age 65 go online for information, compared with 84% of those between the ages of 18 and 29.[13] Accordingly, your veteran patients will benefit from clear explanations of their interventions, supported as much as possible by an evidence-based rationale.

Veterans grew up during a paternalistic time of medicine, where physicians and other health-care providers essentially told them what to do. They will need encouragement to take a more partnering role with their health-care providers. Because this generation grew up in an era where respect for authority and good manners were widely reinforced, they may be more comfortable with the use of more formal titles. It is very helpful to ask them how they prefer to be addressed, for example, "Would you prefer that I call you Mr. Smith?" or "How do you prefer to be addressed?"

Many veterans remember a time when physicians made house calls. Thus, they value compassionate personal contact with their health-care providers and use this as a yard-stick of their satisfaction with their care. A 2002 study at the University of Pennsylvania demonstrated that the three most important expectations of elderly patients were a caring practitioner, technical proficiency, and an efficient, warm office atmosphere. Interestingly, many respondents in this study said they would keep going to a caring provider even if they had been misdiagnosed.[14]

Finally, this generation worked hard to create a loving and supportive family environment for their children, many of whom are now returning this kindness to their elderly parents by serving as caregivers. Thus, family education is an important element of PT intervention for these patients.

Despite the challenges they face, this generation is the first to reach their later years at a time when outdated stereotypes of the elderly are losing their hold. Many veterans remain physically active at levels well above those of much younger individuals. (Sixteen women above age 70 finished the Boston Marathon in 2007!)[15]

Toileting Taboo

Beth, a physical therapist at an acute-care hospital, is providing instruction in toilet transfers to her 83-year-old patient Edith Smith in preparation for her discharge home the following day. Edith, who has severe arthritis that has also begun to limit her hand dexterity, has recently had a total hip replacement. Robert, Edith's husband of 58 years, is present. Edith has now completed the transfer with minimal assistance from Beth. Because Edith is having difficulty managing her pants, Beth asks Robert to assist, explaining that she might also need help with wiping. Robert's eyes widen visibly. When Beth asks him if he is all right, Edith manages a nervous giggle and says, "This is a first for us. Each of us has always gone to the bathroom in private."

Questions

1. Is this a generational issue? What values and traditions might be guiding this behavior for Edith and Robert?

2. How might Beth address this issue with Edith and Robert?

3. How does empathy come into play?

4. What other communication approaches might Beth use to help Edith and Robert feel more comfortable?

5. What alternatives might exist?

Clinical Scenario

Talking Points/Field Notes

The Veterans' Generation: Understanding Their Perspectives on Health Care and Communication

The purpose of this interview is to obtain the veterans' generation perspective on the changes they have experienced in health care in the course of their lives. The following questions can be helpful:

1. If you had to describe your earliest memories of health care in one or two sentences, what would you say?

2. What do you think are the biggest positive health-care changes in your adult experience?

3. What changes in health care concern you the most?

4. What are the most important things a health-care professional can do to secure your trust and confidence?

Compare and discuss the results of your interviews. What themes emerge? What can you learn from these interviews to help you communicate more effectively with members of the veterans' generation? Reflect on your observations in your field notes.

Veterans as Colleagues

A tendency toward respectful formality and a preference for face-to-face communication are general characteristics of veterans in the workplace. Veterans enjoy small talk and place great value on collegiality. They tend to place significant emphasis on proper spelling, grammar, and punctuation in written communication. Many veterans are also habituated to respecting the chain of command and the importance of working one's way up in an organization. Thus they may not understand the desires of their younger colleagues to ascend the career ladder quickly, achieving success through merit rather than rank.

Appropriate dress, language, and demeanor are important to them; they may therefore be critical of their more casually dressed younger colleagues. They may be less comfortable with multitasking, preferring to start one project before taking on another.

Despite their traditional approach to work, veterans can be benevolent and inspiring mentors. Their wealth of knowledge and experience, along with their historical perspective, can provide a rich and valuable element to any workplace in which they find themselves.

Communication Resources From the Veteran Age

Many veterans were influenced by Dale Carnegie's 1937 book *How to Win Friends and Influence People*.[16] It gave detailed suggestions for making good first impressions, engaging in enjoyable conversation, and managing conflict. These suggestions have retained their value over the years. Carnegie also wrote numerous other books on workplace communication and established a training institute, which has educated over 7 million persons worldwide.[16]

Micromanaging or Mentoring?

Robert is a 24-year-old new graduate physical therapist who has just taken a position in a clinic that sees many patients with occupational injuries (requiring extensive documentation related to Workers' Compensation claims). The clinic does not use a computer for documentation.

Robert's clinic director is Adam Jenkins, a 75-year-old physical therapist who started his career in the military. Adam greatly enjoys mentoring younger staff and has earned their respect. However, he requires that all new staff submit their handwritten notes to him so that he can check and correct spelling and grammar. Adam is known to return these notes with numerous suggestions. Robert is annoyed with this requirement, particularly because he would rather spend his time treating patients than revising notes. Furthermore, Robert feels that the clinic's efficiency would be greatly enhanced if they could use a computer template for their notes (of course, use of a computer would also allow checking of spelling and grammar).

Questions

1. How might Adam's request be related to his generational perspective?

2. How might Robert address Adam's request?

3. What can Robert learn from Adam in this situation?

4. How might Robert suggest computer documentation to Adam? How might he offer to assist Adam toward the transition to computerized documentation?

Talking Points/Field Notes

The Veterans' Perspective on Communication

Interview a member of the veterans' generation who is still in the workforce. The goal of this interview is to understand his or her perspective on generational communication. The following questions might be helpful:

1. When you were growing up, what was the nature of generational differences between you and your parents/grandparents? Which issues were prevalent?

2. What key experiences contributed to your attitudes about education and work?

3. How have these attitudes affected your life and work?

4. How do you think communication has changed in your lifetime? What societal changes have affected this the most?

5. What are the most important things younger generations can learn about effective communication?

6. What are some ways to enhance communication between colleagues of different generations?

Compare and discuss the results of your interviews. Were there any prevalent themes? Use the results of your interview to compile a list of suggestions for optimizing communication with the veterans' generation. Reflect on your observations in your field notes.

The Boomers 1943 to 1960: Consensus Builders

Historical Perspective

Coming of age in a time of tremendous economic prosperity and guided by diligent, hard-working parents, the 79 million members of the "baby boom" generation were told that all things were possible. Many boomers grew up in an almost surreally idyllic suburban environment, free from today's prevalent concerns about child kidnapping and street crime. The majority of young boomers lived in predominately two-parent homes where they where heavily nurtured, particularly by their mothers. With the majority of mothers staying at home to raise their families, only 2% of boomers attended institutional day care.[2]

During their elementary school years, the boomers benefited from the support and energetic guidance of their veteran-generation teachers. Many of these educators were intelligent women who could easily have flourished in other professional careers had these been more welcoming to their gender. Not wanting the same limitations for their female students, these teachers encouraged boomer girls toward ongoing education and the attainment of career success. As a result, more boomer women than ever before entered the workforce with college degrees, where they have outearned their veteran-generation counterparts.[17]

As a result of their solicitous parenting and the continuous affirmation of their potential to change the world, the boomers developed a grand idealism along with a preoccupation with self-actualization. Little did they realize that these attributes would result in significant conflict with their elders during their teens and early adulthood, as the ordered predictability of their childhood gave way to the turbulent social atmosphere of the early 1960s.

The historic events of the 1960s began with the assassination of John F. Kennedy in 1963, the first to be captured on film and aired relentlessly on national television. The middle years brought the Vietnam War, along with simmering racial tensions that erupted into fiery street riots and violent antiwar protests in Detroit and Chicago. Then, just when it seemed like the country might gain its equilibrium, the 1960s came to a heartbreaking end with the assassinations of Martin Luther King Jr. and Robert Kennedy within 2 months of each other in 1968.

Observing this senseless rampage, the boomers found themselves becoming increasingly alienated from their elders, which they expressed through rebellious denunciations of the veteran "establishment."

While the college campuses of the veteran generation were genteel and sedate, those of the boomers became national theaters for raucous antiwar demonstrations. A tragic culmination of these occurred at Kent State University in 1970, where National Guardsmen who were called in to halt such a demonstration killed four students.

All of this social turmoil transformed the boomers from well-behaved kids to "anti-establishment" adults, who renounced their parents' values and sought their identity through contentious gatherings such as the 1967 "Summer of Love" and the 1969 Woodstock Music Festival.

To further demonstrate their disaffection, young boomers also challenged societal proscriptions about sexual behavior and preached a new gospel of free love. This attitudinal shift was conveniently facilitated by the development of the first FDA-approved birth control pill in 1960 and the 1973 *Roe versus Wade* decision legalizing abortion.[18]

In the 1970s and 1980s, things seemed to quiet down for the boomers as the Vietnam War ended and a new wave of conservatism emerged within the ranks of national leadership (heralded by Presidents Nixon, Ford, and Reagan). Boomers finished college and entered the workforce, shifting their focus inward and looking for the sense of spiritual connection that had evaded them in their years of social agitation.

As adults in the workforce, the boomers have retained their idealism and zeal for self-realization, with varied results. On one hand, they are competitive and hard-driven for career success; on the other, their passion for "feel good" consensus can bog down these hard-driven efforts.

Nevertheless, the boomers have helped to shape many of the key social justice policies that are in place today. These include the Equal Employment Opportunity Act (1972),[19] the American Hospital Association Patient Bill of Rights (1973),[20] and the Education for All Handicapped Children Act (1975).[21] These boomer initiatives have had significant societal benefits, but according to their critics, they have also produced a tangle of bureaucracy that obscures their effectiveness.

Contributions to the Physical Therapy Profession During the Time of the Boomer Generation

Despite their sometimes misdirected idealism, the boomers' passion for personal and societal betterment, along with their sheer numbers (almost 80 million), has placed them at the "focal point for American society as a whole."[2] With such a sense of self-importance, it is no surprise that boomers tend to be image-conscious. John Molloy's 1975 book *Dress for Success* (which was updated in 1988) set the standards for Boomer workplace attire.[22]

Boomers also place high value on their relationships. Although technological forms of communication have been a consistent part of their work lives, they grew up largely without this and thus tend to prefer face-to-face dialogue. Accordingly, a common boomer criticism of their younger peers is that their communication skills have suffered owing to their reliance on impersonal technological methods.[2]

With their inclinations toward team building and decision making through consensus, boomers enjoy camaraderie and small talk. The boomers have made significant contributions to the PT profession, as shown in **Figure 9-2**.

Boomers as Patients

Because of their large numbers, aging boomers are beginning to make an unprecedented impact on the health-care industry as they require increasing services. Thus their needs and concerns have been surveyed and analyzed more than those of any other generation.[2]

These surveys reflect a highly diverse group (in terms of educational level, race, and socioeconomic status) whose health-care needs are likely to be equally complex.

Figure 9-2. Changes in PT profession during the time of the boomer generation.

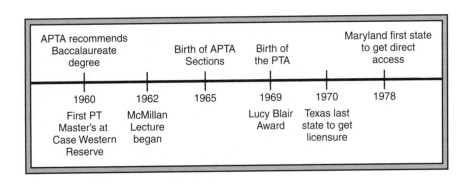

The boomers' hard-driving work ethic has taken its toll on the health of many of its members. According to the American Association of Retired Persons 2004 "Boomers at Midlife" survey,[23] only 30% are "very satisfied with their physical health," and 20% state that their physical health is the one thing they would most like to change. Having spent the bulk of their adulthood pursuing career success, many boomers admit to not having enough time for exercise or the preparation of healthy meals.

As a group, there appears to be a direct relationship between the boomers' education, socioeconomic status, and perceived quality of life. Boomers with college degrees and a good standard of living are more likely to be satisfied in both domains. They are also more confident of their ability to maintain optimal health than their less educated and poorer counterparts.[23]

The first boomers will turn 65 in 2111. By 2030, the number of adults over age 65 in the United States will double, reaching 20% of the entire population. This burgeoning elderly population will require services for which our current health-care system is ill prepared.

In 2008, the Institute of Medicine (IOM) published *Retooling for an Aging America: Building the Health Care Workforce.*[24] This report makes three prominent recommendations for the health-care system: (1) increasing the number of geriatric specialists across all health-care disciplines, (2) improving recruitment and retention of geriatric health-care specialists, and (3) improving cost-effective care.

The IOM report has significant implications for physical therapists. Although geriatrics has long been a recognized specialty area in our profession, physical therapists will see increasing numbers of geriatric patients in all settings and thus must be knowledgeable about their needs. In short, you can expect to see boomers and their older cohorts wherever you practice.

As older adults, the boomers retain much of their idealism and will thus have high expectations for their medical care. Awareness of their needs, in addition to their generational attitudes, will thus be essential if we are to meet these expectations.

A 2007 report by the American Hospital Association[25] outlines several facts pertaining to the boomer's expected health-care needs. Chronic conditions such as diabetes, arthritis, and hypertension are expected to affect at least 60%, and over 30% will be overweight. Total knee replacements will increase by a factor of eight, along with other orthopedic procedures to maintain the joints of one of the most physically active generations to date.

As patients, boomers are generally wise consumers; many will eagerly research their conditions and arrive at their appointments bearing articles about medications and treatment approaches. They are more comfortable with managed care but will also challenge it in order to get the best value for their dollar. Accordingly, boomers will want to know all of their options, along with the evidence for each, before making a decision. Many will demand an equal partnership with their health-care providers, rejecting those who take a paternalistic, "doctor knows best" approach.

Unlike the veterans, who placed their trust mostly in traditional approaches to health care, 70% of boomers have tried alternative therapies.[25] Thus you may need to coordinate your care with providers from a broader spectrum of disciplines.

Boomers have also grown up during a time of ongoing public education about the importance of maintaining good lifestyle habits for optimal health. Many are actively pursuing healthy lifestyles and will be eager to work with their health-care team to maintain these. Boomers may also be more interested in exploring preventive options for health maintenance.

Like the veterans, boomers will seek health practitioners who are willing to take the time to engage in face-to-face dialogue. If they find a practitioner whom they like, they are likely to maintain an ongoing relationship through their remaining years. Finally, boomers are likely to be less formal and more understanding of generational differences provided that they are treated with genuine care.

In summary, the boomers will present health-care practitioners with an engaging and interesting challenge, which will likely reshape the face of health care. In turn, their presence in the health-care system is likely to result in continued opportunities for our profession.

Clinical Scenario

New Age Nightmare?

Justin is a therapist in an outpatient clinic in a small town that has an active "new age" community. He is evaluating Mary, 59 years old, who has just been referred for cardiac rehabilitation following a mild myocardial infarction (MI) and balloon angioplasty. Mary is 30 pounds overweight, with metabolic syndrome and mild hypertension. She lives with her husband, who is also overweight.

When Justin discusses an intervention plan consisting of aerobic exercise, Mary is resistant. She states that her new age "crystal healer" told her that her MI was partially the result of a blockage in her "heart center" and that she needed "nurturing touch" to promote her healing process. Mary thus asks that Justin perform massage as a part of her treatment. She shows Justin an article from the Internet that supports the use of massage in reducing stress after heart surgery. Mary also states that her insurance will cover therapeutic massage from a licensed physical therapist, which will enable her to use her money to join the local health club where she plans to take aerobics classes.

Justin's clinic has stringent productivity guidelines that typically involve seeing between two and four patients per hour.

Questions

1. How might Justin respond to Mary's request for massage? Is it a reasonable one?

2. Should Justin support Mary's desire to join a health club for her exercise?

3. How might Justin reconcile the productivity guidelines of his clinic with Mary's request?

4. What alternatives might exist? What role might Mary's husband play in her treatment?

Talking Points/Field Notes

The Boomer Generation: Understanding Its Perspectives on Health Care and Communication

The purpose of this interview is to obtain the boomer generation's perspective on the changes they have experienced in health care in the course of their lives. The following questions can be helpful:

1. If you had to describe your earliest memories of health care in one or two sentences, what would you say?

2. What do you think are the biggest positive health-care changes in your adult experience?

3. What changes in health care concern you the most?

4. What are the most important things a health-care professional can do to secure your trust and confidence?

Compare and discuss the results of your interviews. What themes emerge? What can you learn from these interviews to help you communicate more effectively with members of the boomer generation? Reflect on your observations in your field notes.

Boomers as Colleagues

Boomers currently comprise the largest generational group in the workforce (45%), driving up the average age for many professions. For example, the American Association of Colleges of Nursing reports that 40% of all U.S. nurses will be over age 50 by 2010.[26] Boomer physical therapists have also increased the age of the average practitioner in our profession to 42. In addition, the number of physical therapists over the age of 50 has doubled since 1999.[27]

The trend toward an aging workforce is expected to continue in the coming decades as retirement benefits become less certain. As of 2006, over 50% of boomers felt that they did not have enough money to retire comfortably at age 65 (at which point it is estimated that they will need at least $2 million in savings to support them for the remaining 20 to 25 years of their projected lives). Consequently, 80% of boomers plan to work past this age.[28]

Therefore you are virtually certain to have boomer colleagues and supervisors in your workplace, and that is likely to be an advantage. As a whole, they are very satisfied with their work lives (40%), with many returning to school and changing careers in order to maintain their engagement.[23] Because work satisfaction is important to them, they are likely to contribute to the high morale and empowerment of their colleagues.

For boomers, work is a large measure of self-worth. Like their parents, they have a strong work ethic but want to accomplish something of value that will create a legacy. Thus many of them retain high levels of ambition and competitiveness and greatly appreciate being recognized for their efforts. Their devotion to work is likely to be a source of conflict, with their younger colleagues desiring a better work-life balance. Boomers may also be more formal in terms of workplace dress, as they view this as an observable measure of professionalism. Because they value consensus, they may also frustrate their independent younger colleagues who value efficiency over "talking things out."

Experienced boomers can be valuable mentors, as they tend to be eager to teach what they know. Many are eager lifelong learners who enjoy demonstrating their knowledge. They enjoy team building and small talk and may become frustrated with younger colleagues who choose technological approaches over more personal ones.

Finally, boomers want to be seen as inclusive but fair and impartial. This has spawned a propensity toward the development of well-intended "politically correct" initiatives, regulated through sometimes cumbersome bureaucratic layers.

Communication Resources from the Boomer Age

Given the boomers' preoccupation with self-actualization and peak performance, it is no accident that the 1970s and 1980s saw an explosion of "self-help" books (which were promoted by a cadre of author "gurus"). These books were meant to inspire excellence among young boomers entering the workforce. Not surprisingly, they all contain suggestions for optimizing communication. *The Greatest Salesman in the World* (1968) by Og Mandino[29] uses a Christianity-based, parable-like style to promote effective internal and external success. This theme had wide appeal to many boomers' spirituality and idealism. A popular quotation from Mandino—"Love doesn't sit there like a stone, it has to be made, like bread: remade all the time, made new"[30]—is an example of the appropriation of gospel-like themes to the cause of self-improvement.

The One-Minute Manager (1982) by Ken Blanchard (a psychologist) and Spencer Johnson (a physician)[31] became a bible for new boomer managers during the 1980s and 1990s. This book promotes the value of setting clear goals and delivering specific praise and reprimands to employees. The books' buzz term "catch them doing something right" spoke to the boomers' emphasis on recognition.

A Difference in Perspective

Kelsey and Brian are young physical therapists working in a federally funded clinic for children with developmental disabilities. Kelsey and Brian like to decorate the walls of their examining room with their patients' artwork. They believe that this helps to create a cozy atmosphere that puts patients and families at ease.

The clinic has just hired a new administrator, Joan, who has 30 years of experience in similar positions. During her first week at the clinic, Joan visits Kelsey and Brian in their examining room. Upon seeing the artwork on the walls, she informs them that it must be removed because it might offend parents whose children are too disabled to draw.

Questions

1. What issues might be behind Joan's concern with the drawings? How can Kelsey and Brian acknowledge these concerns in a supportive manner?

2. How might Kelsey and Brian discuss their perspective (that the drawings put families at ease) in a way that might appeal to Joan's ideals?

3. How might Kelsey and Brian negotiate a solution that honors all perspectives?

Talking Points/Field Notes

The Boomer Perspective on Communication

Interview a member of the boomer generation. The goal of this interview is to understand their perspective about generational communication. The following questions might be helpful:

1. When you were growing up, what was the nature of generational differences between you and your parents/grandparents? Which issues were prevalent?

2. Which key experiences contributed to your attitudes about education and work?

3. How have these attitudes affected your life and work?

4. How do you think communication has changed in your lifetime? What societal changes have affected this the most?

5. What are the most important things younger generations can learn about effective communication?

6. What are some ways to enhance communication between colleagues of different generations?

Compare and discuss the results of your interviews. Were there any prevalent themes? Use the results of your interview results to compile a list of suggestions for optimizing communication with the members of the boomer generation. Reflect on your observations in your field notes.

Generation X , 1961–1981 (Also Known as the 13th Generation): Masters of Change

Historical Perspective

Generation X, comprising 49 million members, is the smallest of the four generational groups.[32]

Parented largely by younger veterans and older boomers, generation X children were born in one of the most "blatantly antichild phases in history,"[2] where many were considered "obstacles to their parents' self-exploration."[33] Strauss supports these contentions, stating that no other generation has been affected more by divorce.[2]

Accordingly, almost half of all generation X children were raised in one-parent families. In addition, as more women entered the workforce in the 1970s and 1980s, their absence from the home spawned the term *latchkey child* to describe the growing numbers of children who came home to an empty house after school.

Left alone without supervision, with many living in unstable families, some teenagers of generation X succumbed to depression. Strauss states that during the 1980s, the suicide rate among children was the highest ever recorded.[2]

On the positive side, many members of generation X became fiercely independent and resourceful, learning to take care of themselves in the absence of family support. The first generation to grow up with the widespread use of technology, they amused themselves with electronic entertainment such as Music Television (MTV) and Pac Man video games. As computers became more prominent, young Gen Xers were among the first to develop a high level of skill, spawning the first "techno geeks," who eventually became the pioneer employees in the exploding field of information technology.

In the face of the many contradictions of their time (e.g., the sexual revolution, leading to the emergence of the AIDS epidemic), Gen Xers also became independent thinkers who viewed the events around them with growing cynicism. Their attitudes about work were profoundly affected when their parents' zealous efforts were rewarded by the layoffs that characterized the 1980s' round of corporate downsizing. In addition, as the cost of living rose (with interest on home mortgages reaching 15% in 1981), young Gen Xers watched in dismay as their hard-working parents struggled to make ends meet. By the time they had grown to young adulthood, many Gen Xers found that they could not afford to buy their own homes; by 1990, some 75% of young men between the ages of 18 and 24 were still living with their parents.[2] A recent survey of the financial status of this generation indicates that 47% live from paycheck to paycheck, with nothing left for savings.[34]

Despite these challenges, generation X is the most educated generation in American history thus far, with 60% of its members having attended college and 30% having a bachelor's degree. Interestingly, generation X is also the first generation whose women outnumber men in terms of college degrees.[33]

Thus, well educated, independent, and rejecting the "work as a reflection of worth" ideology of their parents, members of generation X tend to seek balance and autonomy in their lives. Their experiences have taught them the importance being prepared, educated, and flexible. They are action-driven and intolerant of bureaucracy. Most of all, they are willing to think beyond convention, unafraid to take risks or try new approaches. As they move toward becoming the generation in power, they will have a profound societal influence as they bring their collective values to bear. **Figure 9-3** shows the continued evolution of the PT profession during the time of generation X.

Figure 9–3. Major changes in the PT profession during the time of generation X.

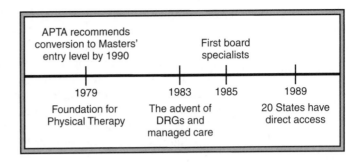

Gen Xers as Patients

As the generation ascending to power, the Xers are confronting adult responsibilities during a period of significant economic downturn. The impact of this is widespread, affecting this generation in several important ways related to their overall health.

First of all, they are more likely than their boomer colleagues (who will soon have Medicare benefits) to lack adequate health insurance, a trend that has steadily worsened in the face of rising health-care costs and decreasing employer health-care coverage. According to the 2007 Kaiser Foundation annual report on Americans without health insurance,[35] 47 million Americans were uninsured, a figure representing 18% of the total nonelderly population (those under age 65) and an increase of 2 million in just 1 year.

A major contributing factor to this rising statistic is an increasing number of employers who have either discontinued or dramatically increased the cost of health care benefits for their employees. Lack of employer-sponsored health insurance is particularly devastating for adults between the ages of 19 and 64, who do not typically qualify for government-subsidized health care. These programs currently include Medicare coverage for the elderly and Medicaid; these provide coverage for nonelderly disabled adults and about 25% of all indigent children.

No government health insurance programs exist for adults between the ages of 19 and 64; some 80% of all uninsured adults fall into this age range. Furthermore, employers are not required to provide health-care benefits to their workers, and 70% of Americans without health insurance are engaged in full-time employment. Individuals in low-paying technical jobs (or those not requiring a college degree) are most likely to be uninsured. However, even in higher-paying jobs where health insurance is offered, some workers may not be able to afford their share of the premium, which can be several hundred dollars per month. As a result, in 2007, some 40% of the uninsured population came from households earning $50,000 or more yearly.[36]

The impact of inadequate health insurance is of particular concern to the nation's 40 million Gen Xers, all of whom are entrenched in the early to middle parts of their careers and acquiring the typical (and increasingly expensive) trappings of the American dream. As members of this generation contend with rising health-care costs against the gloomy backdrop of a depressed national economy, financial stress abounds. Sadly, much of this stress is related to difficulties paying medical bills. A recent report by the Commonwealth Fund[37] explored these difficulties and reported that 21% of working-age adults, both insured and uninsured, are paying off accrued medical debt, with 44% owing $2,000 or more.

It is therefore likely that compared with their older cohorts, Gen Xers will be more cost-conscious consumers of medical care, selecting only the most critical interventions. As a result, you may see patients whose financial situations compel them to forego treatment of chronic health conditions such as diabetes or hypertension. According to the

Commonwealth report, 18% of insured adults and 59% of those without insurance chose not to fill a prescription related to the management of a chronic condition.

The issue of chronic health conditions affects all Americans, and generation X is no exception. Gen Xers are currently the generation with the fastest-increasing rates of obesity. If this trend continues, it is predicted that 75% of Americans will be obese or overweight by 2015.[38]

A recent report on the health habits of the American workforce singled out Gen Xers as being the most likely to eat unhealthy snacks at work and to engage in a sedentary lifestyle that precludes regular exercise. Other studies of generation X have suggested that they are more likely than their older cohorts to suffer from stress-related complaints such as depression and anxiety.[39]

Along with their younger millennial cohort, Gen Xers are also more likely to take sick days for "mental health" reasons and to have difficulties with eating disorders and substance abuse.[39] Perhaps these health concerns are related to the challenges of living in stressful times, and it will thus be important to identify the nature your of patients' particular challenges in your future practice.

Generation X has also shown that they are survivors who have a strong sense of their priorities. They are less likely to tolerate what they view as time-wasting bureaucratic processes such as insurance paperwork or extensive medical intake forms. You will need to be able to provide clear and sensible explanations for these, along with anything related to your plan of care. On the positive side, because of their higher levels of education and their pursuit of life balance, your generation X patients may also be committed to their long-term health and thus willing to undertake advantageous lifestyle changes.

Gen Xers are a computer-savvy group likely to demand evidence for your suggested interventions, particularly if their financial situations demand frugality. They may also develop their own unique approaches to their treatments, working them in as best as possible into the context of their busy lives. In other words, these patients are unlikely to have time for extensive exercise programs, especially if they lack functional context.

Finally, because of their stressful lifestyles, Gen Xers stand to benefit significantly from programs related to health promotion. Physical therapists are in a prime position to play a crucial role in their quality of life through the design of programs related to fitness, weight control, and stress reduction. It is likely that the exercise programs of the future will also incorporate technology, enabling our patients to exercise with computer-generated images, pacing, and feedback.

A Difference in Perspectives

Clinical Scenario

Garrett is a 26-year-old physical therapist in a busy outpatient facility. He has just greeted his new patient, 37-year-old Jake Peters. Jake, a trucker, is being referred to PT after a minor work-related road accident that resulted in a back injury.

Garrett first asks Jake to complete the facility's medical intake form. Jake protests, stating that paperwork is a "bureaucratic waste of time" and that Garrett should have gotten his medical record from the referring physician. When Garrett politely repeats the request, Jake grudgingly complies, doing little to hide his irritation.

When Garrett reviews the intake form, he notes that "hypertension" is checked among the list of chronic conditions. Garrett then asks Jake if he is taking antihypertensive medications, and Jake embarrassedly admits that he is not because of their expense. Garrett then asks to take Jake's blood pressure, and again Jake is resistant, stating "I'm here for my back, not my blood pressure!" However, Jake's blood pressure turns out to be 210/150.

Garrett tells Jake that his blood pressure is dangerously high and that he therefore cannot be evaluated. Garrett also tells Jake that he must immediately go to the nearest hospital emergency department. Upon hearing this news, Jake becomes angry, stating that he feels fine and that the visit to the emergency department is going to cost him money he doesn't have.

Questions

Throughout this scenario, Garrett and Jake demonstrate differing perspectives that are likely in impact their therapeutic partnership. Jake appears to have significant concerns about his financial situation. In addition, he exhibits irritability and impatience toward activities that he considers irrelevant or time-wasting. These issues may arise with your generation X patients.

1. How might Garrett explain to Jake the significance of his elevated blood pressure, along with the potential consequences of leaving it untreated? How might Garrett also explain his decision to withhold the examination?

2. How might Garrett express empathy to Jake related to financial concerns about his medication?

3. What information will Garrett need in terms of Jake's insurance situation, particularly in light of Jake's financial concerns?

4. What responsibility does a physical therapist have in terms of knowing about patients' insurance coverage? What responsibility does the physical therapist have in terms of educating patients about the limits of their insurance company's services? For example, many insurance companies will authorize only a set number of PT sessions.

5. How should Garrett proceed with respect to scheduling a follow-up visit with Jake?

6. Should Jake not have any medical insurance, what are Jake's options?

Talking Points/Field Notes

Generation X: Understanding Its Perspectives on Health Care and Communication

The purpose of this interview is to obtain generation X's perspective about the changes they have experienced in health care in the course of their lives. The following questions can be helpful:

1. If you had to describe your earliest memories of health care in one or two sentences, what would you say?

2. What do you think are the biggest positive health-care changes in your adult experience?

3. What changes in health care concern you the most?

4. What are the most important things a health-care professional can do to secure your trust and confidence?

Compare and discuss the results of your interviews. What themes emerge? What can you learn from these interviews to help you communicate more effectively with members of generation X? Reflect on your observations in your field notes.

Gen Xers as Colleagues

As the generational group moving toward the assumption of power, Gen Xers currently comprise 30% of the workforce, a number that will continue to increase as their older cohorts retire. As they move toward dominance in the workplace, they are likely to reshape its environment according to their own values.

A major difference between Gen Xers and their older cohorts is the Xer's rejection of time- or loyalty-based career advancement. Rather, this group values education and preparation as the strongest measures of merit. Furthermore, while their older cohorts tend to remain for many years in a single career and even in a single setting, the average Gen Xer is likely to have 10 to 12 jobs during his or her life and up to four different careers.[33] Gen Xers are mostly likely to leave jobs where there is limited potential for advancement, poor treatment from managers, or a stressful environment.[33]

Of all the generations in the workforce, Gen Xers are most comfortable with change. This is evidenced by the fact that they created 70% of the start-up companies in the 1990s.[39] Furthermore, their creativity, independence, and technological expertise make them ideal leaders in the implementation of new ideas. Their comfort with technology often positions them to make related changes that increase efficiency and market visibility.

Although they are known for their independence, Gen Xers are also comfortable working in teams, as long as their opinions are heard and their contributions sincerely acknowledged. This desire for acknowledgment was poignantly summarized by one Gen Xer who said "Create a team. Give us the family we never had."[39]

Work does not equal worth for this cohort, as it does for the older cohorts. Instead, Gen Xers place a high value on efficiency, so that they can attend to other aspects of their lives. As a result, they are unlikely to share in their boomer colleagues' enthusiasm for long, face-to-face "let's talk it out" meetings.

Gen Xers thrive on support, feedback, and encouragement, but they dislike being micromanaged or having their ideas deflected by false promises or fear of change. They are also likely to challenge any directive that is justified purely by "That's how we have always done it" or "Because I said so."[39]

The Gen Xers' tendency to question the rationale of decisions and policies is not disrespectful (as it is sometimes interpreted to be by their older colleagues) but rather from a genuine need to understand how these affect their contributions.

Because Gen Xers prize life balance, they want their work to be enjoyable and even fun. "Casual Fridays" are their invention. However, when the workday is done, they are likely to be off and running to their next activity.

In contrast to many of their parents, Gen Xers are proving to be highly involved with their families; many are simultaneously caring for elderly parents and young children. Thus they may seek employment situations that permit flexible work hours or even the option to work at home periodically.

Gen Xers are less formal and less impressed by titles and power players, especially if the latter are less than competent. They value accountability but are also quick to forgive misunderstandings if this favor is returned.

Despite Gen Xer's often maverick perspective and their unfortunate "slacker" label, they show considerable promise in the workforce and have already had a significant impact on the PT profession. Gen Xers currently make up the age group with the highest membership in the American Physical Therapy Association (APTA) (15%, compared with 10% for boomers and 2% for millennials).[4]

*Clinical Scenario*

A Question of Balance

Julie, age 36, has just completed her Ph.D. and accepted her first PT faculty position. She will be the youngest of her five colleagues, the rest of whom are in their late forties and early fifties. Julie is intelligent and eager to learn. She has also worked hard to balance her numerous responsibilities, being a single mother with two young children. She is involved in many of their school activities and is the "den mother" to her daughter's Brownie troop.

When her department chair distributes the schedule for the fall semester, Julie is dismayed to see that the department faculty meetings are scheduled for 5 p.m. on the night of her daughter's Brownie meetings. As Julie talks more to her colleagues, she learns that they stay late most evenings and often arrive at work as early as 7 a.m. In addition, all of them maintain an uninterrupted open-door policy whereby students may stop by anytime to address concerns or even just to chat.

While Julie has no problems working long hours, she needs flexibility in order to spend time with her young family. Because of these demands, Julie must "work smart," which means limiting distractions in preparing for class. Julie feels torn, because as the newest member of the faculty, she doesn't want her colleagues to view her as a poor team player or, even worse, a "generation X slacker." She also appreciates their tremendous enthusiasm and wants to learn from them.

Questions

1. How might you describe the work culture of Julie's department? How might Julie begin to explore ways of working within this culture while maintaining the balance she so desires?

2. How might Gen Xer Julie build camaraderie with her boomer colleagues?

3. What might Julie have to offer her colleagues? What might they have to offer her?

Talking Points/Field Notes

Understanding the Generation X Perspective on Communication

Interview a member of generation X who is in the workforce. The goal of this interview is to understand his or her perspective on intergenerational communication. The following questions might be helpful:

1. When you were growing up, what was the nature of generational differences between you and your parents/grandparents? Which issues were prevalent?

2. Which key experiences contributed to your attitudes about education and work?

3. How have these attitudes affected your life and work?

4. How do you think communication has changed in your lifetime? What societal changes have affected this the most?

5. What are the most important things younger generations can learn about effective communication?

6. What are some ways to enhance communication between colleagues of different generations?

Compare and discuss the results of your interviews. Were there any prevalent themes? Use the results of your interviews to compile a list of suggestions for optimizing communication with members of generation X. Reflect on your observations in your field notes.

Communication Resources from the Age of Generation X

As a generation characterized by pragmatism, independence, and the pursuit of career expertise, this cohort has embraced communication resources that promote these values. Among these is motivational guru Anthony Robbins, whose book *Awaken the Giant Within* explores internal communication strategies (which he calls "transformational vocabulary") that facilitate self-efficacy over every aspect of one's life.[40] Although the fast-paced, "sound bite" approach of this book has earned Robbins a fair amount of criticism, he nonetheless has shown the ability to effectively translate previously little known concepts of neurolinguistic programming (NLP), such as empowering self-talk, for a broad public audience. A masterful public speaker, Robbins also has an effusive enthusiasm, which generates attention and attracts proponents of his ideas.

Another book focusing on the development of empowering internal communication is Steven Covey's *The 7 Habits of Highly Effective People*.[41] As an experienced veteran with many years in the business community, Covey forged a connection with his younger cohorts, and perhaps generation X in particular, by promoting the importance of an independent character ethic as the first step in personal success. Accordingly, the first three of his seven habits pertain to having self-awareness, ordering priorities for personal success, and formulating goals. The remaining goals build on the first and lead the reader toward interdependence and the ability to work effectively with others. The seven habits appear to include concepts from emotional intelligence and NLP as well as positive psychology, all of which, as we have discussed, have a significant impact on internal and external communication. The widespread popularity of both books is a telling affirmation of the value of these concepts in life success, regardless of how different authors may deliver them.

Millennials, 1982 to 2000*: The Great Connectors, or the Next Hero Generation

Historical Perspective

Tolerant. Diverse. Optimistic. Engaged. Enter the millennial generation. Each of these speak to what is likely to be the largest cohort ever (estimated between 83 and 90 million),[42,43] who, like the boomers, will become the societal focal point at every stage of their lives. Although some of them have yet to reach high school, collectively they have already made a substantial impact in key societal areas. They are more politically active than their older cohorts, as evidenced by their 49% voter turnout in the 2004 elections.[43] Because this generation is showing every indication of being among the most civic-minded ever to emerge in American history, it is expected that their impact will reshape every sphere of society.

Millennials will likely replace generation X as the most educated generation. Members of this cohort are attending college at the highest rate of all generations thus far, with 57% selecting their academic institutions on the basis of academic reputation.[44]

The millennials have already reordered the conventional racial demographic of the United States. They are the most diverse generation, with almost 40% belonging to a minority group; 18% are Hispanic. According to 2006 census data, the remainder are non-Hispanic whites (62%), blacks (14%), and Asians (5%).

As a result of this diversity, the millennials lack many of their parents' judgments about race. Accordingly, the 2003 Pew Gen Next study reported that 89% of millennials agreed

---

*There does not appear to be agreement on the actual year span of this generation, with some sources defining it as early 1978–1996.[43] Strauss and Howe[2] determined 1982 as the start of the Millennial Generation, but because their book was published in 1991, they did not define its end. This text will use the span identified by Lancaster and Stillman.[44]

with the statement that "it is all right for blacks and whites to date each other" and 60% reported actually having done so.[45]

The Pew report also indicated that millennials as a group have similarly tolerant attitudes to other related issues, including gender equity and gay marriage. Nevertheless, perhaps as result of a childhood overshadowed by the AIDS epidemic (which led to school programs emphasizing sexual abstinence and drug abuse resistance), the millennials are also more avoidant of these high-risk behaviors.

Despite their general characterization as optimistic and confident of their ability to effect positive change in all their spheres of influence, the millennials lived out their childhoods amid the disenchanting years of the Oklahoma bombing, the Columbine shootings, and the 9/11 terrorist attacks. Nevertheless, a 2007 Pew report found that they are the most optimistic of all generations, with 84% stating that their lives are excellent or good.[45]

Perhaps the millennials' optimism was a result of the solicitous protection of their boomer and generation X parents. Each of these older generations, once having assumed the responsibility of parenthood, devoted their full attention and resources to the careful nurturing and support of their offspring. But ironically, they did so for entirely different reasons. The boomers, who were largely raised in the tranquil environment of a suburban utopia, sought to recreate a similarly affirming experience for their children.

In contrast, many Gen Xers sought instead to provide the stability, empowerment, and sense of community that were denied them in their formative years. Despite these differences, both parent groups have insinuated themselves into the lives of their children in ways that previous generations would have considered unnecessary at best ("In my days, kids were kids," said one veteran father) and intrusive at worst ("If my parents would have shown up at one of my baseball games, I would have been *mortified*.").

Because of their attendance at all the little events, some of which were engineered entirely for their benefit (e.g., kindergarten graduation ceremonies, complete with little mortarboards), the millennials' parents have become collectively known as the "helicopters."

The renewed enthusiasm and concern for the welfare of the nation's children that began in the late 1980s was a dramatic contrast to the prevalent "antichild" attitudes of the previous two decades. Millennial children were treated as precious commodities, protected at every turn. Beginning with their births, ubiquitous "Baby on Board" stickers adorned their parents' cars, loudly (and proudly) exhorting other drivers to be mindful of the priceless human cargo within.

When the millennials ventured out of their cribs, parental fear of kidnapping prompted the careful arrangement of play dates, which were supervised in an unbroken line of sight. As preoccupation with the growing millennials usurped their parents' energies (as well as the contents of their wallets), commercial entities took notice. For example, the movie industry, which in previous decades had limited the availability of children's fare largely to the annual Disney release, burgeoned with smart and creative G-rated films. Offerings such as *Shrek, Antz,* and *Chicken Little* were peppered with catchy boomer-era music and clever double entendres that made them truly enjoyable for millennial children *and* their parents. Parent–child togetherness was further reinforced by "mommy and me" exercise classes at the local fitness club, along with carefully orchestrated family vacations at Knotts' Berry Farm or Six Flags (where young-at-heart parents joined their children on the rides).

Millennial children suddenly had a vote, and it mattered. Thus insulated and affirmed by their parents, school-age millennials devoted their emerging energies to realizing their parents' dreams of being the "best kid on the block."

High parental expectations along with the increasing demands of a global market have contributed to making the millennials the busiest generation ever, earning them the title of "masters of multitasking." From the time they could walk, they were enrolled in increasingly competitive preschools, sports teams, and chess clubs. To further escalate the parental ante, George W. Bush's educational initiative entitled "no child left behind" instilled the nation's elementary schools with an obsession for higher test scores; he also promised that students in the high school class of 2000 would be "the first in the world in science and mathematics achievement."[2]

The level of preoccupation with high achievement, from both parents and teachers, has been a source of stress for young millennials as they face the increasingly competitive demands of college and the workplace. As young adults, many millennials have found that they cannot easily let go of the need to succeed. In a recent report on millennials from Northwestern University,[46] one 20-year-old sophomore commented, "Sleep is for the weak." This student, along with many of her millennial peers, has a double major, whereby "8 years of college work are crammed into 5." The Northwestern report describes other aspects of millennial college life based on several group interviews of students living in the campus dormitories. Although the authors are careful to disclaim their results as a comprehensive overview of the entire generation, it nonetheless highlights many of the prominent trends that have elsewhere been ascribed to millennials.[2,43,44]

Of greatest significance for this cohort are its expertise, comfort, and dependence on technological forms of communication such as computers, cell phones, and digital music devices. Because these appliances have been a prominent part of their educational and social lives from the very beginning, many millennials have developed an astonishing ability to become "brilliant multitaskers"[46] who use these devices simultaneously. As an illustration, the Northwestern report describes the daily campus scenario in which students, who are presumably studying, sit with their laptop computers ("I will have 10 different web pages open at one time" says one) while listening to their digital music, checking text messages, and taking the occasional glance at a open textbook.

While many older cohorts might shudder at this level of stimulus, the millennials appear to thrive on it. According to another Northwestern graduate student, her peers "are learning from a young age how to handle a lot of distraction, which is going to bode them well, because once you graduate, all (of) life is multitasking."[46]

While the use of technology has in all probability enhanced the lives of the millennial generation in particular, it is creating some new ethical challenges. Having accustomed themselves to the lightning speed of computer-delivered information, some college millennials admit that they avoid conventional forms of library research, thus relying entirely on questionably accurate Internet sources.[46] However, Manjoo[47] cautions that reliance on technological sources for factual information may "keep us tightly coiled in a world in which digital manipulation is so effortless that spin, myth, and outright lies might get the better of us."

Another concern is the speed with which numerous sources of Internet information can be appropriated for personal gain. Accordingly, concerns about Internet plagiarism have begun to emerge across college campuses, where millennials make up a large number of students. Researchers at Coastal Carolina University found more than 250 sites where students could download entire term papers.[48]

In reading about these ethical challenges, it is important to realize that the issues created by technology for the millennial generation are simply another example of how emerging societal trends create tension between freedom (to choose a course of action) and responsibility (to address the consequences). For example, when the boomers went through their young adulthood, the birth control pill forced a similar challenge with significant societal implications for that generation.

On the positive side of the millennials' love of technology is their connectivity with friends and family. Computer sites such as MySpace and Facebook enable online interactions with literally endless numbers of individuals and provide a wide audience for the sharing of information, both personal and otherwise. Despite the communication pitfalls of anonymous personal disclosure that were discussed in Chapter 1, many millennials enjoy the rich variety of dialogue that is available in these venues.

The most important relationships of the millennial generation are not rooted in the Internet, however. Perhaps because of the nurturing roles of their ever-present helicopter parents, many millennials enjoy deeply engaged relationships with their mothers and fathers, forged through their protracted togetherness. Now, even with many of their lives unfolding in separate places, technology affords continual contact between parent and offspring. Thus, for many millennials, life is a colorful web of relationships that unfold through equally varied forms of contact.

All in all, by their own admission, life is full of promise for this generation, even though they, like the older cohorts, face significant societal challenges that may stretch their dollars, restrict their health care, and threaten their sense of safety. No strangers to these challenges, the millennials have already weathered the storms of terrorism, war, and recession. Their ultimate historic contributions as they transcend these challenges are yet to be realized but brightly anticipated.

During the time of the millennial generation, the PT profession has evolved toward an almost complete acceptance of doctoral-level preparation. As the millennials come to power, it will be exciting to see how our profession continues its long history of growth. **Figure** 9-4 shows some of the contributions to the PT profession in the time of the millennial generation.

Millennials as Patients

Although still too young to have a significant history as consumers of health care, early indications suggest that the millennials are facing some of the same issues as their older cohorts. This includes lack of adequate health insurance (according to a 2007 report of the Kaiser Foundation, 39% of the 47 million uninsured Americans are between the ages of 19 and 34).[36]

The millennials are also poised to join their older cohorts' contributions to the growing population of obese Americans. In 2008, some 57% of men and 52% of women between the ages of 20 and 34 were overweight or obese, as were 16% of children and adolescents between the ages of 9 and 19.[49] If these rates continue to rise, it is expected that there will also be a concurrent rise in obesity-related conditions such as type 2 diabetes and hypertension.

In their research on millennials, Howe and Strauss[50] suggest that the three major health issues facing this generation will be obesity, asthma, and attention deficit disorder (ADD). Although the authors do not propose definitive reasons for these conditions, they allude to the contributing factors of a steady flow of rapid-paced stimulation and decreased physical exercise (with more time spent indoors engrossed in technological forms of entertainment).

The fast-paced, pressured lives of many millennials have also led to an increase in stress-related disorders such as anxiety, depression, and substance abuse,[51] although

Figure 9–4. Major changes in the PT profession during the time of the millennial generation.

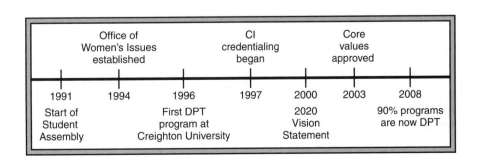

substance abuse among members of this generation is less in comparison to that of their older cohorts.[43]

A recent report at the University of California Santa Barbara reported an increase in binge drinking, along with a steady increase in the numbers of students seeking on-campus counseling services.[51] Stress is a part of life for all generations, but a fast-paced, demanding lifestyle can certainly make this a more prominent concern.

On the positive side, the millennials have shown the ability to work hard and face life's challenges with enthusiasm. These attributes can also serve them well in the pursuit of lifelong wellness, particularly through the adoption of health-enhancing behaviors such as regular exercise and stress reduction.

Physical therapists are poised to make a considerable impact on the health of this generation. In our efforts to be the consumer-recognized practitioner of choice for the treatment of conditions affecting function and quality of life, we should promote an ongoing professional relationship with our patients in the manner of a family physician or dentist. Younger millennials are likely to come to appointments with their parents in tow, giving us the opportunity to develop health-promotion programs for the entire family. In addition, with their love of technology, millennials can be encouraged to monitor their progress through a growing number of on-line resources for the monitoring of health behaviors.

Dancing Dominique

Clinical Scenario

Elaine is a physical therapist in a sports medicine clinic that has just developed a comprehensive wellness/fitness program targeted at adolescents. Her newest patient is Dominique, a 15-year-old high school freshman who has just returned from a summer weight-loss camp, where she lost 30 pounds. Dominique arrives at the clinic in the company of her 49-year-old mother Rachel, who is well known in the community as a competitive triathlete. Dominique is a beautiful young girl who appears to be about 10 pounds overweight.

As Elaine begins her intake interview with Dominique, it becomes apparent that she is at the clinic mostly at the behest of her mother, who does a good deal of the talking. Rachel states her concerns that Dominique's weight distribution (mostly in her waist), puts her at risk for metabolic syndrome, a factor related to the development of type 2 diabetes. Rachel wants Elaine to develop a supervised fitness program for Dominique to complete after school 3 days a week. Rachel is very concerned that Dominique will gain back the weight she lost at summer camp and states "I was an overweight kid and I don't my daughter to go through the same heartache that I did."

The following week, Elaine sees Dominique for their first session, which will involve a circuit of treadmill, stationary bike, and a few resistance machines. After walking on the treadmill for 15 minutes, Dominique abruptly stops the machine and turns to Elaine, saying "I'm not going to do this! It's way too boring and besides, I would rather be hanging out with my friends!"

Questions

1. Do you think most 15-year-olds would really enjoy a program such as the one described above? How might Elaine empathically address Dominique's concerns? What questions might she ask Dominique in order to explore other fitness approaches?

2. How might Elaine address Rachel's concerns related to the health of her daughter? What other resources/disciplines might be helpful?

3. How might Elaine work with Rachel to develop a program of incentives and rewards to encourage Dominique's investment and participation?

The Rest of This True Story—To Be Read After Discussion

Dominique, a self professed "computer junkie," wanted to explore some technologically enhanced exercise programs. She discovered an interactive computer-based program called Dance Dance Revolution (DDR), which provides guidance and feedback for several different dance routines.[52] At first, Rachel was skeptical about Dominique's idea, thinking it would be a waste of time. Elaine then volunteered to look for evidence-based support for this device and found one research study promoting its value for weight loss in postmenopausal women.[53]

Rachel then enthusiastically purchased this device and Dominique agreed to use it three times a week for 30 minutes. She also agreed to come to the facility once a week for strength training with Elaine, who rewarded her with a points system that could be redeemed for prizes. Dominique enjoyed the DDR so much that she even used it beyond the agreed upon time. Two months later, Dominique had lost the remaining weight and Elaine decided to purchase a few DDR games for the adolescent fitness program at her facility. Dominique has since recruited three of her friends to exercise with her at Elaine's facility.

Talking Points/Field Notes

The Millennials' Perspective on Health Care

The purpose of this interview is to obtain the millennial generation's perspective on the changes they have experienced in health care in the course of their lives. The following questions can be helpful:

1. If you had to describe your earliest memories of health care in one or two sentences, what would you say?

2. What do you think are the biggest positive health-care changes in your adult experience?

3. What changes in health care concern you the most?

4. What are the most important things a health-care professional can do to secure your trust and confidence?

Compare and discuss the results of your interviews. What themes emerge? What can you learn from these interviews to help you communicate more effectively with members of the millenial generation? Reflect on your observations in your field notes.

Millennials in the Workplace

The oldest millennials are just beginning to enter the workforce, where they currently make up about 21% of the population.[51] Their unique attitudes, abilities, and perspectives are promising to challenge some of the long-held notions of their older colleagues.

First, millennials will bring many of their fast-paced habits to the workplace. They will work hard but expect it to enhance their professional development more quickly than their older cohorts would. Accordingly, the concepts of "paying dues" and following the chain of command mean very little to the millennials, whose sense of time is much faster ("every second is stretch, and a year is long-term").[4] Thus, millennials' expectations for opportunities, advancement, and salary may seem unrealistic to their older colleagues. Millennials live in the moment and may need help seeing the big picture. They will not be afraid to question policies and procedures, not out of disrespect but rather to understand why these considerations are important right now.

Millennials have grown accustomed to technological "drop-down menus" to guide choices; they will benefit from clear instructions for the completion of work-related tasks.[4] Millennials tend to be more informal with respect to clothing, language, and interactions. Thus they may need guidance in appropriate ways of dressing as well as professional means of addressing patients, colleagues, and supervisors. As consummate multitaskers who become bored quickly, they may need assistance with time management for big projects. In providing guidance to millennial colleagues, it is helpful for their older colleagues to realize that these differences are not intentional affronts to professionalism but rather indicative of real generational differences.

Because millennials do a great deal of communication technologically, they may need assistance with proper grammar and spelling for professional written documentation. Even though they need lots of guidance and support, millennials don't want to be treated like children but rather respected for their contributions.

On the positive side, millennials are also accustomed to change, diversity, and teamwork. With their love of social networking, they can become enthusiastic participants in their workplace. Their civic-mindedness can make them tremendous potential ambassadors for their respective professions, where they are poised to make significant contributions.

Communication Breakdown

Clinical Scenario

Ryan, age 22, is on his first internship at a busy acute-care hospital. His clinical instructor (CI) is Dan, a 36-year-old experienced physical therapist who is well respected for his knowledge and skill. Two weeks into the internship, Ryan calls his school academic coordinator, saying that he is having "communication difficulties" with Dan. He describes the following concerns:

1. Ryan feels that Dan is not giving him enough positive feedback, reporting, "Whenever I ask Dan how I'm doing, he says "fine." But I need to know *why* I'm doing fine!"

2. Dan wants Ryan to build his caseload, but Ryan wants time to observe Dan treating patients. Ryan says "I feel like I'm just a warm body here; after all, I'm here to learn!"

3. Ryan told Dan that he wanted to end his internship 2 days early so he could attend his best friend's wedding. Dan said that he would allow this only if Ryan worked on two Saturdays. Ryan has a job as a waiter on Saturdays and doesn't want to lose money. He thinks Dan is being unreasonable.

4. Dan told Ryan that he expects all his notes to be turned in without a single spelling or grammatical error. Ryan says, "How can I possibly do this if my notes to be handwritten? I'm used to computer spellchecking!"

Questions

1. Identify the specific issues related to each of Ryan's concerns.

2. How might generational differences contribute to the communication issues between Dan and Ryan? (Which generation does each of them represent?)

3. How might you explore Ryan's concerns with Dan?

4. What suggestions do you have for Ryan?

5. What suggestions do you have for Dan?

Talking Points/Field Notes

Understanding the Millennial Perspective on Communication

Interview a member of the millennial generation who is in the workforce. The goal of this interview is to understand his or her perspective on intergenerational communication. The following questions might be helpful:

1. When you were growing up, what was the nature of the generational differences between you and your parents/grandparents? Which issues were prevalent?

2. Which key experiences contributed to your attitudes about education and work?

3. How have these attitudes affected your life and work?

4. How do you think communication has changed in your lifetime? What societal changes have affected this the most?

5. What are the most important things this generation can learn about effective communication?

6. What are some ways to enhance communication between colleagues of different generations?

Compare and discuss the results of your interviews. Were there any prevalent themes? Use the results of your interviews to compile a list of suggestions for optimizing communication with members of the millennials. Reflect on your observations in your field notes.

Communication Resources from the Millennial Generation

As we discussed previously, stress is a prominent feature of the millennial generation. The hectic pace of their lives can challenge adequate time for reflection and enjoyment of the present moment. Recently, two books by Eckhart Tolle, *The Power of Now: A Guide to Spiritual Enlightenment* [54] and *A New Earth: Awakening to Your Life's Purpose,* [55] have received widespread attention for their insights and guidance on living joyfully in the moment. Each of these books promotes the examination of sabotaging self-talk that keeps us in a perpetual state of urgency. Both books are highly spiritual, without subscribing to any particular religion. Their practical, encouraging, and insightful messages are useful in retooling internal communication toward greater equanimity.

Parting Comments: Generational on Professional Behavior in Physical Therapy

In view of all the generational differences we have discussed, an interesting question is whether there are also related differences with respect to the prioritization of important professional behaviors.

A recent study by Gleeson and May[4] found no significant differences in the descriptions of professional behaviors cited by study respondents of different generations. This study found that arriving at work on time and wearing professional dress were important behaviors described by all age groups. In addition, other research has demonstrated that similar values are shared by all generations. As Gleeson[4] states, however, "many clinicians and employers have noted differences in how the generations demonstrate these areas."

Implication for Physical Therapy Practice

Generational perspectives are but one element of the broad spectrum of diversity which characterizes individuals. In the context of physical therapy, awareness of these can provide rich opportunities to learn from our patients and colleagues. Furthermore, this awareness can help us optimize our communication with persons of all ages. Most importantly, by understanding the cyclic nature of generational types (i.e. civic, adaptive, idealist and reactive), we will be more appreciative of the gifts and challenges which repeatedly confront all persons as history unfolds.

Chapter Summary

1. Today's workplace includes members of four different generations: Veterans (1922–1945), Boomers (1946–1960), Xers (1961–1981), and Millennials (1982–2000).

2. Each generation has its own social culture. Thus, generational differences in attitudes, perceptions, and experiences may contribute to possible communication challenges. Awareness of generational differences can enhance external communication and promote effective interactions with members of all groups.

Take-Home Menu

1. Professional archives: Many state APTA chapters have a historical archive that includes recorded histories of older chapter members. Check with your chapter to see if you can assist in this effort. It can be a great way to learn about the history of your chapter and even to develop a friendship with one of its older members. (This can also be an enjoyable activity with an older friend or relative.)

2. Time capsule: Create a PT class time capsule for your academic program. Include news clippings, music, and interviews with students and faculty. Interesting questions can include "What will you hoping in the year 2020?" "What are you most looking forward to in your professional life in the next 10 years?" The capsule can be opened at a future date, perhaps during a class reunion.

3. Life-span movies: With a classmate, find and view a film that depicts persons facing "age appropriate" developmental issues rooted in various historical periods. Discuss how these characters' issues are affected by the historic times in which they were living and how these might be affected if circumstances had been different.

Examples of such movies include the following:
   – *October Sky* (1991). Based on the true story of Homer Hickam, a pioneer of the 1960s space race. A coming-of-age story that addresses intergenerational conflict between parent and child as well as the impact of differing educational backgrounds and economic conditions.
   – *Harold and Maude* (1971). A lonely, eccentric young man develops a deep relationship with a fun-loving and equally quirky elderly woman during the 1970s. Addresses issues of death and loss. References to the political climate of the 1970s.
   – *Bend It Like Beckham* (2002). Two adolescent girls face issues related to cultural differences, competitive sports, and the meaning of friendship during the 1980s. Addresses the influence of culture and tradition, adolescent rebellion, and intergenerational conflict.
   – *Away From Her* (2006): A man must cope with the many challenges of institutionalizing his wife due to deterioration from Alzheimer's disease. Set in the mid-2000s. Addresses issues of marriage, aging, and loss.

References

1. Reinhold M. *Studies in Classical History and Society.* London: Oxford University Press; 2002.
2. Strauss W, Howe N. *Generations: The History of America's Future, 1584–2069.* NewYork: William Morrow; 1991.
3. Rediff.com. Get ahead Q and A: http://qna.rediff.com/ Main.php?do=getanswer&catid=28&questid=6468576. Accessed April 8, 2008.
4. Gleeson PB. Understanding generational competence related to professionalism: Misunderstandings that lead to a perception of unprofessional behavior. *J Phys Ther Educ.* 2007;21(3):23-28.
5. Civic-minded millennials prepared to reward or punish companies based on commitment to social causes. Corporate Social Responsibility Newswire: http://www.csrwire.com/PressRelease.php?id=6641. Accessed April 8, 2008.
6. Generation Watch: News and views of America's living generations: http://home.earthlink.net/~generationwatch/gw_background.html. Accessed April 10, 2008.
7. Boychuk D, Judy E, Cowin L. Multigenerational nurses in the workplace. *J Nurs Admin.* 2004;34(11):493-501.
8. Katz M. The invention of welfare. *J Policy Hist.* 1998;10(4):401-418.
9. Drake D. *Reforming the Healthcare Market: An Interpretive Economic History.* Washington, DC: George Washington University Press; 1994.
10. Selim A, Berlowitz DR, Fincke G, et al. The health status of elderly veteran enrollees in the Veterans Health Administration. *J Am Geriatr Soc.* 2004;52(8):1271-1276.
11. Schoenberg NE, Hyungsoo K, Edwards W, Fleming S. Burden of common multiple morbidity constellations on out of pocket medical expenditures among older adults. *Gerontologist.* 2007;47:423-427.
12. National Institute on Aging. One in seven Americans age 71 and older has some type of dementia, NIH-funded study estimates. October 30, 2007: http://www.nia.nih.gov/NewsAndEvents/PressReleases/PR20071030ADAMS.htm. Accessed April 14, 2008.
13. Pew Internet and Family Life Project: http://www.pewinternet.org/. Accessed April 11, 2008.
14. Elderly expectations of health care easy to satisfy but complicated. *EurekAlert:* http://www.eurekalert.org/pub_releases/2002-03/ps-eeo031402.php. Accessed April 10, 2008.
15. 111th Boston Marathon. 2007 finishers over age 70: http://www.boston.com/sports/marathon/runners/over70women/. Accessed April 14, 2008.
16. Dale Carnegie. Dale Carnegie Training Website: http://www.dalecarnegie.com/. Accessed April 17, 2008.
17. Earl L. Baby Boomer Women—Then and Now. University of Toronto: http://prod.library.utoronto.ca:8090/datalib/codebooks/cstdsp/71f0004xcb/2003/pe_archive_sa/english/1999/pear1999011003s3a03.pdf. Accessed April 15, 2008.
18. DeNoon D. The history of birth control. Web MD: http://www.webmd.com/content/Article/71/81244.htm. Accessed April 15, 2008.
19. EEOC. United States Equal Employment Opportunity Commission. The law. Available online: http://www.eeoc.gov/. Accessed April 15, 2008.
20. American Hospital Association Management Advisory. Patient Bill of Rights: http://www.patienttalk.info/AHA-Patient_Bill_of_Rights.htm. Accessed April 15, 2008.
21. Pardini P. The history of special education. Rethinking schools online: http://www.rethinkingschools.org/archive/16_03/Hist163.shtml. Accessed April 15, 2008.
22. Molloy JT. *John T. Molloy's New Dress for Success.* New York: Warner Books; 1988.
23. American Association of Retired Persons. Boomers at midlife: The AARP life stage study: wave 3. 2004. AARP: www.AARP.org. Accessed April 17, 2008.
24. Institute of Medicine. Retooling for an aging America: building the health care workforce. Report brief. April 14, 2008: http://www.iom.edu/CMS/3809/40113/53452.aspx. Accessed April 16, 2008.
25. When I'm 64: How boomers will change health care. 2007: http://www.aha.org/aha/content/2007/pdf/070508-boomerreport.pdf. Accessed April 16, 2008.
26. AACN Media Relations Fact Sheet. American Association of Colleges of Nursing. 2002: http://www.aacn.nche.edu/media/backgrounders/shortagefacts.htm. Accessed April 17, 2008.
27. APTA 2007 Demographic Survey: http://www.apta.org/AM/Template.cfm?Section=Home&Template=/MembersOnly.cfm&ContentID=46077. Accessed April 30, 2008.
28. Growing old, baby-boomer style experts examine impact on society as boomers approach retirement: CBSnews.com. Accessed April 17, 2008.
29. Mandino O. *The Greatest Salesman in the World.* Westminster, MD: Bantam; 1968.
30. Brainyquote. Og Mandino quotes. http://www 237 html. Accessed April 18, 2008.
31. Blanchard K, Johnson S. *The One-Minute Manager.* New York: William Morrow; 1982.
32. NAS insights: http://www.nasrecruitment.com/TalentTips/NASinsights/GettingtoKnowGenerationX.pdf. Accessed April 18, 2008.

33. American Institute of Architects. *Practice Management Digest*, 2007: http://www.aia.org/nwsltr_pm.cfm?pagename=pm_a_20030801_genx. Accessed April 18, 2008.

34. MSN Money. Supremely confident to super stressed: Landmark gen X study from Schwab uncovers six distinct financial mindsets. February 11, 2008: http://news.moneycentral.msn.com/ticker/article.aspx?Feed=BW&Date=2080211&ID=8171101&Symbol=SCHW. Accessed April 30, 2008.

35. The Henry J. Kaiser Family Foundation. The uninsured: A primer. Key facts about Americans without health insurance. October 2006: http://www.kff.org/uninsured/. Accessed April 29, 2008.

36. DeNavas W, Proctor CB, Smith J. Income, poverty, and health insurance coverage in the United States: 2006. U.S. Census Bureau, August 2007: http://www.census.gov/prod/2007pubs/p60-233.pdf. Accessed May 1, 2008.

37. Collins SR, Davis K, Doty MM, et al. Gaps in health insurance: An all American problem. The Commonwealth Fund. April 26, 2006: http://www.commonwealthfund.org/publications/publications_show.htm?doc_id=36786. Accessed April 30, 2008.

38. Nationwide: Better health on your side. As obesity rates continue to rise, is the workplace a source of or a solution to unhealthy lifestyle habits? http://www.nwbetterhealth.com/docs/press-releases/obesitpress-release.pdf. Accessed May 1, 2008.

39. Generation X born 1965–1980: http://www.valueoptions.com/spotlight_YIW/gen_x.htm. Accessed April 30, 2008.

40. Robbins A. *Awaken the Giant Within: How to Take Control of Your Mental, Emotional, Physical and Financial Destiny!* New York: Fireside; 1989.

41. Covey S. *The Seven Habits of Highly Effective People.* New York: Free Press; 1991.

42. Lancaster C, Stillman D. *When Generations Collide: Who They Are, Why They Clash, How to Solve the Generational Puzzle at Work.* New York: Harper Business; 2002.

43. New Politics Institute: The progressive politics of the millennial generation. June 20, 2007: http://www.newpolitics.net/node/360?full_report=1. Accessed May 1, 2008.

44. University of California Los Angeles, Higher Education Research Institute. 2006 American Freshman Survey. Available online: http://www.gseis.ucla.edu/heri/PDFs/pubs/briefs/brief-081707-CollegeRankings.pdf. Accessed May 5, 2008.

45. Pew Research Center. A portrait of generation next, released January 2007: http://people-press.org/reports/pdf/300.pdfhttp://people-press.org/reports/questionnaires/300.pdf. Accessed May 1, 2008.

46. Northwestern University. For alumni and friends of Northewestern University. Millennials: Always on. Summer, 2006: http://www.northwestern.edu/magazine/summer2006/cover/millenials.html. Accessed May 1, 2008.

47. Manjoo F. *True Enough: Learning to Live in a Post-Fact Society.* Hoboken, NJ: John Wiley & Sons; 2008.

48. Shulman M. I have a question: Is it web research or technology assisted plagiarism? *Santa Clara Magazine,* Fall 2004. Santa Clara University: http://www.scu.edu/scm/fall2004/research.cfm. Accessed May 3, 2008.

49. The Endocrine Society and Hormone Foundation. Obesity in America: http://www.obesityinamerica.org/childhoodoverweight.html. Accessed May 5, 2008.

50. Howe N, Strauss W. *Millennials Rising: The Next Great Generation.* Westminster, MD: Vintage Books; 2000.

51. Young M. Managing Generations in the 21st century workplace. University of California Leadership Institute: http://www.ucop.edu/ucli/presentations_10_06/young.pdf. Accessed May 5, 2008.

52. Dance Dance Revolution. http://www.ddrgame.com. Accessed May 6, 2008.

53. Experts at 2008 American Geriatrics Society Annual Scientific Meeting reveal how popular video dance game helps postmenopausal women: http://www.americangeriatrics.org/news/video_game042204.shtml. Accessed May 6, 2008.

54. Tolle E. *The Power of Now: A Guide to Spiritual Enlightenment.* Novato, CA: New World Library; 1999.

55. Tolle E. *A New Earth: Awakening to Your Life's Purpose.* New York: Penguin; 2005.

CHAPTER 10

Communication for Empowering Therapeutic Alliances

"Let no one ever come to you without feeling better and happier."

Mother Teresa of Calcutta (1910–1997),
Humanitarian and Nobel laureate

Chapter Overview

Our patients' achievement of optimal quality of life can be greatly facilitated by supportive therapeutic alliances with their health-care practitioners. This chapter explores the application of effective communication in the context of building such partnerships, the components of which include understanding the challenges of the illness experience and applying the principles of patient-centered care.

Key Terms

Self-efficacy

Illness

Therapeutic alliance

Patient-centered care

Person-first language

What Does It Mean to Be a Patient?

Pain and Suffering

What is a patient? *The American Heritage Dictionary of the English Language*[1] provides eight different definitions of the term. Five of these are adjectives, relating to the bearing of pain, annoyance, or difficulty. The most ancient use of the term, however, is as a noun, meaning "one who suffers." Accordingly, a guiding assumption in health care relates to the concept that *patients come to us because they are suffering on some level.*

The concept of suffering as a subjective experience of pain derives from many sources. Accordingly, Cherney describes suffering as "a state of severe distress with events that threaten the intactness of the person."[2] Cicely Saunders, who is credited with being the founder of the hospice movement, was one of the first physicians to identify (and then treat) the numerous sources of distress confronting patients at the end of life. Saunders coined the term *total pain* to describe the sum effect of these multidimensional contributions to patients' suffering. According to Saunders (who, in 1967, established the world's first medically based hospice in London), these sources include not only physical, emotional, and spiritual elements but also other potent stressors such as family responses, financial concerns, and coping with the increasingly obfuscating demands of the medical bureaucracy. In summarizing the patient's perspective, Saunders wrote: "The whole experience for a patient includes anxiety, depression, and fear; concern for the family . . . and often a need to find some meaning in the situation, some deeper reality in which to trust."[3,4]

Figure 10-1 illustrates some sources of total pain.

The degree to which each of our patients suffers depends on many factors. Not surprisingly, any loss of function is likely to be stressful; our patients are thus likely to experience one or more elements of total pain. Although the extent of this distress will vary, even patients with minor injuries are likely to face challenging consequences that affect their daily lives. To illustrate this concept, read the exercise contained in **Box 10-1** on page 242 and reflect on the questions that follow.

Figure 10–1. Elements of total pain that contribute to patient suffering. *(Adapted from Saunders.[3,4])*

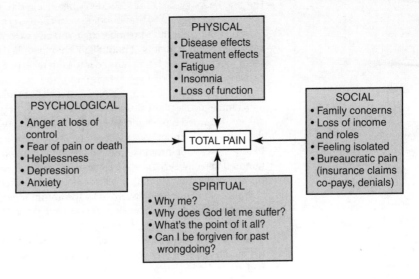

BOX 10-1:   Experiential Exercise in Total Pain

The purpose of this exercise is to reflect on the experiences that face an individual who suddenly and unexpectedly becomes a patient.

This exercise is most effective if done as an entire class, with one person reading the scenario out loud. It can also be done in a small group. It is helpful if the script is read slowly in a calm, unemotional tone of voice. If it is not feasible to complete this exercise in a large or small group setting, you can read it yourself.

> This scenario will guide you through the experiences that face many of our patients. You are asked to sit in a comfortable relaxed position with your eyes closed. Take a few deep breaths and direct your awareness to the present moment where you can mindfully attend to the following scenario.
>
> As I read the following description, you are asked to listen with mindful attention, as you acknowledge the feelings and thoughts that arise as you imagine yourself in this situation.

IDENTIFYING WITH TOTAL PAIN: A LIFE-CHANGING IMPACT

> The first beginnings of dawn cast a warm glow through the windows of your room, heralding a beautiful spring day. As you stir to a heavy consciousness, your first thought is the 8 a.m. exam you are supposed to be taking this morning. Then, feeling the surging pain in your leg along with a rising panic, you suddenly remember.
>
> You are not a physical therapy student comfortably resting in your bed at home. You are in a hospital bed with your right leg immobilized as the result of a car accident the previous night. As you struggle to reconstruct the events of the past 12 hours, you are increasingly overwhelmed by the throbbing in your leg, which is heavily stabilized by open reduction and external fixation.
>
> The covers have fallen off your bed and you are cold. To add to your frustration, you discover that instead of your favorite pajamas, you are wearing a thin hospital gown that is twisted around your waist, leaving you exposed. Despite your embarrassment, you know that it will hurt to dislodge the gown, so you don't even try.
>
> As this cascade of unpleasant sensations invades your attention, you realize that you really need to go to the bathroom. But because your leg is immobilized, you quickly recognize that you will not be able to do this alone. Thus, with a growing sense of frustration, you ring the nurse's call button.
>
> As you wait, memories of the previous night pierce your consciousness through a sharp and painful series of dissonant flashbacks: Ending work at 11:00 p.m. after a long day at school. Feeling exhausted. Getting into your car. Driving the long stretch of interstate. Fighting heavy eyelids. Then, suddenly being jolted to awareness as your vehicle weaves off the road and screeching tires bringing your car to a slamming halt against a guard rail.
>
> After that, you can't remember anything else except vague mental images of an ambulance ride, with lots of bright lights and people darting in all directions around you. You seem to recall papers being pushed into your face for a signature and someone asking if you had an "advanced directive" (a living will). Your last memory is something about "emergency surgery." Breathing into a mask. And that is all until this moment.
>
> As these recollections sink in, your mind reels with questions cloaked in a rising tide of anxiety. How bad is the injury to your leg? How long will you be disabled? How will you finish the semester at school? Will you even be able to graduate? How will you pay for this treatment without insurance? Are your parents coming from your hometown, several hundred miles away? Will you be able to go through with the wedding you had planned at the end of the semester? How will your fiancé (or fiancée) react to this news?
>
> Your painful reverie is disturbed by the abrupt arrival of a nurse, who enters your room with a brief knock. As he stands over your bed, you become painfully aware that you are half naked. "What do you need?" he asks. Despite your own discomfort, you can't help but notice his slightly impatient tone of voice. You know he is busy and you don't want to be a demanding patient, but you hurt and you need help. As the nurse raises the head of your bed, you fight back tears of pain and frustration.

BOX 10-1:   Experiential Exercise in Total Pain—cont'd

Questions

1. As you read or listen to this scenario, reflect on it as if it were actually happening to you in the context of your current situation. Without stopping to censor yourself, quickly write down several of the feelings that it provokes for you.
2. Go over your list of feelings and consider why you might have them. What role might your health-care providers play in helping you address these?
3. As the patient in this situation, what sources of "total pain" might be an issue for you? Refer to Figure 10-1 if needed.
4. How might the nurse interact with you in a more helpful way?
5. If you were to receive a physical therapy consult, what concerns and goals might you have for therapeutic intervention?

As the scenario in Box 10-1 suggests, despite incurring a relatively minor, non-life-threatening injury, this patient would likely experience many elements of total pain. Furthermore, this injury is likely to result in several challenges related to pain and mobility restrictions. Most likely, the focus of this patient's treatment would be directed toward these musculoskeletal limitations. Thus, in the absence of unforeseen complications, a full recovery from the physical trauma would be expected and this patient might return to school in a matter of a week or two. Would all be well? What other sources of "total pain" might this person experience, even after his return to everyday life? In order to answer this question, consider the following information: Recent research on the long-term effects of motor vehicle accidents suggests that there are other potentially disabling consequences that require attention and support. In situations of such accidents resulting in trauma (which number some 3 million a year in the United States), between 10% and 45% of those injured will experience symptoms of posttraumatic stress disorder (PTSD).[5] This is defined by the *Diagnostic and Statistical Manual of Mental Disorders*[6] as "the development of characteristic symptoms following exposure to an extreme traumatic stressor involving direct personal experience of an event that involves actual or threatened death or serious injury."

Symptoms of PTSD include flashbacks (where the traumatic event is reexperienced), heightened arousal, a numbing of general responsiveness, and future avoidance of stimuli associated with the traumatic event (such as avoidance of driving).[6] Such patients need emotional support from friends, family, and health-care providers. They also benefit from early access to psychological counseling and medication if needed.[5]

As this discussion suggests, the total pain of our patients may go unrecognized by busy health-care providers. For example, in a typical acute-care setting, a physical therapist would likely see this patient for brief instruction in ambulation with no weight bearing on the fractured lower extremity. Considering this intervention from a purely task-specific point of view, it would be considered as a relatively straightforward process that should take about 30 minutes. Furthermore, in a busy acute-care setting, most physical therapists would likely have several other patients also needing their intervention (in addition to the documentation required for each visit).

With such a busy schedule, it is possible for health-care providers to develop a process-oriented tunnel vision that reduces the focus of patient care to the management of involved body parts. This "part-specific" approach overlooks the psychological and emotional needs of our patients, limiting the effectiveness of our therapeutic communication, our engagement with patients, and even, quite possibly, the effectiveness of our interventions. As you will learn in the coming sections of this chapter, an empathic awareness of the patient's perspective can keep the door open to meaningful interactions, even in the presence of time restrictions.

Disruption of Quality of Life

As we have discussed thus far, our patients come to us because they are experiencing a stressful change in health that disrupts their functional quality of life. The concept of "patient experience" is critical here, because regardless of the nature or severity of this health change, the patient's subjective perception of self-efficacy is disrupted.

Self-efficacy relates to the beliefs and expectations that people have regarding their ability to accomplish important life tasks. For each of us, meeting our daily responsibilities is a prerequisite for effective and satisfying function in our various societal roles.

As an example, let's supposed that you sustained a severe ankle sprain while trail running. Although this would not be considered a serious injury, it could pose significant challenges affecting your everyday experiences. Obviously, you would not be able to run for awhile, and you might experience pain that would interfere with other pursuits giving your life pleasure and meaning. Deprived of a major form of stress control, you might find yourself becoming irritable, leading you to snap at friends or loved ones. Your lack of mobility might challenge your basic activities of daily living (bathing, home care, shopping, etc.). You might restrict social events or outings into the community because of the "hassle factor."

Thus, with a single injury, your self-efficacy is challenged in virtually all of your customary roles, with resulting consequences for your physical, emotional, and psychological well-being. If you have ever had an experience such as this, you can surely begin to understand some of the multifaceted concerns that face our patients.

The acknowledgment of such concerns is reflected in The World Health Organization's *International Classification of Disability and Health* (ICF). A major construct of the ICF model is the impact of a health condition on the physical, social, and environmental elements that contribute to self-efficacy. Thus the ICF model, which is gaining wide acceptance in PT,[7] views the sequelae of a health condition in terms of their impact on the patients' body structures, personal and environmental contexts, and the degree to which participation in customary activities is affected. Accordingly, Steiner suggests that this model can be used as an evaluation tool to enhance communication between patients and their health-care providers.[7] When used in this manner, the ICF can help interdisciplinary team members elicit important information about their patients' perspectives, needs, and goals.[8]

Societal Attitudes Toward Persons With Illness

Another way of contextualizing the impact of a health condition is to examine the psychosocial changes that result. The term psychosocial addresses the psychological and societal consequences of a given life situation. In turn, these consequences may contribute to widely held attitudes about disease and illness.

For example, in the early 1980s, infection with the human immunodeficiency virus HIV was first found among persons who engaged in sexual activity with others of the same gender. This finding led to a widespread societal assumption that HIV was a "gay disease" (even as evidence grew to support other forms of transmission). Furthermore, for persons who condemned the gay lifestyle, HIV became a disease associated with "immoral lifestyles" and "promiscuity." These early attitudes had upsetting psychosocial consequences for persons affected by HIV. The example of HIV is a particularly unfortunate one in that these widespread societal attitudes had a destructive impact on the care of those affected. Nevertheless, negative social attitudes prevail about most health conditions.

The term *sick role* was first used by Parsons in 1951[9] to describe societal concessions and expectations toward a person with illness or injury. Many of these attitudes still prevail today.

According to Parsons, the societal prerogatives of being sick include excusal from the performance of social duties and exemption from blame for the illness. In exchange for such social indulgences, sick persons are expected to make every attempt to recover fully, to seek competent assistance, and to cooperate with their health-care providers. Accordingly, even today, health-care providers are likely to become frustrated with persons who abuse "sick role" prerogatives. Examples of such abuses would be persons who refuse care, who fail to comply with therapeutic interventions, or who pretend to be ill to escape work responsibilities.

Despite our distaste for such practices, unconditional positive regard requires that we suspend judgment, and with good reason. In our current health-care system, restricted access to care and limited patient resources may both contribute to our patients' inability to meet societal expectations. Thus the patient who does not comply with treatment interventions may simply not have the financial resources to do so.

The effectiveness of any societal system depends on its ability to adapt to the needs of the persons it serves. Interestingly, Parsons' theory has also contributed to a rather persistent societal view of health care as a power hierarchy dominated by the physician. Accordingly, Parsons suggests that the primary role of physicians is to "reinforce the societal goal of wellness and to judge the legitimacy of illness for the patient."[10,11]

However, as our health-care system expands to meet the needs of an increasingly diverse population requiring progressively more sophisticated levels of care, such a hierarchical system is not likely to be as effective. Furthermore, technological advances have changed the power differential between patients and their physicians, so that "patients' power to direct care pushes the relationship towards greater equity."[12]

As a physical therapist, you will be expected to abide by the seven Core Values for Professional Behavior of the American Physical Therapy Association (APTA), which include a mandate for societal responsibility. This will include working with members of an increasingly diverse interdisciplinary health-care team in order to meet your patients' goals. One of the ways in which you can prepare for this exciting opportunity is to learn as much as you can about the roles and responsibilities of other health-care professionals.

The Concepts of "Illness" and "Disease"

In order to center the following discussion on the patient's subjective experience, it is useful to distinguish between two descriptors related to a health condition.

The term *disease* pertains strictly to a pathological process that disrupts body organs and systems. In this context, a stroke pertains to the disruption of blood flow within the cerebral arteries with resulting ischemia of the surrounding cortical tissue. Because the disease process occurs at the organ level (the brain in the case of stroke), the nature of its consequences is somewhat predictable and sometimes irreversible.

The other term, *illness*, pertains to the *uniquely subjective experience* of body sensations, emotions, beliefs, and altered behaviors that manifest themselves in a person who feels unwell. The experience of illness can be highly variable, depending on a variety of factors such as attitude, outlook, pain, and the presence of social support. For example, one person undergoing a total hip replacement for severe arthritis may optimistically view this surgery as a new lease on a pain-free life, while another may pessimistically see it as the first of many future surgeries as their condition progresses.

Regardless of such differences, it is most helpful to provide empowering support that minimizes the subjective illness experience for each patient according to his or her needs. Accordingly, Gerteis states, "It is the experience of illness that brings patients to the health care system . . . and it is from illness that they seek relief."[13]

The Personal Challenges of the Illness Experience

We all experience illness at some point in life. Although many illnesses are self-limiting and without long-term effects, others are insidious, gradually taking a toll on body systems and function.

The transition from health to illness-related decline has been studied at considerable length,[13] and there is much support for the concept of the illness experience as a series of psychological challenges affecting the patient, family, and health-care team. Awareness of these challenges can enhance our communication with patients at various points in their experience and are thus worthy of discussion.

Stewart and colleagues[14] describe a three-stage "developmental process" that accompanies the evolving illness experience as well as the subsequent decision to seek medical care. These overlapping stages of *awareness, disorganization,* and *reorganization* provide helpful insights into what the author calls "normal human responses to disaster," which emphasize "how the humanity of an ill person is compromised."

The duration and impact of these stages is related to the nature of the pathological process and is most likely to be extensive in chronic conditions that affect health over time. Because chronic diseases such as heart disease, cancer, and diabetes are the leading causes of death and disability in the United States,[15] it is likely that you will encounter patients in the midst of these challenges.

These phases are briefly explored below, along with the impact of the health-care environment. This will provide the foundation for a discussion of patient-centered care later in the chapter.

Awareness

The first stage of the illness experience pertains to the growing realization of a decline in health. This stage is often characterized by ambivalence.[14] As the person grapples with symptoms, the desire to understand what is wrong coexists with a reluctance to acknowledge that there is actually a problem. The onset of awareness might be underscored by functional changes that are noticeable to the patient and his or her family members (e.g., discovering that an aging mother has recently fallen several times). In the face of growing awareness, the person may vacillate between maintaining independence and accepting care from others. Then, as symptoms become more consistent, the individual may begin to feel vulnerable, fragile, and defenseless. These feelings may intensify as the individual seeks medical care and receives a diagnosis, particularly in the case of a chronic or progressive condition.

In other pathological processes, especially if caused by trauma (such as spinal cord injury or traumatic brain injury), the onset of symptoms may be sudden and undeniable. Nevertheless, a similar sense of vulnerability may arise as the patient becomes more aware of the extent and nature of his or her impairments. In the case of progressively degenerative diseases such as multiple sclerosis and amyotrophic lateral sclerosis, each exacerbation evokes a new awareness of functional decline.[16,17]

Disorganization and Coping

The acknowledgment of declining functional independence resulting in the need for medical care is a stressful life event that threatens self-efficacy. As a person faces these changes, feelings of confusion, frustration, sadness, and anger may contribute to a sense of disempowerment. In response, psychological coping mechanisms come into play.

Susan Confronts a Health Challenge

Susan and Jim Staley are a married couple in their mid-fifties. Their three children have grown up and left home. The Staleys have always been physically active, enjoying outdoor activities such as hiking, biking, and canoeing.

In the past 2 months, Susan has had to confront a noticeable decline in her functional abilities. When she was in her forties, she developed the first signs of osteoarthritis in her hips. Although she considered the accompanying pain bothersome, she was able to control it with nonsteroidal anti-inflammatory drugs (NSAIDs), which allowed her to continue her activities. In the past 2 months, however, the pain has slowly gotten worse, and at times she experiences painful grinding in her hip joint while walking. Now Susan finds herself unable to enjoy her outdoor activities with Jim. She is also noticing some range-of-motion (ROM) limitation at her hips, which makes it difficult to lean over in order to put on her socks or to lower herself into the bathtub.

As a result of her activity limitations, Susan has gained 15 pounds during this time (which further stresses her hip joint). On a recent visit to her family physician, she mentioned her concerns and was given a referral to an orthopedic surgeon. Susan knows that the likely recommendation for her will be total hip replacements, but she is anxious about surgery and would like to postpone it as long as possible. Her concerns are heightened by the fact that her older sister developed a life-threatening deep vein thrombosis following knee replacement surgery (also because of osteoarthritis) 3 years earlier.

Thus, instead of immediately going to the orthopedic surgeon, Susan first decides to seek PT intervention from your clinic for pain control and exercise. Your examination reveals slight weakness in her abdominals, hip stabilizers, and lumbar spine. Susan also has ROM deficits in bilateral hip external rotation and flexion. You are now at the point of recommending an exercise program.

Questions

1. What information do you need from Susan in terms of the impact of her hip pain on her quality of life? How would this information be useful to both of you?

2. How might you explore Susan's concerns with her regarding total hip replacement surgery?

3. Would you recommend that she see the orthopedic surgeon? How might this be useful?

4. How could you partner with Susan's orthopedic surgeon to assist her in her goal of nonsurgical approaches to pain management?

5. How might you support Susan as she comes to terms with the eventual need for surgery?

We all use coping mechanisms when we confront difficulties and the related emotional stress. According to Lazarus, coping is defined as "ongoing cognitive and behavioral efforts to manage internal or external demands that result in psychological stress."[18,19]

Feelings of stress result from conflict (a perceived mismatch between what is desired and what occurs) and include feelings of disgust, jealousy, anger, envy, guilt, shame, anxiety, and sadness. Coping strategies help the individual address two important questions related to the distressing event. These are, "What is at stake?" and "What can be done about it?" When our coping is effective, we are able to maintain positive feelings that enhance self-efficacy[20] and promote recovery.

Table 10-1 illustrates the eight major coping styles identified by Lazarus.[18] They are presented in descending order in terms of their impact on producing positive emotions.

Table 10–1. Coping With Stress*

Approach	Description	Effect on Emotions
Positive reappraisal	Finding the good in the situation Optimistic self-talk Being open to growth	Significant relationship to positive emotions
Planful problem solving	Taking constructive action to address source of problem	Significant relationship to positive emotions
Escape-avoidance	Wishful thinking Avoiding anything related to conflict	Variable relationship to positive emotions
Accepting responsibility	Owning the problem Being accountable for problem	Variable relationship to positive emotions
Seeking social support	Seeking advice and counsel Seeking information Seeking emotional support	Variable relationship to positive emotions
Self-controlling	Not being impulsive Not telling others Keeping feelings to oneself	Variable relationship to positive emotions
Distancing	Making light of situation Trying to forget situation Distracting oneself	May result in negative emotions (approaches significance)
Confrontational coping	Expressing needs/emotions Negotiating/persuading Self advocacy	May result in negative emotions (approaches significance)

*In descending order of effect on producing positive emotions. Adapted from Lazarus RS. Coping theory research: Past, present, and future. *Psychosomatic Medicine* 1993;55:234–247.

The effectiveness of coping strategies is variable between persons and events, so that different coping styles work for different people at different times. In Lazarus's research, only two of the eight strategies, positive appraisal and "planful" problem solving, showed statistically significant consistency in improving emotions from negative to positive (P values of 0.003 and 0.004, respectively). These are listed at the top of Table 10-1.

The next four strategies were shown to have variable effects between individuals, which supports the idea that there are few optimal approaches for successful coping.[18] However, the last two strategies, confrontational coping and distancing, were associated with a greater likelihood of increasing negative emotions (although at a level only approaching statistical significance). Accordingly, Lazarus reported respective P values of 0.07 and 0.06 for these strategies.[21,22]

The variability of coping styles indicates that the stages of disorganization and eventual adjustment to a chronic condition proceed differently for each patient. In addition, external factors such as availability of compassionate and competent care, family support, educational level, and emotional maturity all affect the ease of this process.[22]

Given our previous discussion about the value of positive psychology, it is interesting to note the power of positive appraisal in producing a positive impact on emotions. Because positive appraisal involves the use of optimistic self-talk, Lazarus's findings provide support for Seligman's research on learned optimism. Further studies will be helpful in establishing a relationship between these coping styles and the achievement of desirable functional outcomes.

Talking Points/Field Notes

Susan Revisited

Because it is likely that our patients will employ a variety of coping strategies, it is interesting to reflect on how these might affect our therapeutic dialogue.

In this exercise, we consider the case of Susan once again in terms of how the use of various coping strategies may be reflected in her communication. An example is provided in **Figure 10-2.**

Strategy	Susan's Application
Positive reappraisal	"Surgery will be difficult, but I will be able to be pain free afterwards." "I am so lucky to be 54 years old and in perfect health other than this."
Planful problem solving	"I will work with my physical therapist to develop an aquatics exercise program that will help me strengthen my hips, and I will join a weight loss support group. That way I am prepared for surgery if it turns out to be the best option."
Escape-avoidance	"Maybe Jim and I should go on a cruise where we can relax and see new sights without having to walk too much."
Accepting responsibility	"I know it's my own fault that I have gained weight. But I can't afford to put more stress on my hips. I need to deal with this before it gets out of control."
Seeking social support	"I am going to join the local arthritis support group. I know a few of their members have had total hip replacements. Maybe they can help me feel more comfortable about this decision."
Self-controlling	"I am going to quit being such a wimp and just get out there and walk with Jim, even if it hurts. I'm not going to tell my children about this either. They have their own lives and don't need to worry about me!"
Distancing	"I am going to knit sweaters for my grandchildren. That way, I won't have time to think about this problem."
Confrontational coping	"I can't believe surgery is the only way to get rid of my pain! She's probably just trying to make money. I'm going to talk to my physician about cortisone shots!"

Figure 10–2. Application of coping strategies to Susan's case. Adapted from Lazarus, 1993.[18]

Directions

Consider Susan's comments as they relate to each of the coping strategies shown in Figure 10-2.

1. Assuming the role of her physical therapist, discuss how you might respond to each of Susan's comments.

2. How do each of Susan's comments and coping strategies highlight different issues and concerns for both of you?

3. How might your course of treatment vary depending on the use of these coping styles?

4. For each of these comments, how might you encourage Susan toward empowerment and self-efficacy?

Regression

A final note on coping styles relates to situations where the level of stress is perceived as extreme. In the early stages of the illness experience, particularly if severe, some persons may become so overwhelmed that they are not able to cope using any of the strategies in **Table 10-1.** Instead, they may react to their stress by engaging in a child-like defense mechanism known as *regression.* Examples of regressive behaviors include becoming either demanding or passive, displaying aggression toward caretakers, withdrawal, and anxiety.[13,14]

As a physical therapist promoting exercise and function, you might occasionally be met with an angry rebuff by a patient who is overwhelmed (perhaps by fear or pain) at the prospect of getting out of bed. Such patients can benefit enormously from nonjudging empathy, support, and opportunities to exert more control in their care (for example, being allowed to choose when to have PT treatment). In working with patients who display these regressive coping behaviors, it is important to recognize them as normal human reactions to loss and not take them personally. Although it can be hurtful when a patient lashes out, our use of positive reappraisal can help us to maintain unconditional positive regard.

Denial

Denial is a form of coping that may involve either distancing or escape/avoidance, but this is not yet clear in the literature.[18] Patients who employ denial may thus appear uninterested in information about their disease. They might also focus on goals that do not appear realistic in light of their situation. They may sleep excessively or not enough, and they may employ negative emotional coping strategies (such as drinking excessively) to distance themselves from the painful emotions evoked by their situation.

Denial strategies might appear entirely counterproductive, and indeed they can provide interesting challenges to the health-care team (e.g., as in suggesting the use of a wheelchair for a patient who denies the need for one). Although consistent denial may prevent a patient from seeking necessary care, research among patients with severe heart disease suggests that the use of denial can provide a temporary sense of "psychological distance" that serves as a reprieve from the painful reality of having a terminal condition. This short reprieve may allow them to marshal the necessary resources to eventually move forward.[22,23]

Denial strategies may also help patients filter out negative information in order to maintain hope for recovery. Rier's first-person account of his recovery from kidney and respiratory failure has been cited as a "welcome view of the critical illness experience."[24] Rier, a medical sociologist, wrote that while in the intensive care unit, he discouraged anyone from giving him information about his condition. He also deliberately chose to be less active in his care, letting others bathe, feed, and turn him in bed so he could conserve his limited energy. In explaining his rationale, he stated that these responses allowed him to get adequate rest so that he could recover more quickly. Rier's account provides compelling evidence for the effective use of denial. It also affirms that we must respect our patients' needs, even if we don't always understand them. This is not to say, however, that you won't find such behaviors challenging. Thus, as a member of a health-care team, you should always feel comfortable seeking the support and assistance of colleagues with expertise in psychosocial domains of function.

Each person tends to develop a general coping style,[17] which they will likely bring to the illness experience. Furthermore, coping dynamics exist within families as well as individuals, and a similar pattern of consistency is also likely to persist when a family member becomes ill. The following case scenario illustrates these concepts.

A Couple's Coping Styles Clash

Andrew, 32 years old, has been admitted for inpatient neurological rehabilitation following a motor vehicle accident in which he sustained a T5 complete spinal cord injury. He also sustained life-threatening contusions to his liver and spleen, which necessitated a 2-week stay in the intensive care unit. A successful computer technology specialist, Andrew had been driving under the influence of cocaine at the time of the accident and reportedly admitted a history of substance abuse in the emergency department. He has been married to Dana for 3 years. They have no children.

After a month-long course of rehabilitation, Andrew is rapidly moving toward functional independence with the use of a wheelchair and assistive devices. However, he has been depressed and irritable and at times has been rude to health-care staff. Dana has made a few visits, but these have been brief. The previous evening, she was seen leaving Andrew's room in tears. Shortly afterwards, a nurse overheard Andrew talking on the phone to a friend and making a casual reference to "partying" on an upcoming evening leave from the rehab unit.

The following morning, at a case conference discussing Andrew's discharge plans, Patrick, the social worker, reported that Dana had initiated divorce proceedings in the weeks before Andrew's accident but had stopped them when she was told that he was not likely to survive. Now that Andrew was medically stable, Dana wanted to follow through with the divorce and had recently informed her husband of her intention to do so. She told Patrick that Andrew's drug abuse was a major contributing factor in her decision and that he had been known to assault her while under the influence. She also reported that Andrew still refuses intervention for his drug abuse because he feels that it does not interfere with his work. Her final comments to Patrick were, "I'm so sad that Andrew has had this accident, but his choices led him here. In the meantime, I want to get on with my life, and that life will be more stable without him."

Despite her decision to complete the divorce, Dana agrees to work with Andrew's health-care team to find an alternative discharge placement, as she would like to claim sole ownership of their home in the divorce settlement.

Questions

1. If you were Andrew's physical therapist, how might you react to this situation? How would you maintain your unconditional positive regard for all involved persons?

2. How can you support Andrew in this situation? As his physical therapist, what will be your major concerns?

3. How can you support Dana in this situation? As Andrew's physical therapist, what will be your major concerns?

4. What responsibility do you think the health-care team has in assisting Andrew and Dana toward an acceptable discharge placement? What needs to be considered toward this outcome?

Talking Points/Field Notes

A Coping Journey

The purpose of this exercise is to reflect on the stages of awareness, disorganization, and coping that might arise in the course of an illness or undesirable life challenge. Consider a time in your life when you became aware of a significant life challenge (perhaps even a change in health) where you successfully employed coping strategies. Then discuss the following and record your observations in your field notes.

Continued

Talking Points/Field Notes—cont'd ■ ▬▬▬▬▬▬▬▬ ▬▬

Balance Check: Please share at your comfort level. The event you select does not have to be deeply personal. For example, it could be the loss of a pet, an injury that affected a sports career, a change of schools, etc. It is suggested that you focus on an event with which you were able to cope effectively. As you reflect on the following questions, consider the coping strategies described in Table 10-2. Which ones resonate for you?

1. In which ways did this challenge make itself evident in your life?

2. What were some of the ways in which you responded as the challenge became evident?

3. In which specific ways did this challenge affect your daily life? How might you have grown stronger as a result?

4. How did you confront the stresses related to this challenge? Which ways were the most helpful? Which ways were not as helpful?

5. What was the nature of your internal communication (self-talk) as you confronted this challenge? Did this change over time?

6. In which ways can your awareness of this impact assist you in understanding your patients' perspectives as they adjust to changes in their health?

7. What do you think are your most useful coping methods in your current life? How did you come to adopt these?

Reorganization

Living with and adapting to a disability or chronic illness is a highly personal and variable journey. Research focusing on the strategies by which individuals reorganize their lives has been conducted on persons with specific types of illness.

For example, research on patients with stroke indicates that higher levels of self-esteem are related to better self-care after discharge as well as improved mobility.[25] Ramini has demonstrated that adolescents with cancer were largely successful in adapting to their illness by using a variety of coping strategies that enabled them to manage symptoms, maintain positive attitudes, and continue with their psychosocial maturation.[26]

Finally, a study of patients with amyotrophic lateral sclerosis (ALS) suggested four different forms of reorganization that are believed to apply in this disease and possibly others of a similar degenerative nature (Huntington's chorea, Parkinson's disease, and multiple sclerosis).[17]

The first is *sustaining*. In this type of reorganization, the person remains positive, focusing more on what can be achieved rather than what is no longer possible. The second type is *preserving*. This involves actively making lifestyle or environmental changes to promote survival and optimal quality of life. One such patient reported taking nutritional supplements and removing toxins from his home. The third type of reorganization is *enduring*, where the person suffers through his or her experience with a level of resignation. "What can I do it about it?" is a prominent question in this approach. Finally, *fractured* reorganization is related to living with significant emotional pain over the many losses involved in a degenerative fatal illness. When patients respond in this manner, health practitioners may feel helpless because of their inability to relieve their patients' distress and may therefore avoid contact. Accordingly, we must realize that not all patients will adapt in empowering ways to their illness. Nevertheless, by listening to their concerns and providing empathy, we may ease their suffering in small but perhaps beneficial ways.

Although research on patient approaches to reorganization is limited, a growing body of evidence suggests that the quality of health practitioner communication has considerable influence. For example, supportive interventions by ICU nurses (such as providing assurance, comfort, contact, and information) have been shown to have a significantly positive effect on patient recovery and on decreasing family stress.[26]

Challenges to Patients Arising from the Health-Care Environment

Unfortunately, some aspects of the health-care delivery system itself can contribute to the patient's sense of powerlessness. These have been described in the literature as "system-induced setbacks" and were identified in a study of stroke survivors during their early poststroke acute care. An example of one type of setback pertained to low patient expectations that are unwittingly conveyed by medical staff. Hart labeled this as a "nothing can be done" setback because of its tendency to increase patient and family perceptions of hopelessness.[27] To that end, as we previously discussed, there is a demonstrated relationship between the recovery expectations of health-care practitioners and the outcomes their patients achieve. Accordingly, in the spirit of the Hippocratic oath to "at least do no harm," we owe it to our patients to reflect a positive expectation for their optimum outcomes.

Ironically, the hospital setting presents a significant "double-edged sword" in that it provides a centralized base for the delivery of high-quality, technologically sophisticated medical care that, in the interests of efficiency and cost-effectiveness, may be delivered in an unintentionally depersonalizing manner.

This process can begin the moment a patient enters the hospital. Consider the impact of having to leave your home and all its comforts to be assigned a diagnosis (which may become the primary identifier for the duration of your admission), and be removed from spontaneous access to friends, family, and the daily prerogatives that add pleasure to your life (e.g., your favorite foods).

To add further to your sense of disconnectedness, a hospital gown is standard issue in the hospital setting. Although this garment is ostensibly helpful for the purposes of easier bedside hygiene and access for examination purposes, little can be said for it in terms of comfort, coverage, or esthetic appeal. The same is true of the hospital wrist band, which prominently (again, for the convenience of the health-care team) displays personal identifiers that many of us choose to reserve for sharing at our own discretion (such as our age).

Along with the relinquishment of clothing choices is that related to meals, hygiene, and schedules. Most hospitals have specific times during which patients are bathed, fed, and monitored. For many of us, such schedules are vastly different from those of our normal everyday lives and can add further to the stress of the illness experience. Imagine the shock of one of my friends, who, during a recent hospitalization, was awakened at 2 a.m. in order to be weighed! This same friend also recounted an episode where a physician came into her room and spoke to her without troubling to make personal contact or looking away from her medical chart. Such actions do little to inspire rapport.

Many hospitals are actively working to improve the quality of the inpatient hospital experience; it is important to remember that the actions of the health-care staff are the most instrumental in this process. Thus you are encouraged to affirm your patients by learning about them in the full context of their lives, especially those details that give them a sense of self-worth and purpose (such as personal accomplishments, interests, and social roles). This effort will be useful in developing both a therapeutic alliance and a meaningful plan of care that will optimize their quality of life upon discharge.

■ The Illness Experience in Social Context

Loss of Role Identity

Role identity is the sense of self derived from the connection between *who we are* and *what we do* in society. Our lives are enriched by the interactions that are played out in the context of our various social roles. Loss of role identity is a well-documented element of the illness experience.[28] Thankfully, its loss can be mitigated in the health-care setting through a "whole person" view of our patients. Furthermore, in working with our patients in the goal-setting process, information about their social roles can greatly enhance the identification of meaningful outcomes.

To illustrate the importance of social roles, consider your own life situation. At this point in your life, you have an important role as a physical therapy student, which involves certain behaviors such as attending class, being respectful, participating in clinics, dressing professionally for patient care, and using the language of clinical practice. Most likely, however, you have several other, equally important roles such as son/daughter, spouse/significant other, athlete, musician, or employee. All of these roles enrich your life by providing opportunities for accomplishment, recognition, and support. Accordingly, your imminent role as a physical therapist will afford you a measure of societal privilege and responsibility, both of which will likely enhance your sense of self as a valuable member of society.

Stigmatization and Shame

Disease processes that alter function in a visible way may contribute to patients' social isolation. Stigmatization is a process whereby persons who are perceived as "abnormal" are negatively labeled, stereotyped, and devaluated. Labels such as *gimp* or *retard* are examples of offensive labels that have been used in reference to persons with disability. Such labels contribute to a sense of shame and social isolation. They can also prevent persons from seeking necessary care.

One on the most commonly stigmatized disease conditions is mental illness. Terms such as *psycho* and *lunatic* are still used to describe persons with severe diseases such as schizophrenia. Sadly, a long history of stigmatization continues to prevail in our society with respect to mental illness and continues to keep many from seeking care.[29]

Ours is a society obsessed with personal appearance and youthful vitality. Thus it is not surprising that those with visibly disabling conditions such as stroke, Parkinson's disease, and multiple sclerosis have reported self-imposed avoidance of social activities because of shame due to their appearance.[30] Sadly, stigma and shame can greatly exacerbate the negative consequences of the illness experience by reducing opportunities for participation in social activities. Over time, these limitations can contribute to isolation, depression, and decreased mobility, further increasing the burden of disablement.

As a physical therapist, you will be in a powerful position to reduce the stigma of disability by advocating for accessible community environments and educating the public about challenges facing persons with disabilities. One of the first ways to do this is to learn about the various community resources for our patients. These resources include support groups, planned activities, and accessible public transportation. As our society ages, such resources will become increasingly important and necessary.

Finally, stigmatizing labels and stereotypes may also contribute to the marginalization of different cultures and races. Accordingly, there is a considerable body of evidence demonstrating significant health-care inequities in the treatment of persons of other races.

Impact of Stigmatization in Health Care

Mary is a PT student on an 8-week internship at an acute-care facility in inner-city Los Angeles. Her CI is Bradley, an experienced and respected clinician.

Mary is assigned to work with Alonzo Guttierrez, 23 years old, who sustained a closed head injury in a recent fist fight. As Bradley reviews Alonzo's chart with Mary, he notes that the patient has sustained two previous closed head injuries as a result of fist fights. Shaking his head, Bradley states, "Here we go, another macho Latino trying to prove himself as a hero street fighter." Bradley then adds, "it really makes me mad that he probably is an illegal resident taking up our tax dollars, like most of these guys."

Questions

1. How does Bradley's statement reflect the use of stigmatization against a specific ethnic group? What impact might this have on Alonzo's care?

2. What approach can Mary use to respond to Bradley's statement assertively and with respect, so as not to harm their working relationship?

3. Mary has never worked with a Hispanic male patient. How might she demonstrate cultural sensitivity when she meets Alonzo?

The Rest of the Story: Please Read After Discussion!

Mary withholds judgment about her CI's statements and seeks to understand his point of view. "What makes you say that?" she asks. Bradley then shares his frustration over having treated several illegal Latino males for assault-related injuries. He states that he feels torn between wanting to give the best care and knowing that this depletes limited health-care funds. He also knows that if these patients are deported, they will not get any care and could die as a result. At that point, Mary responds with empathy and assertiveness. "From your experiences, I can see how you might have these feelings about Latino males. However, as a student, I want to approach all my patients without any preconceived stereotypes that could affect my plan of care." She then asks Bradley to help her learn about cultural issues related to the management of Hispanic patients. Bradley apologizes for his comment and offers to teach Mary some Spanish that can she can use to establish a rapport with Alonzo. They then both go into his room to begin the examination.

The Therapeutic Alliance and Patient-Centered Care

Developing the Therapeutic Alliance

The ability to optimize desirable health changes in our patients depends largely on the quality of our partnership, which is known as the therapeutic alliance. Specifically, this is defined as the "collaboration between patient and therapist in efforts to combat the patient's problems."[31]

In an optimal health-care delivery system, the therapeutic alliance is one of many supportive relationships that collectively define patient-centered care. **Figure 10-3** shows the relationship between the elements of the therapeutic alliance and those of patient-centered care.

In Figure 10-3, the patient and therapist are represented in the context of their respective "whole person" life experiences. This representation is meant to suggest that both individuals should not be defined entirely by their roles in the health-care system. Simply

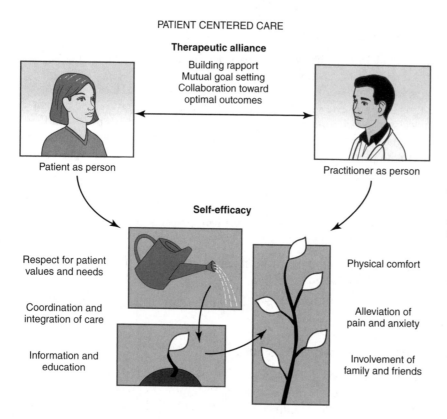

PATIENT CENTERED CARE

Therapeutic alliance

Building rapport
Mutual goal setting
Collaboration toward
optimal outcomes

Patient as person

Practitioner as person

Self-efficacy

Respect for patient
values and needs

Coordination and
integration of care

Information and
education

Physical comfort

Alleviation of
pain and anxiety

Involvement of
family and friends

Figure 10–3.   Integrated model of patient-centered care. The challenges of the illness experience and the health-care environment are ameliorated by empowering communication. In addition, self-efficacy is promoted through the elements of patient-centered care. *(Adapted from Gerteis M, Edgman-Levitan S, Daley J, Delbanco TL, eds. Through the Patient's Eyes:* Understanding and Promoting Patient Centered Care. *San Francisco: Jossey Bass; 1993.)*

put, they are persons first. As we will discuss in the following section, this frame of reference has important implications for the therapeutic alliance.

The Importance of Person-first Language in the Therapeutic Alliance

Mark Twain once said, "The difference between the right word and the almost right word is the difference between lightning and the lightning bug."[32] As we begin this exploration of strategies to promote effective therapeutic alliances, the most important first step is to consider the language we use to describe our patients. Thus far, we have defined such individuals as experiencing a degree of pain which compels them to seek medical care. We have further explored the concept of suffering as a multi-dimensional variant which is felt on many levels. With these factors in mind, how do we describe our patients in a way that acknowledges them as unique, whole human beings despite the presence of disease or injury? Even more importantly, how do these descriptions drive both our internal and external communication as it pertains to our engagement with patients? Consider the following Champ and Blockhead scenario.

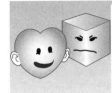

Champ and Blockhead Prepare for the Day

It is just before 8 a.m. in a busy inpatient hospital PT department. Champ and Blockhead are both members of the department's postsurgical team and are scheduling the day's new admissions. As they look over patient diagnoses and consult orders, they engage in the following conversation:

Champ (who is reading a consult): This looks like an interesting patient! She's a 70-year-old woman who fractured her patella while surfboarding! She should be interesting to meet! I'll see her.

Blockhead: Be my guest! I have enough knees on my schedule for now. (He picks up another consult.) This one's a shoulder, I'll take it. I haven't seen one for awhile and I don't want to get rusty. By the way, did you happen to finish that preop hip last evening?

Champ: You know, I was hoping to, but Mrs. Jones had her husband with her, and they had lots of questions about her surgery. She seemed nervous, so I talked to her about the procedure and what she can expect in terms of PT. By the time we got done, it was time for her dinner, so I told her I would see her first thing this morning.

Blockhead: Dude, that's a drag, you're going to be behind today. Why didn't you just tell her to ask her doc about the surgery? That's his job isn't it?

Champ: I suppose I could have, but I put myself in her shoes and decided that she needed information so she wouldn't lose a good night's sleep worrying. Now I think things will go a lot better for her since she knows what to expect. Are there any more patients for me to see this morning?

Blockhead: Yeah, there's a whirlpool for an infected foot. You can have it, I hate doing wounds. They're nasty and they take forever. There are two knees left to do. I'll take them. They're boring but at least I'll have time for lunch.

Questions

1. How would you describe the different approaches used by Champ and Blockhead to select their patients?
2. Consider the language used by both Champ and Blockhead in describing their patients. How would you describe each of their approaches?
3. How might the language used by Blockhead affect his level of engagement and connection with the patients involved?
4. How might the language used by Champ affect his level of engagement and connection with the patients involved?
5. How does it feel when you are described entirely in objective but impersonal terms? (Student, customer, patient, man, woman, Latino, African American, etc.)

How can we use language to promote more inclusive awareness of each person we treat?

As the Champ and Blockhead example suggests, the way we conceptualize and describe other persons can have a profound effect on our attitudes and interactions. On a more critical scale, most forms of prejudice involve the use of depersonalizing labels. Once these are ingrained in our consciousness, their mindless, habitual use can leave a pervasive, negative impact (as you well know if you have ever been on the receiving end).

In the context of health care, "person-first language" involves the use of language that identifies patients as *persons with a disability,* rather than *persons defined entirely by their disability.*[33,34] For example, consider the impact of calling a patient a *quad* as opposed to a *person with quadriplegia.* Thus, in referring to patients, it is important to use a person noun instead of a disability noun. While this may seemed contrived at first, continued use of person-first language over time will help keep you mindful of the diverse human elements that exist in each person. The principles of person-first language also involve avoidance of negative labels (e.g., *mongoloid* to refer to a person with Down's syndrome), disempowering labels (stroke *victim*, wheelchair-*bound*) and the substitution of *disability* (which is a more specific term for a person with restricted function) for *handicap* (which connotes a social or environmental limitation imposed by society on those with disabilities).[9] **Table 10-2** illustrates the use of person-first language.

Implications for Physical Therapy

The American Physical Therapy Association (APTA) requires the use of person-first language in all articles, proposals, and abstracts submitted for publication or presentation. In 1991, the APTA House of Delegates issued the following position statement[35]: "Physical therapy practitioners have an obligation to provide nonjudgmental care to all people who need it."

The statement then directs authors to a publication entitled *Guidelines for Reporting and Writing About People With Disabilities,* which includes specific suggestions for person-first language. You are strongly urged to acquire these guidelines and use them in your clinical documentation.[36]

As we have already discussed, the habitual use of person-first language is instrumental in the development of a therapeutic alliance with our patients. This will help us maintain a perspective of patients as *unique individuals* whose lives have been disrupted by a process that affects their quality of life. Furthermore, the use of the term

Table 10–2. Elements of Person First Language

Instead of These Devaluing Stereotypes	Use These Person First Terms
Stroke patient	Patient with stroke
Cerebral palsy kids	Children with cerebral palsy
The mentally ill	Persons with mental illness
Cancer victim	Person with cancer or cancer cancer survivor
The schizophrenic	Person with schizophrenia
I have two hips to treat today	I have two patients with hip fractures to treat today
She's an epileptic	She has epilepsy, or She has a seizure disorder
He's confined to a wheelchair (are we "confined" to our shoes?)	He uses a wheelchair
Handicapped bathroom	Accessible bathroom
She's retarded	She has a developmental or learning disability
He's spastic	He has muscle spasticity
Invalid, incapacitated, handicapped, cripple	Person with a disability Person who walks with crutches
My grandmother is demented	My grandmother has dementia

Talking Points/Field Notes

The Impact of Labels

For the next 48 hours, be particularly observant of the language used in the media or other sources to describe persons with illness or disability. If you want to broaden your observations, you might be on the lookout for depersonalizing language of any kind. You may quickly find examples in newspapers, magazines, and on-line articles. You may even overhear these in conversation. As you read or hear such language, consider the following, then discuss with classmates and record in your field notes.

1. Describe one or two examples of stereotyping language you have encountered. How long have you been familiar with such terminology? What impact do you think this has had on societal attitudes about the persons involved?

2. What effect does this language have with respect to the development of attitudes about the persons involved? What is typically the nature of these attitudes?

3. How might you rephrase the language you encountered toward nonjudging, person-first terminology? What impact does this have for you?

4. As a future physical therapist, how can you begin now to increase your use of person-first language and to avoid negative terminology in referring to persons with disabilities or backgrounds that are different from your own?

alliance suggests that our role is to provide coaching to empower our patients toward self-efficacy.

Although the deliberate use of this term may seem overstated, it represents a departure from more traditional views of health care as a paternalistic, authoritarian system where the practitioner tells the patient what to do and the patient is a passive recipient of care. As we have discussed, this system is no longer appropriate in a society where patients have unprecedented access to information and the management of widely prevalent chronic conditions (hypertension, obesity, diabetes) requires active patient participation. By viewing our patients as active (and equal) partners in their health-care journey, we will be compelled to adjust our communication in a way that fosters an empowering therapeutic alliance.

The coaching elements of the therapeutic alliance are predicated on the development of an interpersonal bond between therapist and patient. This involves a genuine compassionate concern about our patients as unique individuals whose welfare is important to us. If you have ever received health care from an impersonal practitioner who seemed more concerned with dispensing skills than in understanding their relevance to your life, you can quickly appreciated the value of such a bond.

The therapeutic alliance is central to optimal health-care delivery, and considerable evidence supports the relationship between the strength of the therapeutic alliance and favorable outcomes in physical rehabilitation.[37]

Internal Communication Prerequisites for the Therapeutic Alliance

In previous chapters, we have discussed the importance of internal communication skills such as a positive outlook and mindful presence. These are important prerequisites in the development of an effective therapeutic alliance. Even if we have only a short time to spend with our patients, they need to feel that they have our undivided attention for that duration. To that end, it can be very helpful to begin each patient interaction with a silent affirmation that centers your intention and attention. An affirmation such as "I am here to be as helpful as possible to this patient" or "I will let my interactions with this patient guide me toward the right things to do and say" have proven useful in many of my own clinical interactions, particularly with patients facing the end of life.

If the use of affirmations does not appeal to you, consider Epstein's suggestion to approach each patient with an "attitude of critical curiosity, openness, and connection."[38]

In previous sections, we have discussed the many challenges of the illness experience. These challenges can overwhelm patients to the point where they feel hopeless and pessimistic. They can thus benefit tremendously from our encouragement, which we must generate first from within. Even in cases where a patient is unlikely to recover, you can still maintain an encouraging outlook and confidence in your ability to facilitate their physical and emotional comfort. In my work with dying patients, I have become convinced of the value of therapeutic touch (massage, gentle range-of-motion exercises, and the facilitation of deep breathing for relaxation) in reducing anxiety and pain. These interventions are just as much a part of PT practice as any other.

External Communication Prerequisites for the Therapeutic Alliance

The numerous elements of external communication discussed thus far are all applicable to the patient alliance, which is, first and foremost, an interpersonal relationship. Thus the elements of emotional and social intelligence can be critical allies in our ability to determine the appropriate approach to the establishment of a therapeutic alliance.

Communication Tasks in Establishing the Therapeutic Alliance

Hill describes the therapeutic alliance as a four-stage process in which both the therapist and the patient have specific roles and communication tasks that must be accomplished for optimal outcomes.[39]

Although these were developed for the psychotherapeutic process, they can be easily applied to the relationship between physical therapists and patients. Obviously, exceptions can occur in situations where cognitive impairments prevent patient participation. However, in such instances, the physical therapist must still demonstrate sufficient communication skills to establish a therapeutic alliance with family members and caregivers. The stages and communication tasks of the therapeutic alliance are described in **Table 10-3**.

Impression Formation/Establishment of Rapport

Just as in all relationships, first impressions are of significant importance in building a relationship with our patients. Eye contact and a friendly, open demeanor are cues that we can use to convey our caring presence. Evidence also suggests that a full-contact, firm handshake given with eye contact promotes favorable first impressions that convey extraversion, intelligence, and openness.[40]

One of the first tasks in the development of the therapeutic alliance involves introducing yourself to your patient, learning his or her name, and determining the patient's preferred form of address. This is a critical first demonstration of your concern for the patient as a person. For the patient (who is involved in those first critical moments of impression formation), this authentic concern is a validating experience that can facilitate comfort and promote the establishment of rapport.

The use of your patient's first name should not be assumed. Rather, you should ask directly, "How would you prefer to be addressed?" This negotiation conveys respect and can also be useful when the patient has a nickname that is not in the chart. You may also find

Table 10–3. Stages of the Therapeutic Alliance

Stage	PT Skills	Patient-Related Elements	Desired Outcome
Impression formation *Establishing rapport*	Introduction: Desired form of address Conveying warmth and approachability Small talk skills Putting patient at ease Displaying interest in patient as person Gaining patient trust Professional demeanor to convey credibility	Being open to participating in PT Determining comfort about sharing information Assessing therapist interest Assessing credibility and professionalism	Patient and therapist have mutual feelings of potential for successful therapeutic relationship
Assessment	Creating sense of permission Eliciting patient information in non threatening manner Conveying responsiveness Active listening, not interrupting Displaying competence and skills Determining patient expectations Conveying therapist expectations	Sharing personal and health information Sharing expectations for therapy Sharing concerns	Therapist accepts fiduciary responsibility for patient (e.g., commits to developing plan of care to achieve patient goals) Patient demonstrates readiness to engage in therapeutic process
Intervention	Providing encouragement, support and appropriate challenge to maintain patient engagement Information on task accomplishment Educating patient and family Maintaining appropriate professional Boundaries	Patient/family participates in plan of care Provides honest feedback to therapist about progression of treatment	Goals of therapy are met in atmosphere of mutual goodwill Therapist and patient feel empowered in alliance
Termination	Empowering patient toward optimal self management (instilling confidence)	Accepting responsibility for health behavior change	Patient feels empowered toward self-management

Adapted from Hill C. Therapist techniques, client involvement, and the therapeutic relationship: Inextricably entwined in the therapy process. *Psychother Theory Res Pract Training.* 2005; 42(4):431-442.

that older patients may ask that you address them more formally (e.g., Mr. Jones). Such a preference may be a generational or cultural issue.

The advent of doctoral education in PT has provoked an interesting professional dialogue about how our patients address us. In educational dialogues with over 400 experienced physical therapists enrolled in transitional DPT programs, I have observed an overwhelming preference for the continued use of first names in clinical interactions. These colleagues believe that first-name address facilitates a more personal connection with their patients. However, they also recognize the importance of promoting our profession as one of doctoring practice. Fortunately it is easy to do both. Thus one frequently suggested approach is to begin the introduction using the doctoral designation ("Hello, I'm Dr. Angela Wilson, your physical therapist"), then following it with an invitation for patients to use a first-name form of address if desired ("You are welcome to call me Angela"). Because most patients continue to associate the "Dr." designation with physicians, the reference to being a physical therapist is important to prevent confusion. Furthermore, it provides a powerful opportunity for educating our consumers. Last, this statement provides an easy transition to the patient's introduction. ("You're Mr. John Morgan? How would you like me to address you?")

Assessment Intervention and Termination: The Therapeutic Process in Patient-Centered Care

While the elements of treatment, intervention, and termination are the heart of PT practice, their integration into the greater context of patient-centered care constitutes the soul of health-care delivery.

In 2001, the Institute of Medicine identified patient-centered care as a key element of quality health care for the 21st century.[41] As a result of this initiative, several granting agencies have supported follow-up studies to identify the specific elements of patient-centered care.[42,43] These are shown in **Box 10-2**.

The remaining three stages of the therapeutic alliance (assessment, intervention, and termination) involve sharing the skills of PT practice in the context of these elements.

Elements of Patient-Centered Care

Let us now consider how each of these elements relates to the therapeutic alliance in PT practice.

Superb Access to Care

In many areas of health-care delivery, such as emergency medicine, "24/7" (24 hours a day, 7 days a week) availability is the presumed standard of care. If you have ever been stricken in the wee morning hours with a severe asthma attack or injured in a car accident after usual business hours, you can certainly appreciate the importance of these extended business hours.

BOX 10-2:   Elements of Patient-Centered Care

1. Access to services
2. Respect for patients' needs and values
3. Coordination of care
4. Physical comfort
5. Emotional support and alleviation of anxiety
6. Effective patient education
7. Accommodation of family and friends
8. Continuity of care

Unfortunately, such availability is not as apparent in other areas of health care. Perhaps you have also been frustrated by having to wait days or even weeks for a desired health-care–related service. Should you be fortunate enough to have escaped that experience, perhaps you have warmed the seat of a provider's waiting room chair well beyond your scheduled appointment time. Such experiences are irritating at best and at worst can greatly intensify the distress of the health-care encounter.

In reality, access to health care is a fluid and dynamic process involving not only the initial encounter but also the ability to provide ongoing support, information, and services as needed. Thus we should consider effective methods of providing follow-up access in order to address patient concerns or to provide further interventions outside of our usual business hours as necessary. Thankfully, technological forms of communication such as e-mail or telephone can extend our availability in this fashion. As a profession, we may also need to reconsider our place in a 24/7 schedule of availability, as the following real case illustrates.

Clinical Scenario

Where Were You When I Needed You?

Two days ago Julie, age 48, underwent a thoracotomy with right-upper-lung lobectomy for resection of an encapsulated lung tumor. Owing to this surgery, Julie is in significant pain and finds turning in bed very difficult. Although she gets some relief with opioid medication, she finds that her comfort can be greatly enhanced by getting out of bed for exercise every few hours throughout the day and night. Because Julie requires moderate assistance and vital sign monitoring while out of bed, she began receiving PT twice daily and found this helpful in reducing her pain when she returned to bed. At 3 a.m. the next morning, after a sleepless 2 hours in moderate discomfort despite medication, Julie rings her nurses' call button and asks if she can receive PT. To her dismay, she is told that PT is available only between 8 a.m. and 6 p.m. She then asks for more pain medication but doesn't fall asleep for another 2 hours.

At 8 a.m. Julie is awakened from her much-needed sleep by a knock on her door. A young woman enters her room and says "I'm Jenny, your physical therapist for today." Jenny asks Julie if she would like to get out of bed to exercise. Julie finds herself replying with irritation, "What I really need right now is to sleep. I could have used PT at 3 a.m., but you weren't here!"

Questions

1. Consider the professions that involve 24/7 care: medicine, nursing, pharmacy, radiology. These are considered essential services in health care. Where do you think PT belongs?

2. How would you respond to Julie's comments to Jennie? What underlying concerns would you explore with her? How might you address these?

3. What role might physical therapists have in a 24/7 schedule of care? Consider the four areas of PT practice as outlined in the *Guide to Physical Therapist Practice* (integumentary, cardiopulmonary, neuromuscular, musculoskeletal).

4. Would you support a 24/7 schedule of care in our profession? Consider your position in terms of its relevance to patient-centered care. How might such a schedule affect patient attitudes about what we do?

5. Julie is asking for PT in accordance with her need for service. Should our patients be able to schedule their care in inpatient settings as they do in outpatient ones?

6. Jenny has introduced herself as Julie's physical therapist "for today," which implies that other physical therapists will be sharing the care of this patient. How might Julie's PT care be enhanced through a greater consistency of care?

Continued

7. What are our responsibilities in terms of providing services to our patients beyond the 8-to-5 workday? How do these responsibilities apply to our professional core values (accountability, altruism, care/compassion, excellence, professional duty, integrity, social responsibility)?

The Rest of the Story

A survey of patients on the oncology unit where this situation occurred revealed strong interest in having PT services available for very early morning exercise and ambulation. Two physical therapists agreed to a shift from 11 p.m. to 7 a.m., which was well received by patients, family members, and staff.

Talking Points/Field Notes

Further Communication Considerations to Enhance Access

Discuss the following:

1. How might we increase our availability to address patient concerns that arise after their visit? Do you think it is appropriate to provide an e-mail address or cell phone number enabling patients to contact you after work hours?

2. In cases of day surgery or other painful procedures, it is typical for the patient to receive a next-day follow-up contact (usually a phone call) from a nurse or physician. These contacts are helpful ways of assessing the patient's status and providing support or assurance. Physical therapists sometimes perform painful interventions such as wound care or manual therapy. Do you think it might also be appropriate to provide a next-day follow-up contact? What benefits might this provide for the patient/ family, ourselves, and our profession? Are you aware of PT practice settings where follow-up contacts are routinely provided? What has been the general impact?

3. How do physical therapists reconcile giving their patients a choice in the selection of treatment times while maintaining an optimal schedule, especially in an inpatient setting where patient care begins early in the morning?

Respect for Patients' Needs and Values

In addition to our patients' need for access to care, they also need validation and support for the beliefs, values, and personal traditions that contribute to the spectrum of human diversity. Although our patients bring many such elements to their illness experience, three of these have significant impact. These are culture, spirituality, and health beliefs.

Respect for Cultural Differences

Cultural differences can affect many elements of the illness experience. A recent study examined the attitudes of 61 African Americans, 45 Latinos, and 55 non-Latino whites regarding cultural factors which impact the medical encounter.[44]

Box 10-3 is based upon the findings of this study and illustrates characteristics of culturally competent communication in health care.

The Culturally and Linguistically Appropriate Services Standards (CLAS) were developed to facilitate culturally and linguistically appropriate communication in healthcare settings. These standards were also developed to reduce unnecessary health-care costs or disparities in service provision arising from lack of cultural sensitivity. They are illustrated in **Box 10-4**.

BOX 10-3:   Characteristics of Culturally Affirming Communication in Health Care

1. Responsiveness and knowledge about complementary and alternative medicine (acupuncture, meditation, massage, or herbal treatments).
2. Awareness of the effects of language on access to care and quality of communication. Awareness of the role of interpreters in visits with limited English-speaking patients, not making assumptions based on English proficiency.
3. Avoidance of health insurance-based discrimination: Not making assumptions or differential treatment decisions based on patients' health insurance status.
4. Avoidance of ethnicity-based discrimination: Not making assumptions or differential treatment decisions based on patients' ethnicity.
5. Avoidance of social class-based discrimination: Not making assumptions or differential treatment decisions based on patients' economic or social standing.
6. Sensitivity to presence or absence of ethnic concordance (patient and practitioner sharing the same ethnic background) on quality of the communication, trust, and interpersonal relations.
7. Sensitivity to patients' modesty and inhibitions associated with sharing information about or revealing sensitive body parts.
8. Sensitivity to immigration-related concerns of recently immigrated patients, such as fears of deportation, acculturative stress, changes in dietary practices, and posttraumatic stress.
9. Avoidance of age-based discrimination: Not making assumptions or differential treatment decisions based on patients' age.
10. Acceptance of the role of spirituality in patients' adaptation and response to illness.
11. Acknowledging patient preferences for involving their families in health care decision making.

Adapted from Nápoles-Springer AM, Santoyo J, Houston K, et al. Patients' perceptions of cultural factors affecting the quality of their medical encounters. *Health Expectations* 2005;8:4-17.

The CLAS standards suggest that non-English linguistic competence is a critical element of effective communication in health care. Thus, as American society becomes more culturally diverse, the ability to speak another language besides English will be an increasingly important skill for health-care providers. For example, as of 2008, the United States has the world's fifth-largest Spanish-speaking population. Furthermore, it is also predicted that by 2025, the population of Spanish-speaking Latinos will double, reaching approximately 40 million.[46] Thus, if you are already proficient in Spanish or another language besides English, you are strongly encouraged to maintain this competence. If you are not proficient in another language, you might consider developing this skill as a means of enhancing your patient/family communication skills.

Respect for Patients' Spiritual Needs

Besides the issues of diversity, which we have already discussed, spirituality is an important element of our patients' individuality. Although spirituality and religion are often addressed as if synonymous, they are, in reality, separate concepts. Of the two terms, *spirituality* is the broader one, pertaining to a personal belief system that provides a sense of hope, meaning, and interconnectedness (with others and with a power greater than ourselves). For most of us, spirituality is a deeply felt awareness that can fortify us with hope, gratitude, and inner peace.[47]

Religion is a system of traditions, practices, and rituals that provide an expression of our spirituality. Thus many persons find that their spirituality is enhanced by attendance at a

BOX 10-4: **Culturally and Linguistically Appropriate Standards (CLAS) for Health Care**

1. All patients should receive health care with respect for their cultural health-care beliefs, practices, and preferred language.
   Example: A hospital offers the services of a Navajo medicine man upon request.
   Example: Respecting the rights of patients who refuse blood transfusion.

2. Health-care organizations should ensure that all staff receive ongoing education and training in culturally and linguistically appropriate service delivery.
   Example: Providing a staff in-service about Native American healing.

3. Health-care organizations must offer and provide language assistance at no cost to each patient or consumer.
   Example: Providing an interpreter for a patient who speaks Mandarin Chinese.

4. Health-care organizations must provide written and verbal notification of alternative language services offered.
   Example: Displaying the Patient's Bill of Rights in both Spanish and English.

5. Family and friends should not be used to provide interpretation services unless requested by the patient/consumer. Health-care organizations must also ensure the ongoing competency of individuals providing the interpretation services.
   Example: Requiring competency-based assessments of interpreters' proficiency.

6. Patient-related materials and signs should be provided in regionally prevalent languages.
   Example: A clinic in Flagstaff, Arizona, has patient information in English, Spanish, and Navajo.

7. Health-care organizations must promote, educate, and implement a plan to provide culturally and linguistically appropriate services.
   Example: A clinic provides an annual medically based Spanish language course for staff.

8. Health-care organizations should complete initial and ongoing self-assessments of CLAS-related activities.
   Example: A clinic develops a CLAS-based patient satisfaction survey.

9. Information on a patient/consumer's race, language, and ethnicity should be collected on the patient/consumer's medical records.
   Example: Demographic data are collected from patients during the admitting process.

10. Health-care organizations must maintain a current demographic assessment of the cultural and linguistic community.
    Example: Analysis of demographic data to determine patient representation from various cultures.

11. Health-care organizations should use formal and informal community and patient/consumer involvement to design and implement CLAS-activities.
    Example: A consultant is hired to develop CLAS-based patient education materials.

12. Health-care organizations must ensure that conflict and grievance resolution processes can be used by all individuals regardless of their cultural and linguistic background.
    Example: Establishment of an anonymous system for reporting grievances.

13. Health-care organizations are encouraged to provide information to the public on their progress and success in implementing the CLAS standards.
    Example: CLAS-related resources and outcome data are presented on a facility website.

place of worship or by the performance of various rituals. Access to these activities may be limited during the illness experience, but many facilities provide support for these through onsite places of worship or a well-developed chaplaincy program.

Because of the actual difference in these two definitions, it is important to realize that a person can be deeply spiritual without being religious. It is also possible for a person to adhere to the practices and rituals of a certain religion without having a satisfying and meaningful personal spirituality. Nevertheless, the search for a spiritual belief system is an important part of the human experience. Accordingly, 94% of Americans believe that spiritual health is as important as physical health.[47]

Not surprisingly, the need for a spiritual connection can become particularly acute when our equanimity is challenged by the illness experience. As an element of addressing their preferences and needs, our patients may thus benefit from spiritual comfort and support to minimize the distress of health decline. One study reported that over 75% of patients would like their spirituality to be considered in terms of their medical care but that less than 20% of their physicians actually discuss these issues. Furthermore, there is a growing body of evidence to support the value of spirituality in minimizing the negative impact of the illness experience.[47]

In order to address spirituality with our patients, a direct approach can be useful, such as, "For some people, their religious or spiritual beliefs can be a source of strength in dealing with life challenges. Is this true for you?"[47] If the patient responds affirmatively to this question, it can then be followed by, "Would you like to talk more about this? In contrast, should a patient not express such interest, the conversation can easily be redirected without having been intrusive.

The HOPE questionnaire can provide a means of exploring spiritual concerns with our patients. It was developed in the hospice setting, where spiritual issues often arise. The HOPE questionnaire is worded broadly, allowing for inclusion of the broad spectrum of religious practices and spiritual belief systems.[48] **Figure 10-4** illustrates the HOPE questionnaire.

Figure 10–4. The HOPE approach to spiritual assessment. *(Adapted from Gowri A, Hight E. Spirituality and medical practice: using the hope questions as a practical tool for spiritual assessment. Am Fam Physician. http://www.aafp.org/afp/20010101/81.html.)*

H: Sources of hope, meaning, comfort, strength, peace, love, and connection
What in your life gives you internal support?
What are your sources of hope, strength, comfort, and peace?
What do you hold on to during difficult times?
What keeps you going?

O: Organized religion
Do you consider yourself part of an organized religion?
How important is this to you?
What aspects of your religion are helpful and not so helpful to you?
Are you part of a religious or spiritual community? Does it help you? How?

P: Personal spirituality/practices
Do you have personal spiritual beliefs that are independent of organized religion? What are they?
Do you believe in God? What kind of relationship do you have with God?
What aspects of your spirituality or spiritual practices do you find most helpful to you personally? (e.g., prayer, meditation, reading scripture, attending religious services, listening to music, hiking, communing with nature)

E: Effects on medical care and end-of-life issues
Has being sick (or your current situation) affected your ability to do the things that usually help you spiritually? (Or affected your relationship with God?)
Is there anything that I can do to help you access the resources that usually help you?
Are you worried about any conflicts between your beliefs and your medical situation/care/decisions?
Would it be helpful for you to speak to a clinical chaplain/community spiritual leader?
Are there any specific practices or restrictions I should know about in providing your care?

Spiritual SOS

Irene McGinity, 69 years old, is on Chris' schedule for a preoperative PT consult the day before she is to undergo a left, below-the-knee amputation secondary to lower leg gangrene caused by diabetes-related vascular insufficiency. Irene's chart indicates that she is of the Catholic faith.

Chris' consult with Irene goes well and Irene seems to understand the course of rehabilitation that will follow her surgery. In preparation for ending their time together, Chris asks if there is anything he can do to make Irene more comfortable before leaving her bedside. Irene quickly replies, "It would greatly help my peace of mind if you would sit and pray with me that my surgery goes well tomorrow." Chris does not believe in God or the rituals of organized religion.

Question

1. If you were in Chris's position, how might you respond? How might Chris acknowledge Irene's spiritual needs without betraying his own belief system?

2. Would you be comfortable praying with a patient who asked you do to do so? How might you go about this?

3. Are there ever situations where it is appropriate for a health professional to share his or her own spiritual beliefs with a patient?

Understanding Patients' Health Beliefs

Whether or not we are aware of it, all of us have a system of health-related beliefs that guide our thinking in terms of the etiology (cause), pathogenesis (development), and forms of treatment related to a given disease process. We tend to place great trust in these beliefs and seek practitioners who support them.

For example, the biomedical belief system attributes the cause of strep throat to a bacterial infection. Accordingly we tend to associate specific consequences such as fever, sore throat, and general malaise with this condition. Finally, most of us believe in the value of antibiotic treatment as a cure for this condition.

Despite the prevalence of the western biomedical belief system, it is important to understand that our patients may have different sets of attributions informing their illness experience. Many of these are related to their culture and socialization process (in the same manner as it is for us). Along with health beliefs related to cause, course, and cure, there are other beliefs that have a significant impact on the illness experience.[49]

The "expanded health belief model" incorporates individual psychosocial, demographic, and biomedical elements into a comprehensive perceptual set that has been shown to predict health outcomes. Of particular importance are beliefs related to self-efficacy in making health-promoting lifestyle changes.[50]

The expanded health belief model explores individual perceptions of susceptibility and likely severity of the disease process. It also explores individual access to mediating resources such as preventive knowledge, support, and self-efficacy. Finally, it explores the potential for changes in health behavior by assessing beliefs about their benefits, barriers, and efficacy.

The exploration of patients' health beliefs is an important element of the examination process. Through thoughtful questioning and empathic listening, we can elicit information about our patients' concerns and their impact on function and quality of life.

As we continue this exploration, we can also discover our patients' attitudes and knowledge about their condition, along with their beliefs about what is needed for them to reach their goals. **Table 10-4** illustrates a process of questioning that can be used to elicit this information.

Table 10–4. Exploring Patients' Health Beliefs in the Context of the PT Examination Process

Element	Examples of Appropriate Questions	Considerations
1. Determining patient's problem/concern	*"I understand that you hurt your knee."* *"What sort of problems has this caused for you?"* *"What brings you here today?"* *"What problems are you having?"* *"Which problem is the worst for you?"*	You are most likely to obtain accurate and complete information if you avoid interrupting the patient. Use of empathy can elicit further information ("That must be frustrating!") Determining patient's sense of worst problem. Can assist with prioritization of goals/treatment.
2. Exploring development of the problem	*"Can you tell me a little more about what you were doing when you hurt your knee?* *"Can you tell me more about how you think your back pain started?"*	This question elicits patient's view of factors contributing to his or her condition. Patients of different cultures may have nonbiomedical views of disease/injury causation.
3. Exploring functional implications	*"What sorts of activities are you having difficulty with because of this problem?* *"What kind of difficulties are you having?"* *"What kind of help makes these activities easier for you?"* *"Which activities are you unable to do because of this problem?" "How has this been for you?*	Understanding patient's perspective of limitations. Provides insight about customary activities, hobbies. Provides information about links between impairments and activity restrictions. Provides information about patient efficacy in addressing problems, can help to identify caregivers. Provides clearer information about limits of "participation." Provides insight into patient's psychological and emotional responses.
4. Exploring patient knowledge about the role and scope of PT	*"My role as your PT is to help you do the Important activities in your life with as much ease and comfort as possible."* *"What do you know about PT?"*	Exploring patient attitudes about PT can help educate and reassure patients about our role in their care. Not every patient may need this, but it is often helpful, particularly in settings not traditionally associated with our services (e.g., womens' health, hospice care).
5. Exploring patient views about recovery	*"What would you like to be able to do as a result of treatment?"* *"How do you think I can best help you?"* *"What do you think it will take for you to get better?"* *"How will you know you are better?"*	Provides information about patient goals/priorities and level of realism of expectations. Provides information about patient expectations of the extent and nature of our role. May provide indication of how they view their contribution to their recovery process. Provides information about patient's "conditions of satisfaction" for successful PT intervention. This information can help us direct our intervention toward meaningful patient outcomes.
6. Exploring patient attitudes about exercise (or other interventions involving an active patient role)	*"One of the ways I can help you as a PT is to provide you with exercise to [insert your rationale here]."* *"What have been your experiences about exercise?"* *"How would you feel about having me give you some exercises for this problem?"*	Provides insight into patient's level of motivation for exercise.

The Impact of Culturally Related Health Beliefs

David practices at a busy rural New Mexico outpatient PT clinic that is affiliated with the Indian Health Service. He is performing an examination on Mr. Yellowhair, a 58-year-old Native American who has recently begun experiencing severe low back pain. When David asks Mr. Yellowhair to describe the development of his condition, Mr. Yellowhair replies that he believes that it is a spirit-borne retribution for having betrayed a friend. Furthermore, Mr. Yellowhair also feels that PT intervention will not work unless he can first receive a cleansing from a tribal medicine man.

Questions

1. How does David acknowledge Mr. Yellowhair's beliefs about the cause of his problem?

2. How might David share the objective results of his examination, which indicate a lumbar strain that is likely related to an overuse syndrome?

3. David was hoping to begin his treatment that day so as to meet productivity standards. How does he reconcile this requirement with Mr. Yellowhair's need to receive a visit from his tribe's medicine man prior to receiving care?

Coordination of Care

As we have discussed, the challenges of being a patient are significant and potentially all-consuming. In entrusting their care to the health-care team, our patients need to feel confident that everyone involved is informed and in agreement about the plan of care. Our patients have many measures on which to base their perceptions of quality care; research indicates that a critical element lies in how well their treatment is organized and integrated into a total system.[13]

Lack of coordination of care has also been reported as a major contributing factor to medical errors, wasteful duplication of expensive tests, and the tiresome need for patients to repeat their medical history to numerous practitioners.[51]

Many elements must be in place to ensure the coordination of care at all levels within a health-care facility. At the system level, patient information must be readily accessible by all persons providing care while at the same time guarding against violations of patient confidentiality. Many health-care facilities have expedited the process of patient data management through an integrated computer network that all team members can access for information and documentation. Most of these computerized systems are secured, requiring the use of individualized passwords by all team members. Accordingly, there are usually strict procedures in place to prevent abuse of these passwords or other inappropriate use of these computer systems. When utilized within facility guidelines however, computerized systems can greatly streamline the efficiency of obtaining important patient information to coordinate interdisciplinary care.

The efficient sharing of patient information involves a carefully orchestrated balance that depends on the ethical integrity of the entire health-care team. In addition to computerized systems to share patient data, verbal dialogues between team members are an important way of sharing information. Much of this sharing is done at the interpersonal level, which has the potential advantage of strengthening team alliances for the patient's benefit. In the treatment of difficult patients, these team alliances can provide emotional support to sustain optimal patient care. However, in the sharing of orally based patient information, we must be certain to choose the appropriate setting to assure confidentiality.

To that end, an old memory comes to mind involving a young medical resident who got on a crowded hospital elevator. Upon seeing a colleague, this resident blurted, "I just gave Mrs. Smith an enema and there is going to be one heck of an explosion soon!" It is appalling to consider that any one of the passengers on that elevator could have been one of Mrs. Smith's family members.

The legal and ethical obligation to maintain patient confidentiality has recently been reinforced by federal legislation prescribing the appropriate disclosure of medical information. The Healthcare Insurance Portability and Accountability Act (HIPAA) regards "protected health information" as "any individually identifiable health information created or received by a healthcare provider that is maintained or transmitted in whatever form the information exists, including orally."[52]

HIPAA was enacted in 1996 in order to prevent violations of patient confidentially arising from widespread use of electronically based storage systems for medical information. As a result of HIPAA, health-care providers may access medical information on a "need to know" basis only. In turn, health-care practitioners may share protected health information with other clinicians involved in the management of a given patient as a means of assuring better continuity of care. **Box 10-5** shows HIPAA Protected Health Information.

As a physical therapist, you will be expected to abide by HIPAA-related policy. However, this should not prevent you from working with other members of your health-care team to assure optimal coordination of care. This involves ongoing communication between colleagues so that patients will receive support and information whenever they need it. Patient concerns can arise at any time in the 24-hour day; thus appropriate

---

BOX 10-5:   HIPAA-Protected Health Information

Name

Address, including city, county, and zip code

Dates, including birth date, admission date, discharge date, and date of death

Telephone and fax numbers

Electronic mail addresses

Social security numbers

Medical record numbers

Health plan beneficiary number

Account number

Certificate/license number

Vehicle or other device serial number

Web URL

Internet protocol address

Finger or voice prints

Photographic images

Any other unique identifying number, characteristic, or code

assistance must be available to the greatest extent possible at all times. Keeping our documentation up to date can keep other team members abreast of patients' progress in PT. It can also be helpful to post illustrated instructions of patient positioning, exercises, or the application of splints, casts, or orthotic devices, so that other team members can provide consistency of care in our absence.

Our patients' medical status can also change unexpectedly; thus it is important to be informed of your patients' current status before you begin treatment. You should make it a point to consult the patient's chart or the nurse providing care each day before seeing your patient in an inpatient setting. This simple practice can ensure that you are fully informed about those aspects of a patient's care which will affect your intervention.

Coordination of care is important throughout the patient's stay, but it can be critical in the process of discharge planning. As a physical therapist, you have vital input in terms of your patient's mobility status and safety, which can have significant implications for the discharge planning process. In addition, you may also be a key team player in terms of identifying and obtaining adaptive equipment in a timely manner. As you work with the health-care team in the discharge planning process, it is important that all bases be covered in terms of appropriate discharge destination, delivery of necessary equipment, and education of all caregivers who will help the patient with the transition home. The following case illustrates what can happen if such coordination fails.

Clinical Scenario

Delayed Takeoff

Andrea is a physical therapist working on an inpatient rehabilitation unit. She has been treating Mel, a 48-year-old truck driver, who was injured when his truck rolled over 400 miles away from his home. Mel sustained a femoral fracture that was stabilized with internal fixation; he is now able to ambulate short distances indoors with a quad cane. Without consulting the rest of the health-care team, Mel's physician has determined that he can be discharged, and Mel plans to fly home on a commercial plane in just 2 days.

Mel is 70 pounds overweight and has a pack-a-day cigarette habit. These comorbidities have challenged Mel's endurance, making it necessary for him to sit and rest after walking any more than 5 minutes. When Andrea learns about the physician's decision to discharge Mel, she expresses concerns about Mel's endurance for the flight (being able to get through the terminal with assistance, toilet himself on the plane, etc.).

To support her concerns, Andrea monitors Mel's oxygen saturation throughout his next PT session. She finds that Mel's saturation drops to 85% during ambulation. She thus contacts Mel's physician to recommend that Mel fly home on schedule only if he has a portable oxygen supply and if the airline provides wheelchair assistance for his transport through the terminal. Andrea also asks that Mel's discharge be delayed until these conditions are met, and the physician agrees.

Questions

1. Whose responsibility is it to inform Mel about the discharge delay? Whose responsibility is it to inform the rest of the team? How might this information be conveyed?

2. How might Andrea work with other team members (the physician, social worker, and nursing staff) to make sure that Mel gets the support he needs?

3. What functional skills might Mel need to practice as part of taking a commercial airplane flight? How might Andrea assist him toward success?

Your patients want the best care from their health-care team and may ask your advice about interventions they are receiving from other clinicians. Even if you disagree with these, you should be aware that it is a violation of the APTA *Guide for Professional Conduct* (principle 11) to "undermine the relationship between the patient and other healthcare providers."[53] This can sometimes be a challenge, as the following case scenario illustrates.

Complication Conundrum

Clinical Scenario

Reid is a physical therapist working in an outpatient orthopedic facility. He often treats patients who are referred from a group of orthopedic surgeons in town. Reid has collaborated with these physicians for several years and they share a mutual respect for each others' expertise.

A new physician, Dr. Jackson, has recently joined the practice. In the past 4 months, Dr. Jackson has referred three of his postsurgical patients for the treatment of drop foot following lumbar laminectomy. This is an unusual result among the physicians in this practice, and Reid is concerned. He therefore decides that he will talk to Dr. Jackson to get his perspective on this matter. In the meantime, one of Reid's patients, Mrs. Manning, has been advised to undergo a lumbar laminectomy by Dr. Jackson. She asks Reid's opinion about his skills.

Questions

1. How might Reid respond in a way that empowers Mrs. Manning to make a good decision about her care without disparaging Dr. Jackson?

2. What role does a physical therapist have with regard to a colleague whose patient outcomes are less than optimal? The APTA *Guide for Professional Conduct* addresses this issue in principle 9.1, Consumer Protection.[53]

3. Is it appropriate for Reid to talk first to Dr. Jackson? If so, how might he go about their dialogue?

Physical Comfort

As we have discussed previously, the illness experience, particularly one involving a hospital stay, removes an individual from the comfort of home. Furthermore, many conditions (and their treatments) involve considerable pain and discomfort. Finally, side effects of many medications (particularly opioids for pain control) can cause uncomfortable side effects such as constipation or itching.

Pain control is one of the most important measures of patient comfort. Much of our current understanding about pain control has evolved from research on patients facing the end of life, where up to 45% are in severe pain. Accordingly, in the hospice and palliative care setting, the assessment of pain (using a 1-to-10 subjective scale) is considered a "fifth vital sign."[54] More recently, the impact of inadequate pain control has been linked with several unfavorable outcomes such as decreased immune function, increased physiological stress, and systemic complications such as deep venous thrombosis and pneumonia. A compelling 2006 study of hospice patients reports an increased survival rate of 29 days among those whose pain was adequately controlled. Accordingly, a current patient outcome measure in U.S. hospice programs is the reduction of pain to a comfortable level (3 out of 10 on the subjective pain rating scale) within 48 hours of admission.[55,56] Attention to adequate pain control has become a standard of care in U.S. hospitals as well. In 2000, the Joint Commission on Accreditation of Healthcare Organizations (JCAHO) established pain control standards for the hospitals they accredit.[57]

As a physical therapist, it will be important for you to assess patients' pain and to ensure optimal comfort during uncomfortable procedures such as wound care or manual therapy. In the case of painful interventions such as these, it is often very useful to premedicate patients (having the nursing staff administer pain medications 30 to 60 minutes prior to PT). This can also be effective in improving patients' endurance and exercise tolerance during PT treatment.

We can also promote patient comfort by offering assistance with grooming and dressing. In many facilities, physical therapists see patients at bedside and can easily offer help with activities of daily living such as grooming or toileting. These are not only measures of comfort but also affirmations of dignity. We can also promote comfort and dignity by appropriate draping of patients, particularly when doing bedside treatments.

Finally, the assurance of patient comfort is the job of every member of the health-care team. This may mean that you sometimes engage in activities that are in the domain of other colleagues, as the following scenario illustrates.

Clinical Scenario

This Is Not My Job!!

Valerie is a physical therapist working in a skilled nursing facility. It is 8 a.m. and she is about to see her first patient of the day, Lucy, a woman with stroke and dementia. She finds Lucy in the bathroom, trying to clean herself after toileting. However, Lucy's clothes, shoes, and skin are soiled with feces. She is confused and distressed. Valerie is aware that the nurses and assistants are short-staffed today and that right now they are involved in the morning care of the other residents. As she considers her options, she first thinks to herself, "It's not my job to clean up residents." She then looks at Lucy, who is now in tears.

Questions

1. How would you respond if you were in Valerie's situation? What do you think are her primary obligations in this instance?

2. Which course of action would best promote patient comfort and dignity? How might Valerie justify any assistance to Lucy in terms of "productivity"? Should productivity concerns be important in such situations?

3. What other concerns might arise if Valerie were to leave Lucy's room to seek assistance?

4. What role do physical therapists have in promoting the comfort of patients? How might this include doing things that "are not our job"?

The Rest of the Story

Valerie immediately proceeded to reassure Lucy and help her with cleaning up and changing clothes. As she continued, Lucy's adult daughter, Shelly, arrived. Valerie introduced herself as Lucy's physical therapist and explained the situation. Shelly was greatly relieved and thankful for Valerie's compassion. They were able to discuss Shelly's concerns and Valerie was able to provide much-needed emotional support. Imagine how this scenario might have been different if Shelly had been the one to find her mother alone in her bathroom predicament.

Talking Points/Field Notes

My Comfort "Musts"

1. Consider yourself in the role of a patient in the hospital. Make a list of up to 10 comfort measures that would be important to you. Consider grooming, diet, environment, clothing, or anything else you would want in your room to enhance your overall comfort.

2. As you look over your list, consider how easily you would be able to acquire these in your hospital room. How would you need the support of hospital staff to enjoy these comforts?

3. As you look over your list, what insights do you have that can be useful in providing patient comfort?

Emotional Support and Alleviation of Anxiety

There is a considerable body of evidence supporting the value of support to reduce the emotional distress of the illness experience.[13] To this end, Gerteis states, "providing emotional support could prove to be more curative than some of the high-technology, expensive therapies currently employed."

Research in the area of support indicates that it involves two major elements—emotional support and instrumental support—which are provided by an individual's social support system.[58] For any given person, a social support system encompasses a broad network of encouraging alliances. These alliances may derive from a number of sources, including personal friends, colleagues, neighbors, and community members. Within the health-care setting, everyone with whom the patient has contact becomes a part of his or her network.

Emotional support is made up of comforting gestures that are intended to provide comfort and to alleviate uncertainty, anxiety, hopelessness, and depression.[58] There are many ways to provide emotional support, and many patients state that they derive comfort simply from knowing that someone is available if they need such help. **Box 10-6**

BOX 10-6:   Communication Methods for Providing Emotional Support

1. Letting your patient know that you are available if he or she has any concerns or questions
2. Use of telephone or Internet contact (for support and follow-up after treatment)
3. Active listening
4. Displays of empathy (using reflections of feeling or content)
5. Physical presence (with or without words)
6. Use of humor
7. Sharing experiences or ideas
8. Diverting attention from problems
9. Physical touch (hand on shoulder)
10. Sending cards, letters, or flowers*

---

*This form of support is most likely to be given from patient's social support network. (You can acknowledge these gestures if appropriate.)

illustrates communication methods of providing support that have proven to be useful. Note that this list is inclusive and contains strategies that may be used more appropriately by a patient's social support network (such as sending flowers or cards). We can support these gestures by acknowledging their presence ("What beautiful flowers!" or "I bet it feels good to know that others are thinking about you!").

Perhaps one of the most important challenges in providing emotional support is using our emotional intelligence to assess whether such help is needed or desired. For a variety of reasons (possibly cultural or generational), some patients may not be comfortable in disclosing their feelings. In these instances, we can still support them by providing the respectful and compassionate care that all patients need and deserve.

Particularly in emotionally difficult situations, the most effective form of support can be one's silent presence.

When a patient is dying, for example, there comes a point where allowing this process to proceed (while ensuring patient comfort) is the most compassionate option. Yet for many of us, such situations evoke feelings of helplessness. No doubt you have chosen to become a physical therapist in order to have an active role in the betterment of others' lives. Accordingly, most of us have an enthusiastic "I can make a difference!" attitude that infuses our clinical interactions. However, some situations are simply beyond our therapeutic capacities, and at such times, sitting in silence with the dying patient or with the grieving family member can be more helpful than you may realize.

Instrumental support pertains to tangible forms of assistance as with money, assistance with child care, shopping, and transportation. In the context of health care, this can mean helping our patients to access these resources after discharge. It also involves helping them to secure necessary assistive devices and other adaptive equipment.

Physical therapists have an important role to play in identifying patients' equipment needs.

In many settings, physical therapists are responsible for ordering appropriate wheelchairs, bathroom safety equipment, and ambulation devices for their patients. However, many insurance companies require that a physician verify the "medical necessity" of all equipment ordered for a patient. In such cases, physicians will often consult other team members for their rationale in making such verifications.

For patients who lack medical insurance, you may find yourself providing creative solutions for equipment alternatives. For example, I have learned in my home health experiences that cans of food can be used as weights, bags of frozen peas can serve as reusable ice packs, and slatted lawn chairs make decent shower seats. This information serves as instrumental support in many ways, as it enables patients to acquire devices that facilitate their independence.

The ability to provide effective instrumental support also relates to your ability to identify community resources and assist patients in accessing these. Such agencies can provide everything from in-home assistance to respite care for caretakers who need time for themselves.

Instrumental support also includes the "nuts and bolts" of day-to-day support, which can help patients and their caregivers make the transition from the hospital to their homes. For example, I once had a patient with stroke who was capable of living independently in her mobile home and wanted to do so. However, she was unable to drive and thus needed help getting to appointments and going shopping. By helping this patient access a community transportation service for persons with disabilities, she was able to achieve her goal of returning home.

Support SOS

Jenna is a physical therapist working in a hospital. She has just finished her evaluation of 59-year-old Margaret Hurley, who has a long history of multiple sclerosis. Margaret was admitted to the hospital because of a recent severe exacerbation. As a result of this episode, she is no longer able to walk with a walker. Thus Jenna has been talking to Margaret about the potential need for a motorized scooter. As she finishes this discussion, Margaret suddenly bursts into tears and sobs, "Today is my birthday! Neither my son nor daughter has called or sent a card!" Jenna places her hand on Margaret's forearm reassuringly and says nothing. Margaret continues; "I'm so scared and I feel all alone!"

Questions

1. Margaret is expressing feelings that reflect several concerns. How might Jenna address these concerns?

2. Which of Margaret's concerns involves emotional support? Which involves instrumental support?

3. How might other team members assist Jenna in directing Margaret to the appropriate support?

Effective Patient and Family Education

In the attainment of self-efficacy, patients and their families need education about how to manage their impairments, how to make lifestyle changes that optimize health, and how to optimize their resources. Patient and family education is thus among the most important interventions we can provide to facilitate an optimal quality of life in the face of a health change.

The topic of patient and family education is of critical importance in your role as a physical therapist. Effective teaching skills are a component of instructional communication, which is addressed in the last section of this text. Accordingly, the final chapter of this book is devoted to this topic, particularly from the perspective of managing health behavior change.

Accommodation of Family and Friends

The illness experience affects not only the patient but also those who love and care for him or her. Family and friends are critical and enduring sources of emotional and instrumental support. They can assist the patient in decisions affecting care. Furthermore, in cases where patients are unable to make their own decisions, they may appoint a family member to act as their legal representative (a role known as "power of attorney"). Thus, family involvement is a critical component of patient-centered care; it has therefore been recommended that the family be considered part of the health-care team.[43]

For the purposes of a realistic discussion on this topic, this text defines "family" in terms of those persons who have an emotional bond with the patient and an enduring concern for his or her welfare, regardless of a biological or legal relationship.

As physical therapists, we have a marvelous opportunity to include families in the intervention programs we design. Physical well-being is an important component of quality of life and can become a family pursuit for the benefit of all involved. Families can encourage and motivate patients in their carryover of functional skills training. They can help patients monitor and chart their progress, and provide physical assistance that may expand options for home exercise programs. Whenever possible, family members should be invited to PT treatment sessions and asked for their insights. Scheduling family education sessions earlier during the patient's episode of care may also prevent him or her from being overwhelmed with a barrage of new information at discharge.

However, none of these possibilities will be realized unless we take the time to identify the patient's network of family members and their levels of involvement. This is best accomplished during the initial assessment. The names and contact information for these caregivers can then be recorded and kept available for the duration of the patient's episode of care. While many patients will have one or two consistent caregivers (a spouse or partner, for example), others will have several who share this responsibility. For example, the five grown sons and daughters of a recent hospice patient set up a rotating care schedule where each took 3 weeks care for their mother in her home. In this instance, it was helpful to the continuity of my therapeutic intervention (and much appreciated by the patient) for me to be apprised of this schedule. Thus, each time a different family member arrived for his or her 3-week "rotation," I would call to give a progress report along with an offer for education and support if needed.

As the importance of family members becomes increasingly understood in the context of patient-centered care, many health-care facilities have identified creative and effective ways to involve them. Gerteis[13] provides several suggestions that evolved from the results of a national survey of 2,000 family "care partners." These include (1) scheduling regular times for staff to be available for consulting or education; (2) posting a bulletin board near the patient's bed for family questions, expectations, or goals; (3) inclusion of a family assessment for use at the patient's bedside to help clinicians understand their needs; and (4) encouraging the involvement of family members in providing nonmedical care such as transporting, dressing, and grooming.

At the institutional level, families can also be included on task forces and committees that evaluate patient services or assess education programs. One pediatric facility that serves children with special needs encourages parents to be advocates for their children, to provide peer support to other parents, and to educate clinicians about the families' needs.[59]

A Bicycling Program Built for Two?

Clinical Scenario

Heidi is a physical therapist at an outpatient cardiac rehabilitation facility. She is working with 80-year-old Marvin Goldberg, who underwent a triple coronary artery bypass grafting procedure. Marvin is now ready to begin a stage 2 cardiac rehabilitation program (supervised and monitored aerobic exercise). Marvin's 79-year-old wife, Alma, has faithfully attended PT with her husband, and her presence has been a source of encouragement.

As Heidi begins to describe the exercise program (which includes sessions on the stationary bicycle), Alma asks if she could exercise on a bicycle next to Marvin, both to encourage him and to work on her own cardiovascular endurance. Marvin is enthusiastic and Heidi agrees to discuss it with her department's director. However, the director informs Heidi that having family members exercise with patients is not possible owing to liability concerns and the fact that bicycles must be kept free for patient use.

Questions

1. If you were Heidi, how might you address the director's concerns? How could Alma's interest in exercising with her husband provide a service opportunity for the PT clinic? What impact might this have on other family members?

2. In order to assure Alma's safety during her exercise, what recommendations should Heidi provide?

3. What other services might the PT program provide for families affected by heart disease?

The Rest of the Story

As this clinical scenario suggests, the inclusion of family can provide support to the patient and opportunities for the development of innovative programs. It also suggests that advocating for our patients may include advocating for their families as well.

Heidi saw an opportunity to develop a "healthy families" program in her PT department. Thus, patients could have a family member accompany them and exercise for a minimal cost. In return, the family member would receive a PT assessment and an appropriate exercise prescription. Finally, in order to assure the safety of family members, they would be required to receive clearance from their physicians prior to beginning the program. Such a program was later actually put into effect. It was very successful and eventually expanded to include multidisciplinary involvement of dietitians and psychologists (who provided stress-reduction training).

Continuity of Care and Effective Transitions

Depending on the nature of a given health condition, patients may find themselves transitioning through several different levels of care, each with its own staff of practitioners. Safe and effective patient management depends largely on communication between these providers.

For example, 70-year-old Robert Jenkins is found unconscious on the kitchen floor by his wife. She calls 911 and an ambulance transports Mr. Jenkins to the nearest hospital emergency department, where a computed tomography scan shows evidence of a brain hemorrhage. Mr. Jenkins is now admitted to the hospital and undergoes a craniotomy to relieve intracranial pressure. Next, Mr. Jenkins is transitioned to the hospital intensive care unit until he is medically stable. Within the following 3 months, he receives services on the hospital's acute-care floor and in a community skilled nursing facility. Finally, Mr. Jenkins is discharged home, then to receive rehabilitation services at the hospital's outpatient unit for the treatment of his residual hemiparesis.

Lack of communication at any point in the transition process can contribute to adverse events. One study examined the accuracy and timeliness of communication between hospital primary care physicians and found several deficits (such as discharge summaries lacking test result data or discharge medications) that affected the quality of patient care in 25% of cases.[59,60]

In the above example, the hospitalist should inform his primary care physician that the warfarin Mr. Jenkins had been taking (for a previous deep venous thrombosis) had been discontinued; it should also recommend that the patient remain off this medication. In addition, the discharge summary from the hospital's physical therapist should include information about Mr. Jenkins's neuromuscular and musculoskeletal status and level of function. The physical therapist at the skilled nursing facility would need to know that Mr. Jenkins had fractured his right humerus when he collapsed at home and that this injury prevented him from using an assistive device during ambulation. Other pieces of information could also facilitate an effective transition between settings. For example, during Mr. Jenkins's hospitalization, his wife exhibited signs of severe anxiety and had requested a psychiatric consult. Because of her anxiety, she was unable to provide assistance to her husband. Finally, the Jenkins's grown children had decided that their parents should not be returning to their home and had requested assistance from the hospital social worker to identify a suitable alternative.

Implications for Physical Therapy Practice

As the example illustrates, our patients face multi-dimensional stresses as they navigate through the health-care system. This stress can be greatly increased by the needless duplication of medical tests, requests to continually repeat medical histories, or unnecessary changes in intervention programs. As a physical therapist, you should be committed to assuring the seamless transition between the care settings of your patients, and the most important ally in this endeavor is your communication. The *Guide to Physical Therapist Practice* provides comprehensive documentation guidelines that include important information about a patient's plan of care.

As engaged professionals, we should also feel comfortable requesting and providing information to our colleagues about the patients we share. It can be very reassuring for the patient to know that we care enough to make this contact.

The provision of patient-centered care in the context of a therapeutic alliance will be one of the most important skills of the 21st-century health practitioner. Although we can look forward to continued advancements in the skills and technologies of health care, nothing will ever replace the central role of effective communication in promoting patient self-efficacy and quality of life.

Chapter Summary

1. Patients come to us because they are suffering on some level. Suffering can derive from many sources, the sum which is *total pain*.

2. Health conditions can have a significant effect on our patients' quality of life. Societal factors such as lack of access, stigmatization, and change in roles can add to the stresses of the illness experience.

3. The illness experience is the subjective perception of a decline in health. For chronic conditions, this involves a process of coming to terms with the condition, seeking help, and coping with the changes involved.

4. The therapeutic alliance is a relationship of mutual trust and goodwill between the practitioner and patient. The therapeutic alliance is the cornerstone of patient-centered care.

5. Person-first language involves describing our patients as persons *with* a condition rather than persons who *are* their condition. The use of person-first language provides the appropriate point of reference for the therapeutic alliance.

6. Patient-centered care is and will be a critical element of quality health service delivery in the 21st century. It includes components such as superb access to care, respect for values, the provision of physical comfort, alleviation of anxiety, patient education, support for families, and continuity of care. We can enhance our ability to engage in each of these elements through effective internal and external communication.

Take-Home Menu

Illness Experience Films

In recent years, numerous films have depicted the challenges of the illness experience. You might find it interesting to review some of the older films along with some of the newer ones. Consider selecting one of each, and compare/contrast the depictions of health-care professionals (particularly PTs). Discuss the particular challenges faced by the patients in these films. How have the challenges changed over the years?

Older Films

- *Whose Life is it Anyway?* (1981). Richard Dreyfuss plays an artist who sustains a cervical level spinal cord injury and chooses to end his life. Interesting ethical/legal issues of the times.
- *Terms of Endearment* (1983). With Debra Winger, Shirley Maclaine, and Jack Nicholson. Depicts the impact of family dynamics and the health-care system surrounding a young mother who develops a terminal disease.
- *The Doctor* (1991). With William Hurt and Christine Lahti. An arrogant physician with no bedside manner undergoes a transformation as the result of his own illness.
- *Regarding Henry* (1991). With William Hurt and Annette Bening. A successful lawyer struggles to put his life back together after a brain injury.

Newer Films

- *Wit* (2001). With Emma Thompson. A Ph.D. English professor reacts with acid candor to her health-care providers after a diagnosis of brain cancer.
- *Two Weeks* (2006). With Sally Field. A family comes together for the two week period before their mother's agonizing death from ovarian cancer.
- *The Death of Mr. Lazarescu* (2005). Romanian film starring Ian Fiscuteanu. A man's death in the midst of a burdensome medical bureaucracy.
- *Sicko* (2007). With Michael Moore. A documentary that delivers a scathing indictment on the U.S. Healthcare System.

References

1. *The American Heritage Dictionary of the English Language,* 4th ed. Boston: Houghton Mifflin; 2000.

2. Cherney N. The problem of suffering. In Doyle D, Hanks GWC, Cherney N, Calman K, eds. *Oxford Textbook of Palliative Medicine,* 3rd ed. Oxford, UK: Oxford University Press; 2004:7-14.

3. Saunders C. Into the valley of the shadow of death: A personal therapeutic journey. *Br Med J.* 1996; 7072(313):21-28.

4. Saunders C. Care of patients suffering from terminal illness at St. Joseph's Hospice, Hackney, London. *Nursing Mirror,* 14 February, vii–x. 1964.

5. Blanchard EB, Hickling EJ. *After the Crash: The Psychological Assessment and Treatment of Survivors of Motor Vehicle Accidents,* 2nd ed. Washington, DC: American Psychological Association; 2004.

6. *Diagnostic and Statistical Manual of Mental Disorders IV-Text Revision (DSM-IV-TR).* Arlington, VA: American Psychiatric Association; 2000.

7. Steiner WA, Ryser L, Huber E, Uebelhart D, et al. Use of the ICF model as a clinical problem-solving tool in physical therapy and rehabilitation medicine. *Phys Ther.* 2002;82(11):1098-1107.

8. *ICIDH-2: International Classification of Disability and Health.* Pre-final draft. Geneva, Switzerland: World Health Organization; 2000.

9. Parsons T. *The Social System.* New York: Free Press; 1951.

10. Parsons T. The sick role and the role of the physician reconsidered. *Milbank Mem Fund Q.* 1975;53:257-278.

11. Cockerham W. *Medical Sociology.* Upper Saddle River, NJ: Prentice Hall; 2000.

12. Young JT. Illness behavior: A selective review and synthesis. *Sociol Health Illness.* 2004;26(1):1-31.

13. Gerteis M, Edgman-Levitan S, Dailey J, Delbanco TL, eds. *Through the Patient's Eyes: Understanding and Promoting Patient-Centered Care.* San Francisco: Jossey-Bass; 1993.

14. Stewart M, Brown JB, Weston WW, et al. *Patient-Centered Care: Transforming the Clinical Method.* Thousand Oaks, CA: Sage; 1995.

15. Department of Health and Human Services. Centers for Disease Control and Prevention. *Chronic Disease Prevention:* http://www.cdc.gov/nccdphp/. Accessed May 27, 2008.

16. Edmonds P, Vivat B, Burman R, et al. Loss and change: Experiences of people severely affected by multiple sclerosis. *Palliat Med.* 2007;21:101-107.

17. Brown J, Addington-Hall J. How people with motor neuron disease talk about living with their illness: A narrative study. *J Adv Nurs.* 2008;62(2):200-208.

18. Lazarus RS. Coping theory and research: Past, present and future. *Psychosom Med.* 1993;55:234-247.

19. Folkman S, Lazarus RS. *Manual for Ways of Coping Questionnaire.* Palo Alto, CA: Consulting Psychologists Press; 1988.

20. Van Egeren L. Stress, coping and behavioral organization. *Psychosom Med.* 2000;62:451-460.

21. Falvo D. *Medical and Social Aspects of Chronic Illness and Disability,* 3rd ed. Boston: Jones and Bartlett; 2005.

22. Folkman S. Personal control and stress and coping processes: A theoretical analysis. *J Pers Soc Psychol.* 1984;46:839-852.

23. Buetow S, Goodyear-Smith F, Coster G. Coping strategies in the self-management of chronic heart failure. *Fam Pract.* 2001;18(2):117-122.

24. Rier DA. The missing voice of the critically ill: A medical sociologist's first person account. *Sociol Health Illness.* 2000;22:68-93.

25. Ramini SK, Brown R, Bruckner EB. Embracing changes: Adaptation by adolescents with cancer. *Pediatr Nurs.* 2008;34(1):72-79.

26. Paul F, Rattray J. Short and long term impact of critical illness on relatives: Literature review. *J Adv Nurs.* 2008;62(3):276-292.

27. Hart E. System-induced setbacks in stroke recovery. *Sociol Health Illness.* 2001;23:101-123.

28. Yu DSF, Lee DTF, Kwong ANT, et al. Living with heart failure: A review of qualitative studies of older people. *J Adv Nurs.* 2008;61(5):474-483.

29. Mental health: Overcoming the stigma of mental illness. *Mayo Clinic. Com:* http://www.mayoclinic.com/health/mental-health/MH00076. Accessed May 27, 2008.

30. Pierret J. The illness experience: State of knowledge and perspectives for research. *Sociol Health Illness.* 2003;25:4-22.

31. Sherer M, Evans CC, Leverenz J, et al. Therapeutic alliance in post-acute brain injury rehabilitation: Predictors of strength of alliance and impact of alliance on outcome. *Brain Injury.* 2007;21(7):663-672.

32. Texas Council for Developmental Disabilities. *People First Language:* http://www.txddc.state.tx.us/resources/publications/p1st.pdf. Accessed May 13, 2008.

33. Folkins J. *Resource on Person First Language.* American Speech Language and Hearing Association. 1992: http://www.asha.org/about/publications/journal-abstracts/submissions/person_first.htm. Accessed May 13, 2008.

34. The language of disability: Problems of politics and practice. *J Disabil Adv Council Austr.* 1988;1(3):13-21.

35. American Physical Therapy Association. House of Delegates, Position Statement. Terminology for communication about people with disabilities HOD P06-91-25-34: http://www.apta.org/AM/Template.cfm?Section=Home&CONTENTID=25509&TEMPLATE=/CM/ContentDisplay.cfm. Accessed May 13, 2008.

36. *Guidelines for Reporting and Writing about People with Disabilities,* 6th ed. Research and Training Center on Independent Living. Lawrence, KS. University of Kansas, 2001: http://www.rtcil.org/products/RTCIL%20publications/Media/Guidelines%20for%20Reporting%20and%20Writing%20about%20People%20with%20Disabilities.pdf. Accessed May 13, 2008.

37. Burns JW, Higdon LJ, Mullen JT, et al. Relationships among patient hostility, anger expression, depression and working alliance in a work hardening program. *Ann Behav Med.* 1999;21(1):77-82.

38. Epstein R. Mindful practice. *JAMA.* 1999;282:833-839.

39. Hill C. Therapist techniques, client involvement, and the therapeutic relationship: Inextricably entwined in the therapy process. *Psychother Theory Res Pract Training.* 2005;42(4):431-442.

40. Chaplin WF, Phillips JB, Brown JD, et al. Handshaking, gender, personality and first impressions. *J Pers Soc Psychol.* 2000;79(1):110-117.

41. Committee on Quality of Health Care in America, Institute of Medicine. *Crossing the Quality Chasm: A New Health System for the 21st Century.* Washington, DC: National Academies Press; 2001.

42. Davis K, Schoenbaum SC, Audet AMJ. A 2020 vision of patient centered primary care. *J Gen Intern Med.* 2005; 20(10):953-957.

43. Silow-Carroll S, Alteras T, Stepnick L. *Patient Centered Care for Underserved Populations: Definitions and Best Practices.* Washington, DC: Economic and Social Research Institute; 2006.

44. Nápoles-Springer AM, Santoyo J, Houston K, et al. Patients' perceptions of cultural factors affecting the quality of their medical encounters. *Health Expectations.* 2005;8:4-17.

45. Office of Minority Health. *National Culturally and Linguistically Appropriate Services (CLAS) Standards.* Joint Commission 2007 Standards for Hospitals, Ambulatory, Behavioral Health, Long Term Care and Home Care: http://www.jointcommission.org/NR/rdonlyres/5EABBEC8-F5E2-4810-A16F-E2F148AB5170/0/hlc_omh_xwalk.pdf. Accessed May 31, 2008.

46. *Austin Business Journal.* July 21, 2005. Spanish Speaking Population to Jump 55% in Austin Area: http://www.bizjournals.com/austin/stories/2005/07/18/daily42.html. Accessed June 1, 2008.

47. King DE, Bushwick B. Beliefs and attitudes of hospital inpatients about faith healing and prayer. *J Fam Pract.* 1994;39:349-352.

48. Gowri A, Hight E. Spirituality and Medical Practice: Using the HOPE Questions as a Practical Tool for Spiritual Assessment. *Am Fam Physician.* January 1, 2001: http://www.aafp.org/afp/20010101/81.html. Accessed June 1, 2008.

49. Charron-Prochownik D, Sereika SM, Becker D, et al. Reproductive health beliefs and behaviors in teens with diabetes: application of the Expanded Health Belief Model. *Pediatr Diabetes.* 2001;2(1):30–39.

50. Stretcher V, Rosentock T. The health belief model. In Glanz K, Lewis FM, Rimer B, eds. *Health Behavior and Health Education.* San Francisco: Jossey Bass; 1997.

51. Commonwealth Fund. Medical Errors, Lack of Coordination and Poor Patient-Physician Communication are Pervasive in Health Systems of Five Countries. May 6, 2003: http://www.commonwealthfund.org/newsroom/newsroom_show.htm?doc_id=223545. Accessed June 6, 2008.

52. Oregon Association of Hospitals and Health Systems. Information Protected by the HIPAA Act: http://www.oahhs.org/legal/hipaa/information_covered.php. Accessed June 5, 2008.

53. American Physical Therapy Association. *Guide for Professional Conduct:* http://www.apta.org/AM/Template.cfm?Section=Ethics_and_Legal_Issues1&TEMPLATECM/ContentDisplay.cfm&CONTENTID=14342. Accessed June 6, 2008.

54. City of Hope and American Association of Colleges of Nursing. End of Life Nursing Education Consortium (ELNEC). *Advancing End of Life Nursing Care.* 2000.

55. Portenoy RK, Sibirceva U, Smout R, et al. Opioid use and survival at the end of life: A survey of a hospice population. *J Pain Symptom Mgt.* 2006;32(6):532-540.

56. National Hospice and Palliative Care Organization. NHPCO Facts and Figures: Hospice Care in America. November 2007: www.nhpco.org/nds. Accessed June 10, 2008.

57. Finfgeld-Connett D. Clarification of Social Support. *J Nurs Scholarship.* 2005;37(1):4-9.

58. Phillips D. JCAHO pain management standards are unveiled. *JAMA.* 2000;284:428-429.

59. Williams L. Family matters: The many roles of families in family-centered care. Part III. *Pediatr Nurs.* 2007; 33(2):144-146.

60. Sunil K, LeFevre F, Phillips CO, et al. Deficits in communication and information transfer between hospital-based and primary care physicians: Implications for patient safety and continuity of care. *JAMA.* 2007;297(8):831-841.

Part 4

Instrumental Communication

Engaged professionalism involves the thoughtful and purposeful use of our knowledge, skills, and interactions in order to effect change. As physical therapists, we have both the privilege and the responsibility to make a transformative impact on our patients, our profession, and society at large. Instrumental communication pertains to the skills that facilitate these outcomes.

Because change is best effected in an atmosphere of cooperation, Chapter 11 explores approaches to facilitating consensus, which include assertiveness and negotiation. Chapter 12 explores the concept of transformational teaching—the sharing of information in formal and informal situations as well as in the context of patient education.

Managing Conflict Through Assertiveness and Negotiation: Instrumental Communication for Facilitating Consensus

"Would you rather be right or happy?"

Gerald Jampolsky, M.D., psychiatrist and author of *Forgiveness: The Greatest Healer of All*

Chapter Overview

Conflict is a natural consequence of a diverse society where differences exist in numerous dimensions. Unresolved conflict contributes to stress and negative interactions. This chapter explores strategies for reducing conflict through assertiveness negotiation. These skills are explored in detail, along with exercises for self-reflection, discussion, and clinical application to facilitate learning.

Key Terms

Conflict

Assertiveness

Negotiation

Nonviolent communication

The Complex Nature of Conflict

Conflict is a Regular Feature of Society

Conflict is a common and predictable occurrence among interacting groups or individuals.[1] According to conflict theorists, social conflict results from individual or group inequities in material goods, status, power, and wealth.[2] As individuals vie for dominance, evidence suggests that there is such a significant emotional investment in their positions and judgments ("I am right, you are wrong," "I am smart, you are stupid") that these statements actually become part of one's self concept. As a result, any threat or opposition is viewed as a personal attack, resulting in competitive arguments and hostile exchanges.[3] Successful conflict resolution thus involves separating oneself from the ego-driven need to be right (hence the quotation at the beginning of this chapter).

Not surprisingly, conflict resolution fails when intense emotions or evaluative judgments prevail over respectful dialogue. In such instances, individuals turn to external sources for conflict resolution. The legal, judicial, and political systems of most societies are direct manifestations of an ongoing attempt to enforce cooperation among diverse social groups who are unable to do so themselves. Instead of attempting to address each party's needs, these institutions provide a mandatory directive in the form of a law, court ruling, or legislative policy. When such directives are described in legal terms, such as "punitive damages," they are usually unfavorable to one of the parties.

At the interpersonal level, conflict can occur whenever individuals working toward a similar goal have incompatible approaches or values (for example, one person pursues academic excellence by studying for exams while another cheats). Conflict can also arise when individuals fail to acknowledge differing attitudinal perspectives (for example, consider the often antagonistic dialogues that occur in our society over issues like abortion or gun control). Conflict often results from emotional reactions to social, economic, or material inequities. For example, even today, significant disparities exist in the quality of the health care delivered to racial minorities and persons of lower socioeconomic status.[4] Such inequities do little to advance compassionate understanding among all citizens. Finally, conflict arises when persons with contrary goals must interact (for example, consider the impact on staff morale when one individual works to maintain the status quo while another actively pursues organizational growth and change).

Conflict can be exacerbated when persons interact in close or crowded conditions.[5]

For example, conflict is a prominent feature in the work setting, which is usually a structured environment requiring close, ongoing interaction. Accordingly, several studies have reported that conflicts with colleagues and supervisors are a leading source of workplace stress,[6] and a recent study reported that "unresolved conflict represents the largest reducible cost in many businesses but is largely unrecognized." Accordingly, in one diary study of employees from a variety of occupations, respondents recorded episodes of interpersonal stress on 50% of their workdays.[7,8] In the work setting, unresolved conflict contributes to depression, burnout, and counterproductive work behaviors (cited examples included spreading rumors, leaving early, and taking office supplies for personal use).[6]

Interestingly, the college dormitory is considered one of the most popular environments in which to study the effects of overcrowding on humans (another is the correctional system).[8] As you might know from personal experience, conflict in this setting is common, and one study concluded that "living in these dormitories . . . is having a substantial effect on the mood and behavior of the residents."[9]

Talking Points/Field Notes: Conflict "Diary" ━━━━━━━━━━━━━━━━━

For the next 72 hours, note the number of times you perceive conflict in your communication (where conflict is defined as "a state of mental discord resulting from incompatible or opposing needs, drives, wishes, or external or internal demands").[10]

Rate the emotional intensity of this conflict on a scale of 1 to 10, where:

1	5	10
Minor emotional stress lasting no more than a few minutes	Moderate stress lasting up to several hours	Significant emotional and physiological stress lasting 24 hours or more

Observe the precipitating factors, and your inclinations regarding a suitable course of action. Then, discuss the following questions and note your observations in your field notes.

Questions

1. Describe the general prevalence of stress over the 72-hour observation period. Was there any identifiable pattern of situations, persons, or environments? If so, describe these and why you think this might be the case.

2. Describe the range of your emotional ratings. Again, was there an identifiable pattern to these?

3. How did you consider these conflicts in terms of strategies for resolution? Do you tend to have a typical mode of response?

4. What might be some helpful approaches to minimizing conflict in your everyday life?

Effects of Conflict

The widespread prevalence of unresolved conflict has significant implications for our health and well-being. To that end, one of the most challenging consequences of conflict are the stress-inducing emotions that are often provoked.[1] Because conflict interferes with efficient social operations between persons, it is often perceived as an emotionally stressful threat. Just as a warning light on a car's dashboard foretells a mechanical malfunction, conflict can produce an emotional signal indicating a malfunctioning social interaction.[1] Depending on the nature of the conflict, we may experience the onset of fear, anger, disgust, or guilt. Each of these emotions can produce considerable discomfort and provoke an unfavorable reaction. For example, studies of interpersonal conflict indicate that anger is the most common and pervasive emotional response to conflict.[11] Unfortunately, it is also the response most likely to contribute to a negative outcome, the ultimate example of which is the devastation of war.[1]

Thus humans, by virtue of their entrenched survival instinct, continue to respond to conflict with elements of a fight-or-flight response. Interestingly, emotional reactions to conflict are also exhibited by nonhuman species and are thought to play a role in natural selection and survival (establishing dominance and social order).[6]

While animals may manage their disagreements in direct and irrevocable ways (as by fighting to the death), unresolved conflict among humans contributes to physical and emotional complaints such as insomnia, anxiety, and other stress-related problems.[12]

Conflict in the Workplace

1. Robert is a new physical therapist in a busy PT department. Although he is friendly and competent, he has a rather "casual" approach to personal hygiene. Several patients have complained about his offensive body odor. His supervisor, Jean, must confront him about this issue.

2. Melanie is supervisor of the orthopedic unit of a large teaching hospital. She values the admiration and approval of her staff to the point where she avoids conflict as much as possible. On an annual performance evaluation with Marcie, one of her staff, Melanie fails to offer important constructive feedback. Instead, Melanie assures Marcie that her performance is satisfactory. Melanie then proceeds to write a critical report about Marcie, which she places in her employment file. A few months later, Marcie applies for a transfer to another unit, supervised by Joni. As Joni and Marcie discuss the transfer, Joni is impressed with Marcie's enthusiasm and feels inclined to approve the transfer. But first Joni decides to ask about Melanie's written report and is stunned to realize that Marcie knows nothing about it.

3. Ricardo is a new faculty member in a PT assistant program. He is eager to suggest new ideas. But when Ricardo tries to share his ideas at a faculty meeting, Rita, one of the older staff, constantly cuts him off with a better idea of her own.

4. Bonnie and Sel are colleagues in a small pediatric facility. Bonnie is notorious for not cleaning up the toys and equipment from her treatment sessions; therefore Sel often finds himself doing this. One day Sel is running late to begin a treatment session and sees Bonnie's mess. His pent-up resentment compels him to write Bonnie an angry e-mail calling her a slob and telling her that he is sick and tired of being her babysitter.

5. Frankie and Theresa are colleagues in a PT department. They share a common desk area with several other colleagues. Both like to get to work early in order to catch up on computer documentation, but Frankie often chatters away on her cell phone as she types. Theresa finds this extremely disruptive, and there are no other computers outside the desk area.

6. Nina has just been hired from within staff ranks to a director's position in a large PT department. An energetic and hard-working person, she is younger than several of the staff whom she now supervises. One of the older staff, Margaret, is resentful of Nina's rapid success. At Nina's first department meeting, Margaret is seen rolling her eyes when Nina brings up new suggestions. At one point, Margaret even sighs loudly and says, "yeah, like *that* idea will work!"

Questions

1. What were your major communication challenges in each situation?

2. How did you attempt to address the conflict in a way that would promote a positive outcome for all parties? Describe these outcomes. If they applied to you, would you continue to experience any emotional stress?

Conflict in itself is not negative; rather, it is the *failure to address its consequences* in an effective manner that supports all parties. When conflict is addressed in the spirit of ameliorating the underlying cause to restore interpersonal connections and reduce perceptions of inequity, it can promote positive effects that facilitate collaboration between individuals. To return to the analogy of the dashboard warning light, full automotive function is restored by fixing the underlying mechanical problem rather than ignoring or disconnecting the signal.

Clinical Scenario

Effective resolution of conflict moves us forward in all levels of interaction. Thus, it might be encouraging to know that in the course of human history, some of our most effective initiatives and solutions have resulted from its effective management. The following example involving the impact of managed care on our profession is necessarily oversimplified for the purpose of illustration.

The advent of managed care in the late 1980s produced conflict between health-care payors (who had generally been reimbursing for services with little question) and health care providers (who had been generous in their provision of these). As national health-care expenditures continued to escalate, the government and the insurance industry decided to take action to reduce these. Consequently, the insurance industry instituted cost-reduction programs involving the assumption of unprecedented authority for determining payment to health-care providers. As a result, our professional decisions about what our patients needed were abrogated by representatives of the managed-care industry. A conflict ensued between insurance companies (with their need to control costs) and health-care providers (with their need for autonomous use of clinical expertise to assure high-quality patient care). As the insurance industry sought guidelines for payment allocations, it began to eliminate payment for interventions that could not be proven effective. This produced further conflict with health-care providers, who often relied on clinical observation to assess the value of their interventions.

In the early stages of managed care, many physical therapists had strong emotional reactions to what they viewed as an intrusion in their clinical decision making, particularly the ability to determine an appropriate level of care. Underlying these strong emotions were concerns about losing our professional autonomy, and even our financial livelihood, as insurance companies increased their rate of reimbursement denials (many physical therapists did, in fact, face salary reductions and layoffs, particularly after the Balanced Budget Act of 1996).

In the hope of reaching more reasonable solutions to these problems, the leaders of our profession began to explore the goals of managed care from the perspectives of all sides. After a period of time, we recognized that insurance companies' refusal to pay for interventions that lacked supporting evidence was, in the most positive sense, a timely challenge to strengthen our professional knowledge base and determine objective tests by which to measure outcomes.

Thus, in the course of addressing the conflicts created by managed care over the past several years, our profession has developed policies and initiatives that have strengthened the quality of our education, our knowledge base, and our evidence for what we do. Examples of these include *The Guide to Physical Therapist Practice, The APTA 2020 Vision Statement,* and the *Professionalism in Physical Therapy Core Values Document.* As our profession broadened its knowledge base, physical therapists expanded their competence through ongoing education. Accordingly, as the doctor of PT degree became the preferred entry-level credential, 1,334 practicing physical therapists had completed transitional programs of study in order to obtain this designation as of October, 2007.[13]

The benefits of managed care are evident in other ways, including an increasing acceptance of direct access and autonomous practice. In addition, many physical therapists have discovered new opportunities for service delivery, such as women's health, primary prevention, and end-of-life care. While the tension between insurance companies and health-care providers continues to various degrees, our profession has shown that we can address these challenges in innovative, meaningful ways. As a result, there has never been a more exciting time to be a physical therapist!

As this example illustrates, effective conflict management promotes the growth (and survival) of relationships, professional organizations, and societies as a whole. The key to success is determining and then addressing the underlying needs of each party.

Talking Points/Field Notes

A Conflict Coup

In a small group, describe a situation where you addressed conflict in a productive and meaningful way. Consider the following questions:

1. What was the nature of the conflict?

2. What was at stake for each party?

3. Describe the self-talk and communication processes that led you toward your chosen approach. How did you present this approach to the other parties?

4. What was the outcome? How did this affect each party?

Responding to Conflict

The manner in which we respond to conflict can significantly affect our outcomes and the persons involved. Thus, the skills of effective negotiation are valuable tools for maintaining and strengthening relationships. In situations of conflict with friends, family, or colleagues, our attachments to such persons will hopefully compel us toward thoughtful negotiation, allowing us to move forward with our bonds intact (or even stronger).[14]

However, in busy public spaces where we randomly cross paths with countless others, we may find ourselves in conflict with strangers. For example, a store clerk talks on her cell phone behind the counter while we wait for service. Given the anonymity of these interactions, we might find ourselves reacting less thoughtfully. Although we may not be in relationship with these individuals, the nature of our reactions can leave a lasting impact for better or worse.

Thus, in order to have a positive influence on all areas of our lives, we must be thoughtful in our approaches to conflict management regardless of the circumstances. For many of us, this means developing greater consistency in our responses.

Talking Points/Field Notes

Responses to Conflict

The following two scenarios describe a public, anonymous conflict and a more private, personal one. Read each scenario and discuss the questions that follow. Then record your observations in your field notes.

Scenario 1: Cut-in Conflict

On your way to class one morning, you stop at your favorite campus coffee shop. Having only a few minutes to spare, you are frustrated to see that the line is long and moving slowly. Nevertheless, you take your place and wait. A few moments later, the person in front of you sees two of her friends approach the back of the line and invites them to join her. As these two friends come forward (completely ignoring you), you now realize that you will probably be late for class. This is not an acceptable option. Consider the following questions:

Continued

Talking Points/Field Notes—cont'd ■ ▬▬▬▬▬▬▬▬▬▬▬▬▬▬▬

1. Describe your self-talk during this scenario. How does it change from the time you enter the coffee shop until when the two persons cut in front of you?

2. What is the prevailing emotion that you experience when the two persons cut in front of you?

3. How do you respond to this situation? Be specific in terms of your verbal and nonverbal behaviors.

4. What is the intended outcome of your course of action? Put this in terms of "What I want to happen is. . . ."

5. How might you describe your typical response to events of this sort (being ignored, having strangers act in ways that prevent you from getting your needs met in a timely manner)?

Scenario 2: Group Project Conflict

You are assigned to work with a group of classmates on an assignment involving the development of a 10-page paper and a 30-minute class presentation. This assignment is graded on a group basis (all members of the group receive the same grade) and is worth 30% of the course grade. Because this will be a semester-long project, each group is asked to select a coordinator. The role of the coordinator is to facilitate communication between group members and to keep the course instructor apprised of the group's progress.

When your group meets for the first time, you are asked to be the coordinator. You all work together to develop a meeting schedule along with a plan to distribute the work evenly.

As the semester proceeds (and gets busier), each member is making steady progress on his or her part of the assignment except for the person who is assigned to developing the slides for your presentation. Each time the group meets to discuss their progress, this person always has a compelling reason to explain her failure to complete her expected task (e.g., not feeling well, having to work, a family argument). When the group express concern, this person assures everyone that she will follow through and not to worry.

However, the night before your presentation, when your group meets for rehearsal, this individual informs you that the slides are only halfway done. Furthermore, she informs the group that she is not feeling well but will try to stay up and finish them "well enough to get by." The rest of you have worked diligently to meet the requirements for an A grade. As the coordinator of your group, it falls on you to address this issue. Consider the following questions:

1. Describe the sort of self-talk that might ensue when a group member fails to complete an assigned task. How might this self-talk change when there is "always a reason" for this failure?

2. What is your prevailing emotion when you learn that the slides are not done?

3. How do you respond to this situation? Be specific in terms of your verbal and nonverbal behaviors.

4. What is the intended outcome of your course of action? Put this in terms of "What I want to happen is. . . ."

5. How might you describe your typical response to events of this sort (when classmates, colleagues, or friends don't follow through on their commitments)?

6. Compare and contrast your reactions to each scenario. Are they more similar or more different? Why might this be?

7. How might your answer to question 4 above affect your actions?

As each of these scenarios suggests, you have many choices in terms of how you might respond. In the coffee shop example, you could react with anger, a loud accusatory voice, and an indignant demand for immediate reparation (telling those two "buttinskis" to get back in line *now*). In the group project example, you could berate your laggard classmate in front of the other members, ordering her to buck up and get the slides done.

In each situation, you could also avoid dealing with the problem, letting the others have control. Thus, in the case of the coffee shop, you would let the two persons cut in without comment; and in the case of the class presentation, you would work with the slides that were available (or offer to complete them yourself). While this solution might sidestep a confrontation, you might also harbor some unpleasant emotional stress.

Finally, you could respectfully negotiate, stating your observations about the other person's actions, stating their impact, and suggesting what you would like to see happen to end the conflict. In the coffee shop, this might mean informing the offending parties that their moving ahead of you would make you late for class, and that you would like them to return to their places in line. Your response might look like this: "You may not have noticed, but I was here before you. I don't want to be late for my class, so I would really appreciate it if you would not get in line before me."

In your group situation, it might involve clearly spelling your expectations for the completion of the slides and asserting your desires for this expectation to be met on schedule. Thus, you might say "I am really frustrated that the slides aren't done because our group has been working hard to get an A grade, not just to get by. I would really appreciate it if you would make this a priority and do your best to get these done well."

In each of these responses, there is no emotional outburst or attack. The offending party is calmly and explicitly informed of what would be necessary to end the conflict. Most importantly, the door is left open for the development or continuation of an amicable relationship.

Assertiveness as a Means of Reducing Conflict

Assertiveness: A Misunderstood Behavioral Spectrum

All responses to conflict involve a degree of assertiveness—which is generally defined as a set of behaviors related to the way that individuals speak up for, defend, or pursue their interests. Nevertheless, considerable confusion exists between assertiveness and aggressiveness. One 1978 study presented normative data on an objective rating scale designed to identify the differentiating characteristics of assertive, aggressive, and hostile responses to conflict.[15] The results of this study indicate that *assertiveness* pertains to behaviors either *maintaining control or reestablishing a level of control* that has been breached, while *aggressiveness* involves behaviors intended to *increase one's control at the expense of another person* (cutting in front of a person waiting in line is a good example). Finally, hostile behavior relates to the exertion of control by inflicting harm. Hostile behavior is associated with subjective feelings of hatred.

Follow-up studies in recent years have built on these distinctions, so that assertiveness is now typically defined as a continuum of intensity with respect to control-based behaviors. **Figure 11-1** illustrates features of the assertiveness continuum.

As this continuum illustrates, low levels of assertive behaviors are associated with passivity (low control). Persons who display low levels of assertiveness are often unable or unwilling to state their needs or establish control in a conflict situation. They may avoid conflict by failing to speak up for themselves in a direct manner. They may have difficulty

	LOW PASSIVE	MODERATE ASSERTIVE	HIGH AGGRESSIVE
PREDOMINANT ATTITUDES	Fear of rejection Unworthiness	Respect, empathy, confidence	Anger, self-righteousness
APPROACH TO CONFLICT	Subjugating	Negotiating	Overpowering

FOCUS	Pleasing others
	Manipulating others
		Maintaining respect
		  for self and others while
		  expressing needs
			Getting needs met at
			  all costs. Defending self
			Dominating others

BEHAVIORAL TACTICS	Submitting
	Overcommitting
	Withholding input
	Playing martyr or victim
		Engaging
		Stating needs and requests
		  calmly and firmly
		Accepting responsibility for
		  feelings
		Empathizing
			Bullying
			Berating
			Coercing
			Blaming

PERSONAL CONSEQUENCES	Lowers self-esteem
	Limits self-efficacy
	Limits social effectiveness
	Development of stress
	  related health problems
		Builds confidence
		Increases self-efficacy
		Increases social skills
			Alienation
			Damages relationships
			Achievements are lonely
			  victories
			Development of stress
			  related health problems

Figure 11–1. Features of the assertiveness continuum.

saying "no" to unfair requests and may even make statements suggesting that their needs are less important than those of others.

However, all humans have a need for understanding respect. Thus each of us will attempt to meet these needs in any way we can.[16] In the case of persons who use a more passive approach, oblique tactics such as manipulation (playing the helpless victim to induce guilt and obtain the desired concession) or the development of psychosomatic complaints (which provide a reprieve from unwanted commitments) are common approaches. However, persons on the receiving end of such tactics quickly sense this "foul play," which only escalates feelings of ill will. Hence the combination of low level assertiveness with indirect attempts to gain control is known as *passive aggression*.

Sadly, because of the frequently negative consequences, the chronic use of passive behaviors over time can take its toll on the health and well-being of the individual. Persons who habitually use passive behaviors in response to conflict often experience low self-esteem, chronic illness, poor relationships, and difficulty in reaching their goals.[17]

In contrast, at the opposite end of the assertiveness continuum are behaviors in which a person seeks to meet his or her needs by overpowering others (aggression). Individuals who use aggressive behaviors may attempt to meet their needs in socially negative ways with little regard for the feelings of others. They may bully others into submission through the use of insults, threatening words, and intrusive body language (they "get in your face"). Thus, the message delivered through an aggressive approach is "my needs and rights are more important than yours, and I don't care what you think about it." However, while these behaviors may appear successful in the short term, individuals who use aggression as their primary approach to conflict often lack social skills and suffer from emotional insecurity. Thus they are often defensive and on the lookout for ways of maintaining dominance over others.[18] Ultimately, their heavy-handed approach contributes to damaged relationships and potential social alienation.[19,20] These individuals also suffer deleterious effects on their physical health.

Finally, in the middle of the assertiveness spectrum are behaviors whereby the individual openly, calmly, and objectively states his or her needs to maintain a level of control in the face of conflict. Used in this context, appropriately assertive behavior is defined as "behaviors emitted by a person in an interpersonal context which express that person's feeling, attitudes, wishes, opinions, or rights directly, firmly and honestly while respecting the feelings, attitudes, wishes, opinions and rights of other persons."[21]

Assertive individuals will seek to work with others to find mutually acceptable solutions to conflict if this is possible. Persons who use assertiveness in this manner tend to be more confident, flexible, and spontaneous. They are also more likely to be at ease in social situations and to develop authentic relationships.[12]

As this discussion implies, the appropriate use of assertiveness is a complex communication skill that requires social and emotional intelligence. While all of us likely know individuals whose behaviors typically place them at either end of the continuum, the greater number of persons are probably somewhere in between. In addition, it is likely that most of us are appropriately assertive some of the time, while we struggle in other situations. While there are times when the use of aggressive or passive behaviors might serve us well (fending off a mugger or listening meekly when a police officer pulls us over for a lecture on our driving skills), such incidents are (hopefully) rare exceptions that will not be further discussed here.

Thus we focus on "middle continuum" strategies for developing assertiveness. First, let us begin by assessing your use of various levels of assertiveness.

Talking Points/Field Notes

Assertiveness Self-Assessment: Part I

Complete the assertiveness assessment in **Table 11-1**. Use the assertiveness continuum to determine how you typically respond. Then discuss the following questions with a small group of classmates and record your observations in your field notes.

Table 11–1. Self-Assessment for Assertiveness

Using the assertiveness continuum below, place the appropriate number next to each statement.

A. Professional/Academic: How assertive are you when:	1 2 3 4 5 6 7 8 9 10
	Passive Assertive Aggressive
1. Asking a question in class or in a large group?	
2. Answering a question in class or in a large group?	
3. Stating an opinion or attitude in class or a large group?	
4. Making an appointment with a professor to discuss your grade?	
5. Volunteering to be a demonstration subject in class or in a group?	
6. Introducing yourself to a professionally well known speaker?	
7. Introducing yourself to a peer?	
8. Introducing another person at a professional meeting?	

Continued

Table 11–1. Self-Assessment for Assertiveness—cont'd

9. Making small talk with a new colleague?

10. Volunteering to organize a class/group project?

11. Sharing your ideas in a group or committee?

12. Giving a class presentation?

B. Everyday Situations: How assertive are you in:	1 2 3 4 5 6 7 8 9 10		
	Passive	Assertive	Aggressive

13. Admitting that you have forgotten another person's name in a conversation with that person?

14. Asking for constructive feedback ?

15. Giving constructive feedback?

16. Reacting to constructive feedback?

17. Admitting a mistake?

18. Apologizing to someone you have offended?

19. Giving directions or instructions?

20. Sharing deep emotions (sadness, passion, anger)?

21. Talking about yourself to others?

22. Asking others about themselves?

23. Asserting a difference of opinion?

24. Defending your position in a case of unfair criticism?

25. Responding to a person who interrupts you several times?

26. Protesting unfair treatment or rudeness?

27. Apologizing for a mistake?

28. Asking for help in a challenging or embarrassing situation?

29. Comforting a person who is extremely upset?

30. Giving or accepting compliments?

31. Telling someone that their behavior is rude, thoughtless, or offensive?

32. Responding to an offensive joke or comment?

33. Dealing with an angry person?

34. Asking for forgiveness?

35. Ending a conversation?

Table 11–1. Self-Assessment for Assertiveness—cont'd

C. Conversational Topics. How assertive are you in discussing:	1 2 3 4 5 6 7 8 9 10		
	Passive	Assertive	Aggressive
36. What PTs do?			
37. The state of health care delivery?			
38. Gun control?			
39. Gay marriage?			
40. The death penalty?			
41. Assisted suicide?			
42. Disability rights?			
43. Abortion?			
44. Politics?			
45. Climate change?			
46. Generational differences?			
47. Death?			
48. Financial matters?			
49. Racial differences?			
50. Religion?			
51. Gender roles?			
52. Your accomplishments?			
53. Other?			

Tabulate your scores as follows:

Passive: The number of scores between 1 and 3

Assertive: The number of scores between 4 and 7

Aggressive: The number of scores between 8 and 10

Then answer the following questions:

1. In which situations/areas were your scores in the passive range? How might you explain these scores? Were there common elements?

2. In which situations/areas were your scores in the aggressive range? How might you explain these scores? Were there common elements?

3. In which situations/areas were your scores in the assertive range? How might you explain these scores? Were there common elements?

4. How might you address the areas where your scores were either passive or aggressive? Consider how you might go about this.

Assertive Behaviors

As you completed the first part of the assertiveness self-assessment, perhaps you were surprised by some of the behaviors that were included. Although assertiveness is often described primarily in terms of responses to conflict, its full complement also includes elements that build and strengthen relationships. This means that anytime you respectfully communicate with others in a way that conveys your authentic thoughts and feelings, you are being assertive. Thus giving sincere compliments, sharing information about yourself or your feelings in an appropriate manner (be it in a first patient encounter or on a first date), and asking for help, information, or support are all assertive behaviors. While these may seem easy, many persons struggle with these behaviors. Let us continue our assertiveness self-assessment with an exploration of your comfort with the use of such behaviors.

Talking Points/Field Notes: Assertiveness Self-Assessment: Part II ■━━━

Comfort With Assertive Behaviors

Table 11-2 lists examples of assertive behaviors. Use the scale to assess your comfort with these behaviors as well as your perception of their importance for professional success.

Table 11–2. Self-Assessment for Assertiveness Behaviors

Use the following SUDS scale (subjective units of discomfort) from Chapter 4 to evaluate your comfort with each of the following assertive behaviors. Then assess the importance of each behavior using the "importance" scale.

Comfort

1	2	3	4	5	6	7	8	9	10
Completely relaxed, at ease		Alert, focused			Tense, anxious			Panic, sweating, dry mouth, racing heart	

Importance

1	2	3	4	5	6	7	8	9	10
Completely unimportant for professional success		Fairly important			Very important			Essential for professional success	

Behavior	Comfort Level	Importance for Professional Success
1. Introducing self		
2. Introducing others		
3. Talking before groups		
4. Giving compliments		
5. Accepting compliments		
6. Giving an apology		
7. Accepting an apology		

Table 11–2. Self-Assessment for Assertiveness Behaviors—cont'd

8. Expressing anger

9. Expressing sadness

10. Sharing deep emotions

11. Comforting a person in distress

12. Giving directions or instructions

13. Stating a difference of opinion

14. Admitting a mistake

15. Saying "no"

16. Being said "no" to

17. Giving constructive feedback

18. Accepting constructive feedback

19. Saying "I don't know"

20. Saying "I don't understand"

21. Saying "I don't care"

22. Expressing thanks

23. Asking for help

24. Setting limits with others

25. Lodging a complaint

26. Confronting rude or offensive behavior

After you complete this scale, discuss the following questions and record your observations in your field notes:

1. With which of the assertive behaviors were you most comfortable? Consider how you developed these skills. How can you apply them toward effective PT practice?

2. For each of the behaviors, what was the relationship between your comfort and your level of assertiveness (from Part 1 of the assessment)? How might you explain this relationship?

3. Which behaviors did you consider to be the most important for professional success? If these were areas in which you rated yourself high in terms of discomfort, how might you use assertive behaviors to improve your skills in these areas?

Assertive Rights: Honoring Self and Others

Assertive behavior involves self-advocacy in ways that are respectful of the rights of self and others. *Rights* pertain to the legal or moral entitlement to engage in or refrain from a given action. Accordingly, the U.S. Constitution outlines the rights of all Americans regarding actions of speech, worship, and legal prerogatives. Rights also pertain to a moral entitlement to societal recognition, such as civil rights.[22]

Assertive rights pertain to the entitlements of all individuals in a civilized society. Interactions that threaten these prerogatives can result in significant emotional and physical harm. Accordingly, persons who are effective in the use of assertive skills promote civility and goodwill in their spheres of influence. There are numerous sources detailing these.[23-27]

A summary of these assertive rights is presented in **Box 11-1**.

BOX 11-1:   Assertive Rights

1. You have the right to say NO: Self-responsibility involves making decisions about the use of your time, money, attention, and energy. You have the right to determine the allocation of these resources.

2. You have the right to change your mind: Change is a constant of life; few things are consistent or rigid. You have the right to adjust your decisions in the light of new information or insight.

3. You have the right to make mistakes (but not to blame others for them): No one is perfect, and part of the human growth process involves experiencing the consequences of less than optimal choices.

4. You have the right to judge your own thoughts, feelings, and behavior (and to be accountable for their consequences): Only you know what it is like to live in your body and to have your perspective. Thus you are the ultimate judge of your behaviors. However, because your actions affect others, you must also be willing to take responsibility for their impact. This may mean that you sometimes allow others (employers or those with whom you have a legal relationship) to judge your behavior in terms of role-related expectations.

5. You have the right to withhold justifications, explanations, or reasons for your behaviors: Responsible self-judgment involves making decisions that are in your best interest. You have the right to either share or withhold justifications for your actions. However, attempting to appease others with white lies or excuses undermines this right.

6. You have the right to decide whether or not you will take responsibility for helping others solve their problems. Just as you have the right to direct your life and choose your outlook, so do others. At times you may consciously choose to help others with their problems. However, in offering this assistance, remember that each person holds ultimate responsibility for his or her own life outcome. Thus effective use of your resources may involve selectively offering your help in situations where it is most likely to be beneficial.

7. You have the right to be independent of the goodwill of others. Seeking the approval of others as a measure of self-worth can diminish your self-esteem and make you vulnerable to manipulation. When you lack the goodwill of those with whom you work, you are free to determine how you will interact in order to achieve the necessary outcomes.

8. You have the right to be illogical in your decision making. Not all decisions can be made on the basis of pure facts and reason. In the gray areas of life, you may call on a variety of resources to make a final judgment. Not everyone will understand this.

9. You have the right to say "I don't know."*

10. You have the right to say "I don't agree."*

11. You have the right to say "I don't understand."*

12. You have the right to say "I don't care."*

---

*These statements are reflections of your right to accept your limitations without having to justify them.

Talking Points/Field Notes

How Well Do You Use Your Assertive Rights?

This exercise is designed to help you determine areas in which you can strengthen your assertiveness behaviors through the appropriate exercise of rights. Before you begin, review your answers to the assertiveness self-assessment in Box 11-1. Then discuss the following questions in a small group, recording your observations in your field notes:

1. Why do many people have a problem with saying no to an unwanted (or even inappropriate) request for their resources? How does it feel when another person says no to you?

2. How might a strong need for the approval of others prevent you from being assertive? How realistic is it to think that you can have the approval of everyone you meet?

3. Why is it so hard to admit making a mistake? How does it feel when another person admits a mistake? How easily could you admit making a mistake to a patient?

4. Why is it so difficult for many people to express disagreement without getting aggressive? How might this affect the quality of intellectual dialogue involving different perspectives?

5. Why is it difficult to admit a change of mind? Why do we expect people to be unchanging and predictable?

6. How do you think relationships are affected when all parties exercise their assertive rights while also honoring those of others?

7. What other rights do you believe are important for all persons to hold for themselves and respect in others?

Adversarial Attitudes About Assertiveness

In completing the previous exercise on assertive rights, perhaps you became more aware of attitudes that interfere with your ability to be assertive. Many others have similar concerns that prevent the appropriate use of this skill. Collectively, these concerns could be called adversarial attitudes about assertiveness, because they are forms of self-talk that argue against the use of this skill (see **Box 11-2**).

BOX 11-2: Adversarial Attitudes About Assertiveness

1. If I am assertive, I will make people angry.
2. If I am assertive, others won't like me.
3. If I am assertive and make others dislike me, I will be devastated.
4. If I am assertive, I will hurt other people's feelings.
5. If I am assertive, others will think I am selfish.
6. If I am assertive, others will think I am overbearing.
7. If I am assertive and don't get what I want, I am not doing it right.
8. Effective assertiveness means that I address all conflicts immediately.
9. All of my conflicts can be best addressed with assertiveness.
10. Either you are born assertive or you are not.

Although it can be unsettling to consider that being assertive might upset others, failure to use this skill can instead result in passive or aggressive behaviors that are more damaging to relationships in the long run. Few of us choose to cause another person's upset, but in reality we can only control our own feelings and behaviors. If these include respectful interactions, the reactions of others are beyond our capacity to change or control.

In contrast to our fears that our friends will forsake us if we are assertive with them, appropriate use of this skill instead conveys a desire to remain authentically committed in your relationships. Furthermore, when we respectfully convey our feelings and concerns to others, we offer them the opportunity to respond in kind.

The bottom line is that given the alternatives (aggressiveness or passivity), assertiveness provides the best opportunities for respectful communication that meets the needs of all parties. Thus, an attitude of greater acceptance of the value of assertiveness may be worth pursuing and maintaining. **Box 11-3** shows accepting attitudes about assertiveness.

BOX 11-3:   Accepting Attitudes About Assertiveness

1. If your assertiveness makes others angry, they have chosen this reaction.
2. Assertiveness promotes respectful and authentic relationships.
3. We cannot control the reactions of others toward us. One of our assertive rights is independence from the goodwill of others.
4. Assertive communication does not attack or shame others. Hurt feelings are an individual choice.
5. Assertive behaviors respect the needs of all parties.
6. Stating your needs directly and calmly is not overbearing.
7. Because you can't control the behaviors of others, assertiveness will not always get you what you want. However, you can be comfortable that you have done your best.
8. Taking a "time out" or "cooling off" period to consider your response is an assertive option. You can then come back with a clearer and less emotional perspective.
9. Assertiveness can involve silence or refusal to engage with a highly aggressive or passive person. Honor your intuition.
10. Although we are born with certain dispositions, most of us can benefit from learning and practicing assertiveness skills.

Talking Points/Field Notes

My Attitudes About Assertiveness

Consider the adversarial attitudes in Box 11-2. Then discuss the following and record your observations in your field notes:

1. Which attitudes contribute to your reluctance to be assertive when you want to be?

2. Which of these attitudes contributes most to your reluctance to be assertive?

3. How might you begin to practice assertiveness in ways that are less difficult?

4. How will you progress in your practice?

Practicing of Assertiveness in Nonconflict Situations

As we have discussed, assertiveness also involves sharing thoughts and feelings in nonconflict situations. By practicing these behaviors on a regular basis, we can develop our confidence with speaking up in everyday situations. Once we have developed our "voice," it will be easier to express ourselves in more challenging situations. Box 11-1 shows many of these behaviors, particularly as they pertain to professional and academic environments (1 to 12), everyday interactions (13, 19, 21 to 23, 28 to 30, 34), and conversational topics (35, 36, and 44). The last of these are probably the least emotionally charged for most persons.

Directions:

1. For the next month, make it a point to practice as many of these behaviors as possible in an appropriate context. Use the Subjective Units of Discomfort Scale shown in **Figure 11-2** to rate your stress levels over time.

2. You may find that recording your progress in your field notes will enable you to be more aware of positive change. Having a supportive friend provide feedback can also be helpful.

3. As you become more comfortable with these behaviors, note the impact on your self-confidence, comfort, and enjoyment of your interactions.

1	2	3	4	5	6	7	8	9	10
Completely relaxed, at ease		Alert, focused			Tense, anxious				Panic, sweating, dry mouth, racing thoughts, pounding heart

Figure 11–2. Subjective "Units of Discomfort" scale.

Implications for Physical Therapy

Assertiveness and Leadership

Assertive behaviors are important features of leadership effectiveness, where two related behaviors—consideration and initiating structure—have been determined to be among the most effective management traits.[28] Consideration is related to the social elements of leadership: concern for others, respect, appreciation, and support. Initiating structure is related to organization, delegation, and management of goal-directed activities.

Assertive behaviors affect both of these dimensions in varying ways. For example, an aggressive leader might disregard his employees for the sake of the bottom line, and a passive leader might be more interested in developing relationships than in driving employee productivity. The interplay of these two assertive constructs affects how they are perceived by associates.[29]

Extremely aggressive leaders are perceived as "socially insufferable"[24] individuals who ruthlessly and autocratically pursue their goals without regard for the social implications. These leaders possess a high degree of initiative-taking behaviors, which allow them to accomplish a great deal for their organization—but at considerable social cost.

On the other hand, leaders who are more passive may enjoy a stronger social network, but their inability to deal effectively with conflict renders them "instrumentally impotent"[24] in terms of employing the necessary initiative-taking behaviors to move the organization forward. These leaders can exasperate their colleagues with their passivity and indecisiveness.

Finally, the middle of the curve represents a balance between concern for others and the appropriate measure of initiative-taking behaviors. **Figure 11-3** illustrates the bell-shaped curve of assertiveness behaviors.

As you review **Figure 11-3**, consider the following Champ and Blockhead scenario.

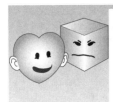

Champ and Blockhead Attempt to Rally the Troops (Another "Truth Is Stranger Than Fiction" Tale)

Champ and Blockhead, both PT supervisors, work for two different branch facilities of Friendly Acres, a large corporate skilled nursing facility. At the last regional meeting of Friendly Acres' supervisory staff, Hector Jones, Friendly Acres' national vice president, informed the group that Friendly Acres had been losing revenue over the previous few months. "This is not good news," stated Mr. Jones. "If we are to keep this business afloat, I need each of you to push staff productivity so that you can meet your projected earnings next quarter. We also need to stop the excessive use of sick time. If you are not able to do this, we will have to look at closing your PT department."

Blockhead has just been promoted to her supervisory position and is enjoying her new respect within the Friendly Acres Corporation. She is terrified of losing face with the regional director. She thus decides that a "no-nonsense approach" is best, and she writes the following memo to her staff.

Our department is losing revenue. This is an embarrassment to me and I can't afford to let this continue. The following policies are in effect immediately:
I need each of you to see at least 10 patients a day, no excuses.
You need to bill for every minute you see a patient, so make it count!
A lot of you have been calling in sick and this must stop. I will need a doctor's excuse from now on for any illness-related absences.
We will be having a mandatory staff meeting on Wednesday at 5 p.m. to discuss this.

Champ returns to her office and thinks about how to convey her concerns without upsetting her staff. More than the revenue-driven emphasis of Friendly Acres, she values the camaraderie of her staff. She also believes that everyone is doing the best they can. Her memo reads as follows:

I have just returned from our regional meeting and there are concerns about loss of revenue. Let's discuss these at a meeting next Wednesday after work, at 5 p.m. Thanks for your thoughts on these issues. Together, I think we can find ways of addressing them.

Questions:

1. What impact would each of these memos have on you as a PT staff member? How might you respond to each?
2. What impact would each memo have on staff morale? How might this affect patient care?
3. What suggestions do you have for both Champ and Blockhead to more effectively engage the staff about this issue?
4. Where might you place both Champ and Blockhead on the bell curve shown in Figure 11-3?

Figure 11–3. Impact of assertiveness levels on colleagues' perceptions of leadership effectiveness in the workplace. Passive leaders tend to be viewed as ineffective at moving the organization forward (instrumentally impotent). Aggressive leaders are viewed as ruthlessly pursuing initiatives without regard for others (socially insufferable). At the top of the curve, concern for others is balanced with task accomplishment (socially and instrumentally balanced). *(Adapted with permission from Ames DR, Flynn FJ. What breaks a leader: The curvilinear relation between assertiveness and leadership. J Pers Soc Psychol. 2007;92(2):307-324. Published by The American Psychological Association.)*

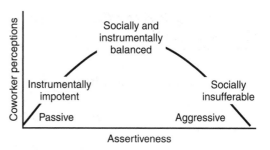

Patient Advocacy

Assertive behavior is an important element of PT practice. In working to promote the best outcomes for our patients, we may need to defend their interests to case managers, other health professionals, and even family members. The ability to clearly articulate our position without aggression, defensiveness, or passivity will help us to be optimally effective in our professional roles.

Supporting Our Patients

As we discussed in the previous chapter, being a patient (or a family member) is challenging on many levels. In addition to the psychosocial stresses of the illness experiences, insurance claims, paperwork, and the bureaucracy of our massive and overextended health-care system can be overwhelming. In the midst of such stress, patients and family members may resort to aggressive or passive behaviors. Patients may act aggressively toward persons in the health-care system for many reasons, including the nature of their condition or their medications. They may also have a history of aggressive behaviors or feel frustrated and angry in light of their circumstances.[30]

In such instances, it is important to recognize these behaviors as attempts to cope with significant stress and not personal affronts. Obviously this can be difficult, especially when you are confronted with "in your face" aggressive behavior. Nevertheless, by maintaining your own calm, assertive focus, you can help to deescalate angry behaviors in order to move toward acceptable solutions to the issues at hand. Assertive mindfulness will also help you to seek assistance if you feel that a situation is beyond your capacities to handle.

Assertiveness as a Tool for Professional Growth

An important element of continued professional growth is the ability to accept constructive feedback without defensiveness. By viewing feedback as helpful information that can help us in our professional development, we can move forward effectively.

Negotiation for Consensus: Strategies for Addressing Needs and Finding Solutions

Needs-Based Conflict Resolution

Theoretical Background

Needs-based conflict resolution involves the mutual acknowledgment of needs and feelings to promote reconciliation (a changed psychosocial orientation between individuals).[31] Needs-based conflict resolution is predicated on the concept that humans share a basic repertoire of needs and that emotional responses to conflict result from interactions where these are dishonored.[32-34]

A theoretical model of universal human needs was originally developed in 1943 by psychologist Abraham Maslow.[35] **Figure 11-4** illustrates Maslow's hierarchy of needs.

As shown in Figure 11-4, universal human needs are arranged in a bottom-up hierarchical order, with the lowest level pertaining to basic survival needs (food, clothing, and shelter). Subsequent levels reflect a progressive repertoire of increasingly sophisticated social needs, such as acceptance, belonging, and esteem. At the very top of the hierarchy are what Maslow called "self-actualization" or "transcendent" needs, which reflect higher-order goals related to spirituality and unique experiences.

According to Maslow, most humans are so engaged in meeting their lower-level needs that few have the luxury of pursuing those related to self-actualization. Furthermore, the unique life circumstances of each individual determine his or her most important needs. For example, persons living in extreme conditions of poverty will direct most of their interactions to securing adequate food and water. To that end, accounts of the aftermath of Hurricane Katrina describe the eruption of violent crime in New Orleans as desperation mounted over the rapid depletion of basic supplies.[36]

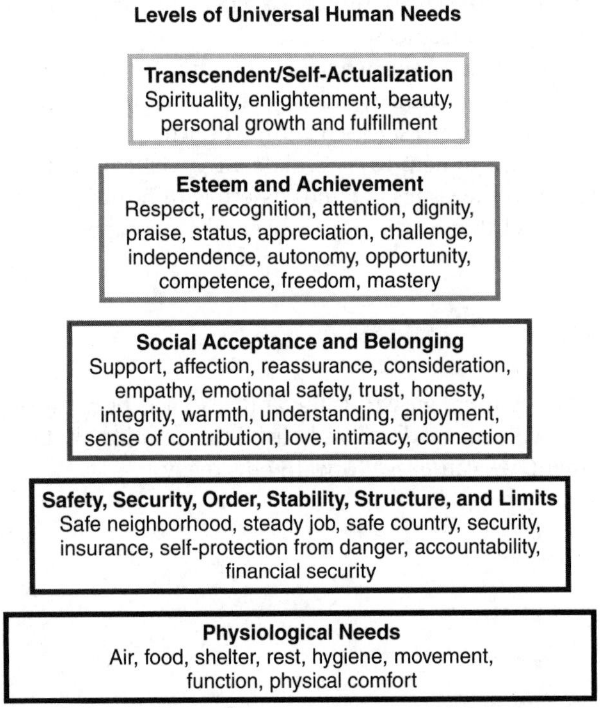

Levels of Universal Human Needs

Transcendent/Self-Actualization
Spirituality, enlightenment, beauty, personal growth and fulfillment

Esteem and Achievement
Respect, recognition, attention, dignity, praise, status, appreciation, challenge, independence, autonomy, opportunity, competence, freedom, mastery

Social Acceptance and Belonging
Support, affection, reassurance, consideration, empathy, emotional safety, trust, honesty, integrity, warmth, understanding, enjoyment, sense of contribution, love, intimacy, connection

Safety, Security, Order, Stability, Structure, and Limits
Safe neighborhood, steady job, safe country, security, insurance, self-protection from danger, accountability, financial security

Physiological Needs
Air, food, shelter, rest, hygiene, movement, function, physical comfort

Figure 11–4. A representation of Maslow's hierarchy of universal human needs.[11]

Since then, other researchers have examined Maslow's original concepts as they apply to the process of conflict resolution.[37,38]

Appreciation, affiliation, autonomy, status, and role have received attention as important core needs that must be honored in the process of successful conflict resolution.

Talking Points/Field Notes

Needs Profile

While the constellation of human needs has been shown to be relatively universal, the importance assigned to these varies between individuals. Thus a person with higher needs in one area (for example, recognition) might be more sensitive to transgressions in that domain. It can be helpful to have a sense of the needs that are more important to us, as this can help us pinpoint potential areas of conflict.

Review the list of needs depicted in Figure 11-4 and make a list of your top five. Then discuss the following questions in a small group. You can also record your observations in your field notes.

1. How do your needs affect your expectations of others in your communication?

2. Which life experiences have contributed to making these needs so important for you?

3. How might your experiences with conflict be related to these needs? Are you more sensitive to conflict in areas of high need?

A Practical Approach to Needs-Based Conflict Resolution

Nonviolent communication, also known as *NVC* or *compassionate communication*, is an internationally recognized needs-based approach to conflict resolution which was developed by psychologist Marshall Rosenberg. As a young Jewish boy growing up in Detroit during World War II, Rosenberg witnessed the devastating impact of a violent racial conflict in his neighborhood, in which over 40 people were killed. A short time later, he was beaten by two classmates who chose him as a target for their anti-Semitic hostilities. These incidents compelled Rosenberg toward the study of human compassion and how to maintain this virtue during the process of conflict resolution. After pursuing doctoral psychology training (where he was mentored by Carl Rogers, the founder of client-centered therapy), Rosenberg developed his practical communication theory of NVC. He subsequently applied his approach in several federally funded school integration projects during the late 1960s and met with considerable success. Since that time, NVC has been used throughout the world as a conflict resolution approach in war-torn countries and has been adopted by government, education, and business organizations. In 1984, Rosenberg established the Center for Non-Violent Communication[39] (http://www.NVC.org), a nonprofit international peacemaking organization that provides training and support for NVC. Interestingly, Rosenberg's choice of the term *nonviolent* was a reference to Mahatma Gandhi's assertion that the natural state of human beings is compassion, but only when "violence has subsided from the heart."[34]

According to Rosenberg, "violent" communication involves thought processes that block compassion between individuals. Such forms of communication involve a "language of domination," which includes moral judgments, blaming, and coercion. This form of communication is damaging because it provokes anger and other negative emotions, thus clouding the underlying issues. Furthermore, its generalized nature ("You're such a slob") heightens defensiveness and alienation between persons.

Accordingly, the major premise of NVC is to avoid the use of evaluative labels. As you are likely to discover, this often involves a deliberate reframing of habitual thought patterns. Accordingly, a related concept of NVC is that all of us are "different but equal." Although this sounds glaringly obvious, our long history of conflicts over differences related to race, religion, gender, and political ideology (to name a few) suggests otherwise. Learning to see individual differences as neither right nor wrong, good nor bad, requires the highest level of compassion, wisdom, and open-mindedness. In turn, these qualities are invaluable in the conflict negotiation process.

Steps of the NVC Process

Rosenberg has defined four key steps of the NVC conflict negotiation process. They include:

1. Observation without evaluation

2. Identification and expression of feelings

3. Taking ownership of needs and feelings

4. Requesting positive actions to meet our needs

Observation Without Evaluation: Just the Facts!

For the purposes of illustrating this step, let us return to the group conflict scenario described previously. Imagine what judgments might evolve in your mind in response to the 11th-hour discovery that one of the group members was completely unprepared with his contribution to the following day's presentation. Terms such as *stupid, irresponsible, lazy,* or *apathetic* might be examples. Let us also say that these labels are accompanied by increasing feelings of anger (and indeed, anger generally escalates when blaming statements are used).[40] Finally, your anger is high enough that you blurt out some of these sentiments to your classmate, who, in turn, becomes defensive and begins firing off one excuse after another. By now, it should be pretty obvious that a peaceful solution to this problem is not forthcoming.

The skill of observation without judging is a seemingly simple but crucial one in the negotiation process. Instead of reacting with emotionally fraught labels, we note the facts of the situation and nothing more. In the case of the group conflict (presented on p. 292), the unprepared group member will be called "member B," and the facts are as follows:

■ The group was given an assignment to prepare and offer as a presentation.
■ All members of the group were to receive the same grade as a measure of the total effort.
■ Each person agreed to assume responsibility for a portion of the assignment.
■ The group met three times over the semester. Each time, member B did not have his share of the presentation done.
■ Member B assured the group that his portion would be done on time.
■ On the night before the presentation, member B did not have his share completed.

These facts, when shared with member B, are much more likely to prevent defensiveness, because there are no personal attacks or condemnations. The facts are as they are, so that member B will hopefully acknowledge these behaviors and move forward productively to resolve the consequences involved.

The skill of observation without evaluation takes practice. **Table 11-3** illustrates guidelines and examples for observing without evaluating; these can help you in this process.

Table 11–3. Guidelines and Examples for Observing Without Evaluating

Guideline	Evaluative Comment	Observational Comment
State specific behaviors rather than generalized personal traits	"Keith is a slob." "Barb is lazy." "Paul is unprofessional." "Jane is rude."	"Keith left dirty dishes in the sink." "Barb was late to work three times this week." "Paul came to work in his gym sweats." "Jane interrupted me."
Avoid use of sweeping generalizations (always never, seldom, frequently, most, all, etc.)	"Maya never answers her e-mails." "Mike is always late." "Most Mexicans are illegal immigrants."	"Maya did not respond to three messages from me." "Mike was late to class four times this month." "In the past 3 months, three of my Mexican patients were undocumented immigrants."
Avoid negative predictions	"If you keep eating like that, you'll get fat." "If Sara doesn't start studying, she'll flunk out."	"If you eat a large pizza for lunch every day, you may gain weight." "If Sara doesn't study this semester, her grades may suffer."
Avoid generalized slang as a form of feedback	"Your service sucks."	"I have been waiting 30 minutes for my appointment."

Talking Points/Field Notes

Evaluation Vacation

The use of evaluative language is such a common feature in everyday communication that most of us are desensitized. The purpose of this exercise is to help you replace such verbiage with more objective and specific language. It is suggested that you try this for at least 72 hours. After you have completed this exercise, discuss the following questions and record your observations in your field notes.

1. Every time you are tempted to use an evaluative label ("He's a jerk"), make a conscious effort to replace it with observations and objective language. ("He yelled at his wife.")

2. Each day, make it a point to compliment at least two persons for a specific behavior. Examples include "I was so impressed at how you listened in that meeting" and "I really appreciate you doing the dishes."

3. Each day, make it a point to describe one emotionally charged event in your day to another person, using objective language: "The traffic coming home was really heavy. One person yelled angry insults and cut in front of me."

4. Observe the use of evaluative language in conversations around you. Note the emotional climate of these. Rather than judging these conversations as good or bad, right or wrong, simply observe without evaluating them.

Continued

Talking Points/Field Notes—cont'd ▬▬▬▬▬▬▬▬▬▬▬▬▬▬

Questions:

1. How did the use of observational language affect your emotional state? In which ways was this different than when you were using evaluative language?

2. What was the impact on your interactions in using observations and objective descriptions?

3. What was the impact of giving specific compliments?

4. How much of a challenge was this exercise? Why do you think this was so?

Implications for Physical Therapy

The use of observations in place of judgments has huge implications for PT practice. Effective leadership involves providing useful, objective feedback that empowers change. To that end, imagine a performance evaluation where your supervisor tells you that your skills are poor. This statement gives no specific information that would enable you to improve your skills, and the word "poor" is likely to provoke a negative emotional response that would damage collegial goodwill. On the other hand, it would be difficult to argue with feedback that identified specific limitations. For example, "When Mrs. Jones fell during her ambulation training with you, I noticed that you were not using a gait belt." Even positive evaluative language does not provide specific information for the improvement of performance. For example, we are more likely to repeat a positive behavior that has been specifically identified in feedback (e.g., "you were very articulate during the discussion" as opposed to "you did a great job").

Effective documentation also requires the inclusion of objective measures. Documentation that a patient is "uncooperative" may invite scrutiny and possible claims denial. In the case of a patient with neurological complications, this term is also inappropriate. Last of all, remember that patients have the right to access their charts at any time. To that end, I remember an indignant phone call from my mother, who had read the following statement in her chart: "Mrs. L.'s husband is a physician, so she will probably have extra high expectations."

Identification and Expression of Feelings

As we discussed previously, the greatest indicator of conflict is an uncomfortable emotional response. We also used the analogy of a dashboard indicator, the purpose of which is to provide a signal of an underlying malfunction. In this context, the feelings that arise in conflict should be welcomed and acknowledged as our body's honest appraisal of a potential problem. The ability to articulate and share these feelings (first to ourselves, then to others) is a potent way of preventing them from festering within. It is also an important step in the resolution of conflict because it involves authenticity and self-responsibility. When a person says "I am frustrated," "I am sad," or "I am anxious," there is really no counterargument, as these statements involve full ownership. And because human feelings are universal, such admissions are likely to introduce empathy into a conflict situation. The result is often a diffusion of antagonism, which promotes resolution.

Just like the language of evaluation described previously, the language of domination does not include statements of feeling. Rather, we substitute thoughts, opinions, and evaluations of how we think others are treating us.[34] **Table 11-4** illustrates guidelines and suggestions for clear feeling statements.

Table 11–4. Guidelines and Examples of Clear Feeling Statements

Pitfall	Example of Pitfall	Example of Clear Feeling
1. Substituting thought for feeling (Evidenced by "I feel" followed by one of the following):		
a. Personal pronoun (I, you, he, she, it, we, they)	"I feel that you don't care."	"I feel frustrated when you don't listen to me."
b. Subordinating conjunction (Examples: that, as if, as though)	"I feel as if I am being judged."	"I feel nervous when you stare at me without talking."
c. Names or personal nouns	"I feel like my professor hates me."	"I feel dejected when I talk to my professor."
d. Labels or judgments of self or others	"I feel like an idiot during practical exams."	"I feel anxious."
2. Replacing feeling statements with statements about how we think others are treating us (Thought words are often verbs, while feeling words are often adjectives)	"I feel ignored when you're with your friends."	"I feel hurt when you don't include me in your conversations."
	"I feel misunderstood at our group meetings."	"I feel helpless when no one asks for my opinions."
3. Replacing feeling statements with thoughts or judgments about what we think we are	"I am a failure in the romance department."	"I feel discouraged in my relationships with men/women."
	"I suck at tennis."	"I am frustrated with my tennis skills."

Talking Points/Field Notes

As you look over the examples in Table 11-4, reflect on your own approach to the expression of feelings. Then consider the following questions and reflect on your observations in your field notes.

1. Are you guilty of any of the pitfalls listed in Table 11-4?

2. If so, what reasons might you have?

3. In which areas do you find it the most challenging to express your feelings?

   a. Intimate relationships

   b. Close friendships

   c. Casual friendships

   d. Work relationships

   e. With superiors

4. Why do you think you might have different comfort levels? How might you appropriately express your feelings in each of these contexts?

Developing a "Feeling Word" Vocabulary

Because many of us are accustomed to using indirect ways of expressing feelings, our vocabulary of these terms may be rusty. **Table 11-5** depicts a list of feeling words.

Talking Points/Field Notes

Use of Feeling Words

The purpose of this exercise is to reacquaint you with the expansive world of feeling words by inviting you to practice their use, as follows. Then discuss with classmates and record your observations in your field notes.

1. Review the list of feeling words in Table 11-5. You might select a few that appeal to you or add your own as desired. If you would like to build your own collection, there are numerous Internet sites that can provide you with extensive lists in response to the search term "feeling words."

2. For the next 72 hours, make it a point to include a direct expression of feeling in at least one conversation a day. You might want to start with more positive emotions and progress to others related to anger, sadness, etc.

Questions:

1. Discuss your experiences using feeling words. How difficult was this? How did you select your opportunities for practice?

2. What were the results of your practice? Were there any changes in the quality of your interactions?

3. How might you continue to develop your practice of using feeling words? How might this help you in future clinical practice?

Table 11–5. **Examples of "Feeling" Words**

Amused	Annoyed	Afraid	Anxious	Appreciative	Angry
Awful	Astonished	Ashamed	Agitated	Anguished	Alarmed
Bitter	Blissful	Baffled	Bewildered	Bored	Buoyant
Confident	Concerned	Curious	Comfortable	Cranky	Contented
Discouraged	Dejected	Delighted	Disgusted	Disturbed	Dumbfounded
Edgy	Ecstatic	Exhausted	Enthusiastic	Energized	Exasperated
Fascinated	Flummoxed	Frustrated	Fearful	Furious	Flippant
Grateful	Gleeful	Gloomy	Glorious	Guilty	Grandiose
Hateful	Happy	Hopeful	Hostile	Horrified	Humiliated
Intrigued	Infuriated	Introspective	Inspired	Isolated	Incensed
Joyful	Jealous	Jubilant	Jittery	Jaunty	Judicious
Kind	Knotted-up	Keyed-up	Knowing	Klutzy	Keen

Table 11–5. Examples of "Feeling" Words—cont'd

Loving	Lonely	Lethargic	Listless	Libidinous	Lighthearted
Melancholic	Marvelous	Miserable	Mirthful	Mellow	Mindless
Nauseated	Naughty	Needy	Nervous	Noble	Nonchalant
Optimistic	Overwhelmed	Outraged	Overcome	Officious	Ominous
Pessimistic	Proud	Protective	Puzzled	Panicked	Peaked
Quirky	Quixotic	Quivery	Quarrelsome	Quiet	Quaky
Radiant	Relaxed	Relieved	Ridiculous	Riveting	Revolted
Scared	Suspicious	Spellbound	Splendid	Scrappy	Sanctimonious
Tremendous	Troubled	Terrified	Touched	Thrilled	Tolerant
Upbeat	Upset	Unassuming	Uncertain	Uncouth	Unsettled
Vexed	Valorous	Vain	Vapid	Vicious	Victorious
Weary	Wretched	Wistful	Whimsical	Woeful	Weepy
Xenophobic	Yearning	Youthful	Zany	Zestful	Zealous

Implications for Physical Therapy

The sharing of authentic feelings in the workplace is an important element of empowerment and collegiality *if done in a nonviolent manner.*[41] Emotionally repressed work environments create job dissatisfaction and employee stress. Interestingly, one of the most important predictors of a feeling-receptive work environment is whether this behavior is exhibited by those in leadership. Not surprisingly, higher levels of employee job satisfaction and personal well-being exist in settings where supervisors demonstrate affective authenticity.[41]

Taking Ownership of Feelings and Needs

A major premise of NVC is that emotions arise in response to needs. Accordingly, negative emotions correspond to unmet needs, and positive emotions pertain to those that are met.

Communicating in a way that links our feelings to our needs is accomplished by the general statement "I feel X (insert emotion) because I need or want Y (insert need)." The "I" component is important in both places as a full acknowledgment of ownership of both our feelings and the needs to which they relate. The most important thing in this statement is that we convey full responsibility for both.

When you note an emotional reaction in response to an observed behavior, you can also include this in your statement, along the lines of "When X happens, I feel Y because I am wanting Z."

When you are including observations in your feeling/need statements, it is helpful to refer to the behavior without direct reference to the person involved. This prevents others from receiving your comment as a judgment or evaluation. For example, a colleague interrupts you several times in a meeting. Rather than saying "When *you* interrupt me, I feel frustrated because I need respect from my colleagues," your statement will be better received with "When *I am interrupted* in meetings...." In this case, no one is being singled out or blamed. Instead, you are merely reporting an observed fact. **Figure 11-5** illustrates suggestions for how to construct such statements.

Scenario #1: A physical therapy staff member often shows up late keeping patients waiting. The supervisor must address this issue.

Pitfalls:

1. **Use of impersonal language to deflect ownership:** "**It** really makes me mad when you show up late! **It** is unprofessional."
2. **Stating a behavior and feeling without linking this to a need:** "When **you** show up late, I feel furious."

Suggestions:

1. "**I feel** angry when members of my staff are late for work **because I need** our patients to be treated professionally."
2. "When members of my staff are late for work, **I feel** helpless **because** our patients have to wait. **I need** accountability from everyone in this office."

Scenario #2: A colleague tells an offensive joke that targets your racial background.

Pitfalls:

1. **Too general, no need stated:** "**That** is really offensive."
2. **Blaming person without ownership:** "**You** ought to be ashamed of yourself!"

Suggestions:

1. "**I feel** discouraged **when** I hear jokes like that **because I need** respect from the people I work with."
2. "**I am** disappointed **when** I hear jokes like that from my colleagues **because I want a** tolerant work atmosphere."

Scenario #3: As a cost containment measure, your new department director asks to approve all staff patient equipment orders.

Pitfalls:

1. **Evaluative judgment of how you think the director thinks:** "**You** must think we're **incompetent!**"
2. **Defensive response:** "**No one** is going to tell me what to do!"

Suggestions:

1. "Are **you concerned because you need** more accountability for our department expenses?" (This response explores the feelings/needs of the director. The word *feeling* is not used, but implicitly inferred.)
2. "**I feel frustrated** when my professional decisions are monitored **because I am wanting** more autonomy in my work."

Figure 11–5. Guidelines and suggestions for statements of feelings and needs.

Needs-based negotiation also involves responding appropriately to the needs and feelings of others. In the NVC process, we need to understand that behind any judgment, label, or evaluative comment, there is an unmet need.[39] Furthermore, each of us communicates in the best way we know how, so that there is really nothing to be gained by launching off on your own counterattack in response to a harshly worded statement of need.

In reality, we have four different responses to such an expression. The first two are not effective and include self-blame or defensiveness and counterattack. The last two involve the examination of feelings and needs. The following example illustrates each of these options.

Let's say that you borrow a friend's bicycle for a quick errand. You park the bike at your destination and, thinking that you will be gone only a minute, forego the lock. The bike is stolen. When you report this incident to your friend, his first response is, "How could you be so stupid!"

In the self-blaming response, you would take your friend's evaluative comment and set off on a negative self-judging spree ("Yes, I know I'm an idiot," etc.). This response simply deflects your friend's judgment toward yourself, which does nothing for your own self-esteem. It may also infuriate your friend, who is probably more interested in getting his bike back.

In the defensive comeback, you would launch a counterattack along the lines of "Don't call me stupid! You're the one who dented my car last year!" This reaction would provoke anger between you and your friend, inviting a further exchange that could cause considerable harm to your relationship.

The third option is to consider the emotions and needs behind your friend's comment. Often these are pretty obvious. In this situation you might say, "I don't blame you for being angry, I know your bike is your only way of getting around." This comment acknowledges your friend's anger over being deprived of a primary mode of transportation (which meets needs for independence, mobility, etc.). It is likely that this response would deescalate your friend's anger and allow you to move forward with a solution.

The fourth option involves examining your feelings in order to assess what needs might lie beneath them. In this case, you might say, "I am so frustrated that this happened because I really try to be responsible when I borrow things." This comment acknowledges your need to be responsible and your feelings when this need is thwarted. When you take responsibility for your needs and feelings, your friend is more likely to be empathetic.

Talking Points/Field Notes

Developing Statements of Feelings and Needs

Below are several situations that require a response. Consider an appropriate feeling/need statement that could be generated. Some situations will be best addressed by exploring the feelings and needs of the speaker. In order to assess the impact of your statement, try role-playing the situation with a classmate. Suggested responses are given after the questions (no peeking!).

1. A patient says "I'm afraid I will never leave this hospital."

2. In response to your request for feedback, your clinical instructor says, "No news is good news."

3. A colleague begs you to work on Saturday for him. It is Friday at noon and you have important weekend plans. Even though you say no, he keeps pestering you.

4. Your roommate keeps interrupting you while you are trying to study.

5. A friend asks for the third time to borrow money. She has yet to follow through on her promise to pay back what she already owes you.

6. For the next 72 hours, use at least two feeling/need statements each day. One statement can be related to your feelings and needs and the other can relate to those of another person.

Continued

Talking Points/Field Notes—cont'd ■

Questions:

1. What was it like to generate these responses? Was it easier to disclose your own feelings and needs or inquire about those of others?

2. Practice observing persons around you and work to reframe judging observations (e.g., "That person who is arguing at the checkout counter is really obnoxious") to needs-based ones ("That person seems angry that the checkout clerk is not making eye contact with her. I wonder if she is wanting more recognition").

3. Comment on your 72 hours of practice. How did your feeling/needs statements affect your communication? How might this aid the negotiation process?

Suggestions:

1. Are you discouraged because you're wanting a faster recovery?

2. I feel apprehensive when I don't get any feedback because I need reassurance that I'm on the right track.

3. I feel irritated when I get repeat requests because I need respect for my decisions.

4. I get anxious when I am interrupted in my studying because I want to be successful at school.

5. I feel disappointed that I haven't been paid back yet because I need trustworthiness from my friends.

Don't be surprised if these exercises seem difficult or artificial at first. The language of NVC takes practice, but as you continue, you will begin to note a more compassionate shift in your observations and in your communication. You may also find that you become more aware of your own needs and feelings. These are positive benefits which make NVC a valuable tool not only for conflict resolution but also for personal and professional growth.[34] Don't get caught up in the exact construction of your statements beyond assuming responsibility for needs and feelings and avoiding the use of judging terms as much as possible.

Requesting Positive Actions to Meet Our Needs

In NVC, the resolution of conflict is a process that begins with the authentic sharing of observations, feelings, and needs. As we have discussed, when this is accomplished with non-judging, self-responsible language, our natural tendency toward an emotionally charged fight-or-flight response will often dissipate. This diffusion essentially resets the interpersonal connection, facilitating effective conflict resolution. Perhaps you have heard this referred to as a "win-win" outcome. In NVC however, the emphasis is more on the mutual satisfaction of needs rather than the equal distribution of resources that the word *win* implies.

In requesting a solution to a situation where our needs are not being met, it is helpful to use what is known in NVC as "positive action language."[39] This first involves stating what we want rather than what we don't want (the positive action). A positive request removes ambiguity from the desired outcome. For example, following a poor report card, an exasperated parent tells his teenager "I don't want you to spend so much time on the Internet!" The teenager then wastes time watching television. In contrast, a request using positive action language would entail a statement like "I would like you to devote 2 hours each evening to your homework." This parent could also state his needs and feelings in making their request, adding "I am worried that your current grades may prevent you from getting into college."

The "action" component involves requesting a specific and observable behavior as a measure of outcome. Thus asking a friend to "be more understanding" does not provide meaningful guidance to your friend. Accordingly, your friend's attempts to fulfill your needs may be completely off base, even creating further tension.

Positive action requests are most effective when they are given a time line. As the mother of a teenager, I have learned that time lines (for chores, curfew, etc.) prevent procrastination and maintain civility in our household. Time lines can be particularly valuable in the work setting. For example, in the clinical education setting, you may find yourself wanting specific feedback from a busy clinical instructor. However, it may not be reasonable for your CI to drop everything the minute you need her insights. Thus, a positive action request might be "I would really like to sit down with you and discuss my patients, but I can see that you are really busy right now. Would it work for you to pick a 30-minute time slot in the next 2 days to review my notes with me?" This request gives your CI the option to meet busy scheduling needs while creating an opportunity for you to meet your needs in a timely fashion.

Finally, in requesting positive actions of others, we must realize that their needs must also be met. Thus it is important to distinguish between requests and demands. Obviously, requests are more likely to engage the cooperation of others for a positive outcome. Thus language such as "Would it work for you to...," "Would you consider...," or "Would you be willing to..." gives others the opportunity to thoughtfully consider your requests and to respond in kind.

In making requests of others, we need to be truly mindful of our expectations. Let's say that we ask our significant other to go to the movies and he responds by telling you that he was looking forward to a quiet evening at home. If you try to lay a guilt trip on him ("Aw come on, you never want to go anywhere!") or criticize ("You are such a bore!"), then your invitation was actually a demand. Demands are often met with aggressive responses such as rebelliousness and are thus not features of compassionate relationships.

There are times when demands are appropriate, especially in issues related to safety. Nevertheless, we must accept that in the final analysis, self-determination is a right and privilege of responsible adulthood (along with accountability for related consequences).

Talking Points/Field Notes

Making Positive Action Requests

Consider each of the following situations and develop a needs-based positive action request. Discuss your answers and role-play them to explore how you might work toward a resolution. Suggested answers follow this exercise (no peeking!).

1. You are irritated when a classmate always asks how you did on an exam.

2. You are embarrassed when a clinical instructor criticizes you in front of a patient.

3. Your best friend is drinking too much and you are concerned about his health.

4. You are angry when a coworker takes all the credit for a project on which you did most of the work.

5. You are humiliated when a patient makes a sexist remark.

6. In the next 72 hours, try to make at least one needs-based positive action request.

Continued

Talking Points/Field Notes—cont'd ▪▪▪▪▪▪▪▪▪▪▪▪▪▪

Note the response you receive and the impact on your communication. Here are some suggested answers:

1. "It embarrasses me to talk about my grades and I wonder if you'd be willing to tell me what need this meets for you?" (This might sound contrived, but it invites introspection from your classmate without making him feel judged.)

2. "I want to perform well on this internship and receiving feedback in front a patient makes me feel overwhelmed. Would you be open to giving me feedback after our sessions?"

3. "I have noticed that at the last three parties we have been to, you have passed out after drinking. Our friendship means a lot to me and I am worried about your health. I am wondering if you'd be willing to talk with me about getting help." Note: Remember that the decision to seek help is your friend's. Your goal here is to provide nonjudging support when your friend is ready to accept this.

4. "I put several hours' worth of time into our project and I feel resentful that my contributions weren't acknowledged. I need some assurance that my efforts were worthwhile, so I wonder if you'd be willing to sit down with me at lunch today and discuss the areas where you think I was helpful. (Note: Once your colleague is able to acknowledge your contributions directly, you can then move to a further request: "I wonder if you'd be willing to share the results of our discussion with our director."

5. An appropriate response here depends on several factors: Whether or not you have an established relationship, the age of the patient, whether the patient has a neurological deficit (in which case, the patient may lack executive function skills such as social awareness. These patients need to be informed that their comments are not socially appropriate). In other cases, simply ignoring the comment, or responding with silence, can also be useful. Another technique involves asking the individual "What do you mean by that?" A direct approach could be to make a direct positive actions request such as, "Comments like that don't work for me. Can we agree to keep our dialogue professional?" Should a patient continue with such comments, it would be appropriate to say "I need to keep my working relationships professional and comments like this make me uncomfortable and less effective as your therapist. I am wondering if your needs might be better met by working with a different member of our staff."

Using NVC in Everyday Life

The four steps of NVC can be invaluable tools for increasing empathy and connections between individuals even in the absence of conflict. As you engage in the process of developing your skills, you might find it helpful to have a few "templates" to guide your formulation NVC components. **Table 11-6** provides a few such templates.

There are times when "colloquial" NVC[42] may be more appropriate than the full four-step process. For example, just before your first presentation at a professional conference, a friend gently notes "Hey, Maura, you're chewing your nails. Nervous, huh?" In this case, this quick empathic observation would likely receive a better response than "Maura, I see you chewing your nails and I know your presentation is in 10 minutes. I am wondering if you are feeling nervous because you need reassurance that you will be successful. Would it help if I told you a few jokes?"

Sometimes, you might even get a cynical response to your early attempts to try NVC in its full four-step entirety. Depending on the nature of situation, it can be useful to acknowledge this. "Are you frustrated because you think I'm using some contrived formula?" I'm just really trying to improve my ability to get beyond judgments in my communication."

Figure 11-6 provides some NVC component templates that can be memorized. You might find this helpful as you incorporate this approach into your communication.

Observations, Feelings, Needs, Requests

Observations

I see_____.
I have noticed_____.
When_____.
I am hearing_____.
Are you saying_____? (when you need clarification)
I am thinking_____ (a way of reflecting a **nonjudging thought** about a direct observation). For example, "I noticed that the laundry was still in the washing machine, and I am thinking that you didn't put it in the dryer." You cannot say "I am thinking that you are a slob."

Feelings

I am_____.
I am feeling_____.
I am wondering if you are_____?
Are you feeling_____?
Are you_____?

Needs

I am wanting_____.
I am needing_____.
I would like_____.
Are you wanting_____?
Are you needing_____?
I am wondering if you are needing/wanting_____?

Requests

Would you be willing to_____?
Would you consider_____?
Would it work for you to_____?
Would you agree to_____?
Would you be up for_____?
Would you like it if I_____?
Would it meet your needs if I_____?

Feelings/Needs

Are you feeling_____ because you are needing_____?
Are you angry because you are thinking_____? (Anger is generally triggered by an evaluative thought.)
I am wondering if you are feeling_____?

The Four Steps in Combination

I am hearing_____ and I feel_____ because I am needing_____. Would you be willing to_____?
I am noticing_____. Are you feeling_____ because you are needing_____? Would it meet your needs if I_____?

Figure 11–6. Templates for NVC components. *(Adapted from: WikiHow: the how-to manual you can edit. How to practice nonviolent communication: http://www.wikihow.com/Practice-Nonviolent-Communication.)*

Talking Points/Field Notes

Workplace Conflict Revisited

Review the six conflict examples that were presented at the beginning of the chapter and reconsider your initial ideas about how you would go about addressing the related issues. Next, reviewing the components of NVC, discuss how you might modify your initial responses using the four steps (observation, identifying feelings, stating needs, making requests). Then answer the following questions and record your answers in your field notes:

1. Compare and contrast your pre- and posttest responses and consider their impact.

2. How might NVC be useful in the professional setting?

3. What impact might NVC have on collegial relationships?

Implications for Physical Therapy Practice

Humans have a fundamental need to be understood and respected. When we communicate in a way that honors this need, we are most likely to build the alliances that facilitate positive change. In the physical therapy profession, we can use the skills of assertive negotiation and NVC to promote desirable outcomes for the good of our patients, colleagues, and our profession at large. Most importantly, these skills will enable us to enjoy more authentic relationships as well as enhanced self-esteem and emotional well-being. Together, these outcomes and benefits will help us enhance our personal and professional engagement as well as our sense of mission.

Chapter Summary

1. Conflict is a feature of a society comprising groups of persons with differing values, lifestyles, and goals. Conflict occurs when there is disregard for these.

2. Conflict can produce negative emotional responses that provoke less than useful approaches to resolution.

3. Unresolved conflict creates stress and contributes to the erosion of interpersonal relationships.

4. Assertive communication is a means of acknowledging the rights of self and others in all interactions. Assertive communication promotes authentic expressions of self, which strengthen relationships.

5. Nonviolent communication (NVC) is a conflict resolution approach involving a four-step process of stating observations, expressing feelings, identifying needs, and requesting positive actions to enrich relationships.

6. A major concept of NVC is that persons are "different but equal." In this approach, differences are not judged but rather honored in the communication process.

Take-Home Menu

1. NVC training is available though conference based training and online. Information is provided on the international website, http://www.nvc.org. This site also has several other NVC resources (books, videos, DVDs) that can be useful.

2. Many university counseling centers have resources for assertiveness training. If you are interested in further developing this skill, you are encouraged to explore this option in your academic institution.

3. The best way to learn the skills of assertiveness and NVC is simply to practice. Many communities have NVC centers that provide guidance and support. You are encouraged to explore these options.

References

1. Van Kleef GA, Côté S. Expressing anger in conflict: When it helps and when it hurts. *J Appl Psychol*. 2007;92(6): 1557-1569.

2. Burton JW. Conflict resolution: The human dimension. *J Peace Studies*: http://www.gmu.edu/academic/ijps/ vol3_1/burton.htm. Accessed July 20, 2008.

3. DeDreu CKW, Knippenberg DV. the possessive self as a barrier to conflict resolution: Effects of mere ownership, process accountability and self-concept clarity on competitive cognitions and behavior. *J Pers Soc Psychol*. 2005;89(3):345-357.

4. Institute of Medicine. *Unequal Treatment: Confronting Racial and Ethnic Disparities in Healthcare*. Washington, DC: Institute of Medicine; 2002.

5. U.S. Forest Service. Social and economic values in natural resource planning. Crowding, conflict, and social norms: http://www.fs.fed.us/rm/value/ Crowding%20conflict%20and%20social%20norms. html. Accessed July 20, 2008.

6. Bruk-Lee V, Spector PE. The social stressors-counterproductive work behaviors link: Are conflicts with supervisors and co-workers the same? *J Occup Health Psychol*. 2006;11(2):145-156.

7. Slaikev K, Hasson R. *Controlling the Cost of Conflict*. San Francisco: Jossey Bass; 1998.

8. Hahn SE. The effects of locus of control on daily exposure, coping and reactivity to work interpersonal stressors: A diary study. *J Pers Indiv Diff*. 2000;29:729-748.

9. Harris B, Klein K. The effect of dormitory design on assertive behavior. Presented at the Southwest Psychological Association, Washington, DC: 1980

10. *Merriam-Webster's Online Dictionary*: http://www .merriam-webster.com/dictionary/conflict. Accessed July 20, 2008.

11. About workplace conflict: The cost of conflict: http://www.conflictatwork.com/conflict/cost_e.cfm. Accessed July 11, 2008.

12. Nueberg SL, Cottrell CA. Managing the threats and opportunities afforded by human sociality. *Group Dynamics: Theory Res Pract*. 2008;12(2):63-72.

13. American Physical Therapy Association. Report on transition DPT programs, October, 2007: http://www .apta.org/AM/Template.cfm?Section=Home&CONTEN TID=44507&TEMPLATE=/CM/ContentDisplay.cfm. Accessed July 20, 2008.

14. Wilson K, Gallois C. *Assertion and Its Social Context*. Elmsford, NY: Pergamon Press; 1993.

15. Bakker CB, Bakker MK, Breit S. The measurement of assertiveness and aggressiveness. *J Pers Assessment*. 1978;42(3):277-283.

16. Rosenberg MB. *We Can Work It Out: Resolving Conflicts Peacefully and Powerfully*. Encinitas, CA: Puddledancer Press; 2005.

17. University of Victoria. Counseling Services. Assertiveness: http://www.coun.uvic.ca/personal/assertiveness.html. Accessed June 25, 2008.

18. Texas Women's University. *Counseling Corner: The Assertiveness Continuum*: http://www.twu.edu/o-sl/ counseling/SelfHelp021.html. Accessed June 25, 2008.

19. El-Sheikh M, Cummings EM, Kouros CD, et al. Marital psychological and physical aggression and children's mental and physical health: Direct, mediated, and moderated effects. *J Consult Clin Psychol*. 2008;76(1): 138-148.

20. University of Iowa, University Counseling Service. Assertive communication: http://www.uiowa.edu/~ucs/ asertcom.html. Accessed July 5, 2008.

21. Galassi MD, Galassi JP. *Assert Yourself: How to Be Your Own Person.* New York: Human Sciences Press; 1977:233.

22. *Stanford Encyclopedia of Philosophy.* Rights: http://plato. stanford.edu/entries/rights/. Accessed June 30, 2008.

23. Jakubowski P, Lange AJ. *The Assertive Option: Your Rights and Responsibilities.* Champaign, IL: Research Press; 1978.

24. Messina JJ, Messina CM. Improving assertive behavior. Coping.Org: Tools for coping with life's stressors: http://www.coping.org/relations/assert.htm. Accessed June 30, 2008.

25. Alberti R, Emmons M. *Your Perfect Right,* 7th ed. Etascadero, CA: Impact Publishers; 1994.

26. Hale R. *Impact and Influence.* Bristol, UK: RHA Publications; 2006.

27. Merill DW, Reid RH. *Personal Styles and Effective Performance.* Boca Raton, FL: CRC Press; 1999.

28. Judge TA, Piccolo RF, Ilies R. The forgotten ones? The validity of consideration and initiating structure in leadership research. *J Appl Psychol.* 2004;89(1):36-51.

29. Ames DR, Flynn FJ. What breaks a leader: The curvilinear relation between assertiveness and leadership. *J Pers Soc Psychol.* 2007;92(2):307-324.

30. Kling R, Corbiere M, Milord RB, et al. Use of a violence risk assessment tool in an acute care hospital: Effectiveness in identifying violent patients. *AAOHN J.* 2006;54(11):481-487.

31. Shnabel N, Nalder A. A needs-based model of reconciliation: Satisfying the differential emotional needs of victim and perpetrator as a key to promoting reconciliation. *J Pers Soc Psychol.* 2008;94(1):116-132.

32. Scheff T. Universal human needs? After Maslow. Foundation of meaning in human life: http://www.soc. ucsb.edu/faculty/scheff/58.htm. Accessed July 16, 2008.

33. O'Connor J, Seymour J. *Introducing NLP: Psychological Skills for Understanding and Influencing People.* Hammersmith, London: Thorsons; 1990.

34. Rosenberg M. *Nonviolent Communication: A Language of Life,* 2nd ed. Encinitas, CA: PuddleDancer Press; 2003.

35. Maslow AH. Toward a universal psychological structure of human values: A theory of human motivation. *Psychol Rev.* 1943;50:370-396.

36. Nossiter A. New Orleans slips into anarchy. Associated Press. September 1, 2005: http://www.cantonrep.com/index.php?ID=240221&r=0&Category=11. Accessed July 21, 2008.

37. Schwartz SH, Bilsky W. Towards a universal structure of human values. *J Pers Soc Psychol.* 1987;53(3):550-562.

38. Fisher R, Shapiro D. *Beyond Reason: Using Emotions as You Negotiate.* New York: Viking Penguin; 2005.

39. Center for Non-Violent Communication: http://www.nvc.org.

40. Klein S, Gibson N. *What's Making You Angry? 10 Steps to Transforming Your Anger so Everyone Wins.* La Crescenta, CA: PuddleDancer Press; 2005.

41. Bono JE, Foldes, HJ, Vinson G, Muros JP. Workplace emotions: The role of supervision and leadership. *J Appl Psychol.* 2007;92(5):1357-1367.

42. WikiHow: The how-to manual you can edit. how to practice nonviolent communication: http://www.wikihow.com/Practice-Nonviolent-Communication. Accessed July 29, 2008.

CHAPTER 12

Instructional Communication for Transformative Teaching

"You must be the change you want to see in the world."

Mahatma Gandhi, Indian spiritual leader, 1869–1948

Chapter Overview

Physical therapists are teachers first and foremost. Engaged professionalism involves the sharing of information in a rich variety of formal and informal contexts. Our audiences include colleagues, members of the health-care team, patients, families, and community members. This chapter explores strategies for "transformative teaching," a form of instrumental communication where information is shared for the purpose of empowering those who receive it.

Key Terms

Behavioral objectives

Mentorship

Transtheoretical model of change

Physical Therapists Are Teachers First and Foremost

What Does It Mean for Physical Therapists to Teach?

Whether or not you realize it, the successful practice of PT involves the *sharing of knowledge* in many contexts to audiences of all sizes and backgrounds. Even if you envision a career that precludes ever standing behind a podium, you have nevertheless embarked upon a professional journey that involves the use of effective communication skills to *empower others* toward a better quality of life. Thus, in the service of that worthy outcome, you will invest a considerable portion of your efforts in the process of teaching. Specifically, that process is defined as "imparting knowledge or intelligence, rules for practice, exhibiting, and inculcating (through frequent repetitions or admonitions)."[1]

This is a broad definition, which suggests that each time you *impart* (i.e., communicate) or *exhibit* (model or demonstrate) *knowledge* (e.g., a fact, suggestion, demonstration, or explanation), you are teaching. In the context of PT practice, your "audience" may be a single colleague who asks your opinion about a treatment idea or hundreds of peers to whom you speak in a professional context. It may be a younger colleague to whom you demonstrate a practicing example of professional behavior in action. Your "presentation" may vary in length from a 2-minute patient progress report at a team conference to a day-long continuing education workshop. It may be a skillful interaction with a difficult patient, which serves as a communication lesson to a physical therapy student under your supervision. Your "audiovisuals" may involve the simple demonstration of an exercise, an elaborate slide-based presentation, or the example you provide to others. As an illustration, consider the following clinical scenario from a physical therapist's workday.

Teaching as a Way of Being in Physical Therapy Practice

Emma is a senior PT on the brain injury unit at a large urban teaching hospital. As a senior PT, Emma provides education to PT students, clinical staff, medical students, and resident physicians in both formal and informal contexts. She is also the liaison to several PT programs in the area. In this role, she schedules student internships and provides guest lectures in neurological rehabilitation courses.

Emma begins her workday at 7:30 a.m., consulting with Randy, a PT intern who is completing an 8-week rotation. Emma provides Randy with feedback from her observations of his previous day's treatment while guiding him to reflect on his own performance. As a seasoned clinical instructor, Emma is highly skilled at the use of directive questions to facilitate learner problem solving. As a result of their discussion, Randy identifies several intervention ideas for his patients.

At 8 a.m., Emma provides one of the monthly staff in-services to the six therapists on the brain injury unit. The staff take turns providing the in-services, which may involve sharing information from a recent continuing education course, leading a discussion on a journal article, or presenting a case study. This morning, Emma shares information from the 2005 American Physical Therapy Association (APTA) *III Step Conference*[2] pertaining to the use of electrical stimulation in patients with neurological deficits.

At the end of Emma's talk, she meets briefly with Riley, her newest colleague, who will be presenting next month's in-service. Riley is a recent graduate, and this will be his first staff presentation. Riley has sought Emma's advice because he admires her clinical, professional, and educational skills. He sees her as a role model and has decided to seek her mentorship. Thus, Riley asks Emma if she would be willing to look over his outline and provide feedback about his organization of the content. Emma is impressed by Riley's enthusiasm for professional development and is more than happy to assist him. As their discussion ends, she also directs

Continued

Riley to APTA's evidence-based website, *Hooked on Evidence,*[3] for further information to strengthen his presentation.

At 9 a.m., Emma sees her first patient, 17-year-old Jeannie, a high school student who sustained a head injury in a car accident 2 months earlier. Jeannie has achieved independence in most of her mobility skills and is being discharged at the end of the week. Jeannie's parents are present for family education in guarding techniques for gait and outdoor wheelchair mobility. Emma instructs Jeannie's parents in these skills and receives a return demonstration from each of them to ensure their competence. Emma also provides Jeannie's parents with written and pictorial guidelines. Jeannie's parents have concerns about her short-term memory loss, and Emma shares information about the cognitive deficits that often result from brain injury. Following Jeannie's appointment, Emma documents the results of her treatment session on the hospital-based communication system, which allows her notes to be read by everyone on Jeannie's health-care team. Emma then telephones Jeannie's case manager and leaves a voice mail indicating that Jeannie and her family will be prepared for discharge on the designated date.

Emma cotreats her next patient, 27-year-old Lucinda, with Allie, the team's speech and language pathologist. Lucinda is emerging from a 2-month coma and is now able to work in the sitting position. In the course of the session, Emma instructs Allie in how to achieve an optimal posture for the promotion of Lucinda's swallowing and mouth closure. By incorporating Emma's suggestions, Allie is able to effectively help Lucinda produce a louder speech volume. For the first time in 2 months, Lucinda's speech can be understood.

Emma then meets with Randy and helps him set up for a wound care session with one of his patients. She reviews the steps of maintaining a sterile field and assists him with blunt debridement and wound dressing.

At 11:30 a.m., Emma and Randy provide verbal reports on their patients at the weekly team conference. As discharge dates are reviewed, Dr. Anne Wallis, the team physician, consults Emma regarding her patients' status with respect to mobility, safety, and equipment needs. One patient's discharge date is changed as a result of Emma's input.

After lunch, Emma meets with a small group of medical students who are completing a clinical rotation in physical medicine and rehabilitation. They are interested in evidence-based practice for brain injury rehabilitation, and Emma introduces them to the *Guide to Physical Therapist Practice*[4] and the *Open Door*[5] search engine on the APTA website. This leads to a discussion about the value of professional organizations, and Emma shares her recent experience as an APTA delegate.

At 2:00 p.m., Emma supervises one of Randy's treatment sessions. As she observes his performance, she formulates her feedback for their meeting the following morning. She is pleased with Randy's efforts in trying some of the treatment ideas he had mentioned earlier in the day. Randy's midterm is at the end of the week, and he has shown consistent improvement in all skill areas. Most importantly, Randy is very "teachable" in that he is open to feedback, self-directed, and eager to learn. Thus Emma plans to encourage him toward greater independence with more challenging patients. This evening, she will document Randy's performance on the Clinical Performance Instrument (CPI),[6] which is the student evaluation tool used by the majority of PT educational programs in the United States. Emma's assessment will ultimately be utilized to determine her recommendation to Randy's PT program for either a "pass" or "fail" of the internship. At 3 p.m., Emma collects patient data for a clinical research project that she is completing as part of her transitional DPT program. Her project is examining the impact of body weight–supported treadmill training (BWSTT) and functional electrical stimulation (FES) on the activation of ankle muscles during gait. Emma will soon be presenting her data at the APTA Combined Sections Meeting. Once her project is completed, Emma also plans to submit it for publication in *Physical Therapy.*[7]

As Emma completes her workday, she returns a phone call from the academic coordinator of clinical education (ACCE) at Randy's school. She leaves a voice mail message in which she responds to the ACCE's request for an update on Randy's progress.

Talking Points/Field Notes

Teaching in Physical Therapy Practice

As you read over the previous description of Emma's workday, jot down the examples of teaching (again defined as the delivery of information) that occurred. Note the situational context, audience, and purpose of each of the teaching interactions.

For each of the teaching interactions you identified, consider the following questions and reflect on your answers in your field notes.

1. From the perspective of the audience member(s), what immediate and long-term outcomes may result from Emma's teaching? For example, how might Emma's family instruction affect the patients and their family members in the short and long term?

2. Comment on the preparation involved in each teaching interaction. What must Emma consider in order to be organized and clear in each situation?

3. What types of teaching methods might be appropriate in each situation? Consider visual aids, handouts, demonstration, discussion.

4. How might Emma involve her audience in each situation? How important is audience involvement in each context?

5. Consider the more informal methods of information delivery such as one on one, e-mail, and voice mail. How can Emma optimize the effectiveness of her message delivery in each of these situations?

As you discuss these questions, it should be apparent that regardless of the context, purpose, or audience size, effective teaching involves thoughtful consideration and preparation.

Despite these similarities, many individuals who teach effectively in small, informal contexts become anxious in larger, formal ones, when in reality the same skills apply. Once you begin to see the similarities involved in each context, you should feel more confident of your ability to teach effectively regardless of the context.

The Contexts of Teaching in Physical Therapy

As the description of Emma's workday suggests, even physical therapists in full-time clinical practice spend a significant part of their time engaged in teaching. **Box 12-1** illustrates a list of common teaching interactions in PT practice.

Successful Teachers Use Effective Communication Skills

As we have already discussed, teaching involves the *effective delivery of information*. Along these lines, perhaps you have noticed that the most effective teachers present their information in a conversational manner. They are relaxed, open, and connected with their audiences. *They convey the same elements of effective external communication that are essential for effective one-on-one interactions.*

In a professional context, whenever physical therapists share information related to their body of knowledge, they are teaching. In a broader sense, it may be useful to consider that *every time you communicate, you are delivering a message, which is the essence of teaching.* Accordingly, everyday interactions provide countless opportunities to practice important skills of teaching. These skills include organization, clarity, and appropriate voice projection. In addition, nonverbal communication such as eye contact, smiling,

---

BOX 12-1:   Common Teaching Interactions in Physical Therapy Practice

1. Instructing technicians and aides about patient care issues through written materials, face-to-face interactions, and demonstrations.
2. Instructing physical therapist assistants about plans of care and related treatments through face-to-face interactions, phone calls, electronic media, documentation, and demonstration.
3. Instructing nursing staff about patient mobility status through written and verbal instructions, and demonstration.
4. Instructing patients and family members about mobility status, evaluation, diagnosis, prognosis, plan of care, treatment goals, and outcomes.
5. Instructing members of interdisciplinary team about patient status through face-to-face interactions, team conferences, phone calls, electronic media, and documentation.
6. Instructing physical therapy students through the identification of goals, providing feedback, direct sharing of information, questioning, demonstration, and assessment.
7. Instructing colleagues during face-to-face interactions, patients' cotreatments, staff in-services, and professional presentations at conferences.
8. Instructing physicians and other health professionals about the role of PT through conferences, phone calls, letters, and e-mail.
9. Instructing case managers and insurance personnel about patient status through documentation, electronic media, phone calls, and face-to-face interactions.
10. Instructing members of the community, such as elementary and high school students, patient advocacy groups, employers, and civic organizations.
11. Marketing about PT to physicians, community members, colleagues, and team members through no-cost screening events, health fairs, presentations, and informal discussions.
12. Writing about PT in newspaper and magazine articles, on websites and blogs, and in journals and books.

---

and an open posture are important elements in all everyday interactions. Accordingly, these are all elements of effective "public speaking." In the words of Timothy Koegel, a media consultant and author, *"Every time you open your mouth to speak in public, you are a public speaker."*[8] **Figure 12-1** illustrates the broader contexts of professional information sharing.

The importance of communication as the hallmark of effective teaching was demonstrated in a study exploring important teaching skills in PT education.[9] In this study, 102 PT students were asked to assess 43 clinical instructor behaviors (previously identified in the literature) in terms of perceived importance and the frequency with which these were demonstrated by their clinical instructors. Not surprisingly, the two most important behaviors pertained to communication and interpersonal relations. Related behaviors included providing useful feedback, actively listening to students, showing empathy for patients, and establishing a comfortable learning environment. Ironically, the study also found that a large number of students felt that these important teaching skills were lacking in some of their clinical instructors. The author, Michael Emery, attributed this disconnect to the lack of formal training opportunities for PT clinical instructors. Subsequently Emery, along with several colleagues, went on to develop the APTA Clinical Instructor Credentialing Program, which began in 1997.[10]

Phone calls	"I just wanted to see how you were doing after our session yesterday."
Conversations	"Have you had any success with taping the shoulder?"
Patient documentation	"Mr. Jones' co-morbidities may limit his progress."
Written memos	"Attention: New Patient Coding Procedure."
Voice mail messages	"Here is an update on Mr. Green."
E-mail messages	"I have reviewed your application."
Interviews	"Here is why I am qualified for this position."
Professional networking events	"How do you treat patients with stroke in your practice?"
Social events	"What do you do for a living?"
Letters	"Thank you for your support of our program."

Figure 12–1. The broader contexts of professional information sharing.

Two more recent reports have supported Emery's original findings. One study of the characteristics of an "exemplary" clinical instructor reported five related themes, the first of which was "creating an open collegial relationship."[11] In the second study, the roles of a good teacher were explored in the context of medical education.[12] This study expanded existing research evidence on the elements of effective teaching to include excerpts from medical students' journals (in which they recorded observations of good teaching occurring in their own learning experiences). Twelve teacher roles evolved from this analysis. They included being a role model in both clinical and educational settings and serving as a mentor and learning facilitator. It should be fairly obvious that effective communication underscores each of these roles. Thus, regardless of the teaching context, these studies confirm the old adage that "your students (or patients) won't care how much you know until they know how much you care."

Effective Teaching Is a Powerful Tool for Career Advancement

As you explore the examples in Box 12-1 and Figure 12-1, it should be readily apparent that teaching is a core element of PT practice. Because teaching is grounded in the broader context of interpersonal communication, we can view each interaction as an opportunity to practice our public speaking.

In Chapter 1, we explored evidence for the importance of communication in PT management. In this context, peer recognition for effective teaching skills will afford you numerous opportunities for career development. These can include promotions within your practice setting (many of which, as the case of Emma illustrates, involve teaching). As you develop knowledge and skills in an area of professional interest, you will quickly achieve even broader peer recognition for your expertise if you offer to share it.

The teaching opportunities in our profession are numerous. Many therapists often begin within their workplace, presenting at meetings and in-services. They may then offer to present at an APTA sponsored event. These can include smaller meetings within a state region (e.g., in Arizona, region 5 includes several small communities in the northern part of the state), which broaden to state (the Arizona PT association has two state wide meetings a year) and national levels (APTA Combined Sections meeting in the winter and APTA Conference and Exposition in the summer).

APTA clinical specialization is another valuable way to obtain recognition for expertise. Clinical specialization is offered within eight recognized areas of clinical practice. These specialties include cardiopulmonary physical therapy, geriatrics, neurology, sports, orthopedics, pediatrics, clinical electrophysiology, and, as of 2009, women's health. Many therapists who achieve this distinction share their knowledge by delivering continuing education courses to peer audiences throughout the world. Over 8,500 physical therapists have obtained specialist certification since the process began in 1985.[13]

Recognition for expertise in clinical education is also available through completion of an APTA-sponsored clinical instructor credentialing course. This course provides excellent training in teaching skills for use in both formal and informal settings. As of September, 2008, there were over 19,100 credentialed clinical instructors in the United States.[14] PT educational programs also welcome the involvement of clinicians as adjunct faculty and laboratory assistants. Serving as an adjunct faculty member in these programs is a valuable way of developing your teaching skills and exploring your interest in a future academic career. **Figure 12-2** illustrates the numerous opportunities for career advancement through effective teaching.

Elements of Transformative Teaching

Transformative Teaching Changes Lives

As one experienced colleague has remarked, "It doesn't matter to me whether I am instructing one patient in the PT department or 1,000 colleagues at a conference, I am working towards the same goal. In both cases, I want them to be able to walk out of my talk feeling like they have a new skill, insight, or outlook."

This type of teaching is obviously much more powerful than the dry and soulless lectures many of us have endured in our academic careers. I once heard this wretched experience described as "a one-way dialogue where the notes of the teacher are delivered

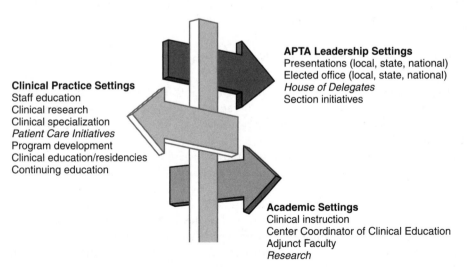

Figure 12–2. Teaching as a path to career advancement.

APTA Leadership Settings
Presentations (local, state, national)
Elected office (local, state, national)
House of Delegates
Section initiatives

Clinical Practice Settings
Staff education
Clinical research
Clinical specialization
Patient Care Initiatives
Program development
Clinical education/residencies
Continuing education

Academic Settings
Clinical instruction
Center Coordinator of Clinical Education
Adjunct Faculty
Research

to the notes of the student without going through the minds of either." Instead of this dismal outcome, we should teach in a way that effects a positive change in our learners. In other words, we should seek not only to *inform* but also to *transform*.

If such an outcome seems daunting, consider that one of the primary goals of everyday PT intervention is to promote patients' motor learning, which is defined as *"a relatively permanent change in knowledge, understanding, or behavior."*[15] Accordingly, if permanent change is the goal of our therapeutic intervention, it follows that it should also be the outcome we strive for whenever we provide any form of "informational intervention." Perhaps our teaching will affect one person in a meaningful way. Or possibly we might engender profound and far-reaching consequences in the manner of the following example.

Randy Pausch was a young professor of computer science at Carnegie Mellon University in Pittsburgh. His brilliant academic career was acknowledged by numerous awards both for his teaching and his innovative contributions to computer technology. Pausch's fun-loving and big-hearted approach to his work earned him the love and respect of students and colleagues alike. Pausch's teaching style involved the development of creative projects that so thoroughly engaged his students that they easily learned many complex principles of computer design. In one interview, Pausch summarized these methods by saying "The best way to teach somebody something is to have them think they're learning something else."[16]

Little did Pausch know how profoundly these words would ring true when he delivered a talk entitled "Really Achieving Your Childhood Dreams" at Carnegie Mellon on September 18, 2007. This presentation was part of the university's "Last Lecture" series, in which top professors were asked, "What wisdom would you try to impart to the world if you knew it was your last chance?" While other "Last Lecture" speakers had enjoyed the luxury of addressing the topic from the safe harbor of conjecture, this was not the case for Pausch, who had been fighting pancreatic cancer for over a year. Although initial treatment had seemed promising, he had just learned that his condition was terminal.

Thus, in Pausch's typical approach of "having students think they are learning something else," the many hundreds of students and colleagues in the standing-room-only audience learned not only about graciously moving one's life forward but also about living with joyful purpose as it comes to an end. ("We cannot change the cards we are dealt, just how we play the hand.")[12]

Within weeks, a videotape of Pausch's lecture appeared on numerous Internet sites, where it was viewed by millions. His poignant message was delivered again on the *Oprah Winfrey Show* a month later, then expanded for a best-selling book in which Pausch addressed the topic of "how to say goodbye." With astonishing ferocity, Pausch's words challenged and inspired a society that is uneasy with the concept of death but often too busy to appreciate the joys and marvels of life. Accordingly, in May of 2008, *Time* magazine listed Pausch as one of the world's most influential people. Pausch died on July 25, 2008, leaving a transformative message whose impact will change many lives.

Talking Points/Field Notes

My Transformative Teachers

Reflect on the transformative teachers in your life. Perhaps you met them in a classroom, or they may have been relatives or friends. See if you can identify at least two such individuals and then reflect on the following questions. You are also encouraged to record your observations in your field notes.

1. What was the context of the learning interactions you had with these persons?

2. Which traits attracted you to their messages? (Consider their communication style, affect, words, etc.).

Continued

Talking Points/Field Notes—cont'd

3. In which ways were their messages transformative?

4. How did you apply these messages in life and what was the impact?

5. How might you apply these approaches to transformative teaching?

Transformative Teachers Speak Forth

Speaking forth is the responsibility of all engaged professionals. Interestingly, *profess,* the root of the word *professional,* is defined by these two powerful words. In the milieu of the PT profession, speaking forth involves defending the values and principles of ethical practice. It means carrying out this role in a way that exemplifies our seven professional core values (accountability, altruism, caring and compassion, integrity, excellence, professional duty, and social responsibility). Accordingly, our profession also requires that we share and deliver information in a variety of contexts, doing so in a way that upholds the societal contract between health-care providers and recipients.[17,18] **Figure 12-3** illustrates the elements of "Speak Forth."

Transformative Teachers Are SOLD on Their Message

If you are sold on your message and deliver it as though it were the most important topic your audience would ever hear, the content is almost irrelevant. Although it is admittedly easier to deliver content to an audience that is intrinsically motivated to receive your message (for example, if your talk were titled "Guaranteed ways to become a millionaire with no effort whatsoever"), transformative teachers can create a learning environment so engaging that even the driest topics spring to life, as the following example illustrates.

S	Transformative teachers are **SOLD** on their message. They truly believe in what they say.
P	Transformative teachers are highly **PREPARED**.
E	Transformative teachers **ENGAGE** their audiences.
A	Transformative teachers are **AUTHENTIC**. They convey an open, genuine approach.
K	Transformative teachers are **KNOWLEDGEABLE** about their subject.
F	Transformative teachers are **FAMILIAR** with the needs of their audience.
O	Transformative teachers are **ORGANIZED**.
R	Transformative teachers are **RESPECTFUL** of their audience.
T	Transformative teachers are **TENACIOUS** in their quest for excellence.
H	Transformative teachers approach their work with **HUMILITY**.

Figure 12–3. The elements of SPEAK FORTH.

A few years ago, after receiving a traffic citation, I was offered the option of either appearing in traffic court (and paying a hefty fine) or attending driving school. In Arizona, attendance at this day-long course (usually held on a precious Saturday) avoids the accrual of points against one's driving license and expunges the offense from the record. Thus the choice is fairly obvious.

On the appointed Saturday, I arrived at my session in a foul humor and hunkered low in my seat with my equally ill-tempered fellow miscreants. Within moments, a jovial looking sixtyish gentleman entered and took his place at the front of the room. He smiled warmly at us and began. "I promise you this won't be the worst day of your life, but I'd be worried about you if it was the best one." With that humorous remark, our icy resistance began to melt. "You just saved yourselves several hundred bucks in insurance costs," he continued, sharing further compelling reasons for us to be thankful for our attendance. Within the first 5 minutes, we were convinced. As the hours went by, the speaker (a retired police officer who taught driving school on a volunteer basis) proved himself a veritable gold mine of helpful tips on driving safely (and legally). He shared his information with humor and with an obvious passion for the importance of his message.

As the day came to end, our instructor finally divulged why he continues to volunteer his leisure time to the education of wayward drivers. "Never use a cell phone while driving," he stated.

"Most of all, if you really care about the safety of those you love, never call them when you know they are behind a wheel." He then shared a story about the night he received a hysterical telephone call from a very dear friend who had just been informed that her teenage son had been killed in a car accident. Apparently the young man had been distracted and lost control of his vehicle, crashing head-on into an embankment. When paramedics arrived at the scene, they found the young man's cell phone in his hand, displaying a "missed call" message. With heartbreaking poignancy, the mother disclosed, "I was the one trying to reach him."

My driving school example is an important testimony to the potency of belief in one's message as a critical ingredient of transformative teaching. Each of us has a passion somewhere in our lives that drives and engages us. No doubt, if you were asked to share this passion with others, you would probably find yourself speaking with great enthusiasm. You might even find yourself sharing poignant anecdotes and experiences illustrating the importance of this passion in your life. If you can capture the essence of this enthusiasm when you share information, you will have gone a long way toward becoming a transformative teacher.

There are many enjoyable ways to make your message come alive. Your own experiences can be powerful. Quotations, stories, and jokes can also add relevance and entertainment value.

Statistics, research articles, and case studies can provide meaningful evidence in support of a given topic. Imagine the impact of telling a group of college freshmen in a health professions survey class, "In a recent Gallup poll, physical therapists had the second highest level of job satisfaction in all professions." When I am teaching my course on professional ethics, I am often able to bring interesting examples of ethical dilemmas fresh from that day's newspaper. Media sources such as magazines, websites, and talk shows provide fascinating information that can add a sense of real life to just about any topic. Movie clips can illustrate content in entertaining and provocative ways. For example, there are numerous movies that provide powerful examples of transformative teaching (you will find some of these in the "take-home menu" at the end of this chapter). Demonstrations are often used to provoke interest in a topic. To that end, they are used widely in the ubiquitous world of infomercials (which may be why infomercials, regardless of length, are more effective than commercials and as effective as direct experience with a given product).[19]

Talking Points/Field Notes

Building a Transformative Presentation: Selling Your Message

Reflect on and discuss the following questions in Part I. Use one of them to select a topic. Then move to Part II to select an appropriate method to bring your topic to life. Discuss how you would go about this in a real presentation. You might also record your observations in your field notes.

Part I: Selecting Your Topic

1. As you have become more involved in your PT education, no doubt you have learned about several professional issues that affect current and future practice (for example, as of 2008, many APTA state chapters have discussed making the "DPT" title a legal designation that is attained with licensure). Which issues have sparked your interest? Which issues would you enjoy learning more about?

2. If you were to identify an important current health-related issue that could be addressed by PT intervention, what would that be? How might you go about developing a professional service project related to that issue? What information would you need? Who would your target audience be? How might you convince them of the importance of this health issue for their own quality of life?

3. Many clinical education sites ask student interns to do staff presentations on topics of interest. Which area of PT practice interests you? Consider areas of practice, diagnoses, or treatments of interest. How might you select an aspect of this practice area to develop a staff presentation?

Part 2: Selling Your Topic and Making Your Message Come Alive

Figure 12-4 illustrates a transformative teaching "sales kit" that includes suggestions for bringing your message alive.

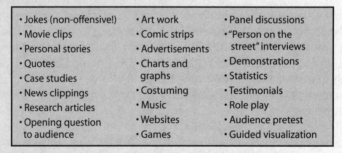

• Jokes (non-offensive!)	• Art work	• Panel discussions
• Movie clips	• Comic strips	• "Person on the
• Personal stories	• Advertisements	street" interviews
• Quotes	• Charts and	• Demonstrations
• Case studies	graphs	• Statistics
• News clippings	• Costuming	• Testimonials
• Research articles	• Music	• Role play
• Opening question	• Websites	• Audience pretest
to audience	• Games	• Guided visualization

Figure 12–4. Transformative teaching "sales kit."

1. Review the list of ideas in Figure 12-4 and consider which ones might be useful in your presentation. How would the tool be used in order to effectively illustrate the importance of your message?

Don't be concerned if you cannot yet identify the best tool from the list in Figure 12-4. As we continue to explore the concept of "Speak Forth," you will gain more clarity and can return to this section.

Transformative Teachers Are PREPARED

Thoughtful preparation is the single most important step in transformative teaching. This is because effective preparation involves assuring optimal connections on three major levels. Figure 12-5 illustrates these three levels.

Figure 12–5. Three levels of connection in transformative teaching.

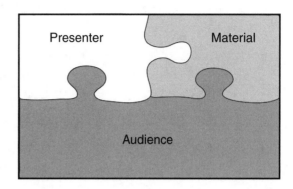

PREPARATION

With respect to preparing a connection between yourself and your material, it is helpful to consider a few important questions. The first is simply "What is your take-home message?" What do you want your audience to do as a result of your presentation? For example, in presenting a talk on childhood obesity to an elementary school parent-teacher organization, you might encourage parents to engage in 15 minutes of activity each day with their children. Perhaps you would donate several pedometers to the group and encourage a walking competition for a period of a time.

In preparing your material, keep in mind that transformative teaching provokes behavioral change. For example, Grammy Award–winning violinist Joshua Bell describes the impact of seeing Randy Pausch's "Last Lecture" video. A compulsive worrier over the possibility of performance mistakes, Bell's attitude changed after seeing Pausch's presentation. He summarized this shift by writing, "You must be willing to take risks if you really want to live. Go for it, and the music will be much more meaningful." As a result of this insight, Bell is now more relaxed during performances, which has enabled him to do some of his best work ever.[20]

Another important question for transformative teaching is, "Why would your audience want to change their attitude or behavior as a result of your presentation?" In order to answer this question, your material should be organized and presented in a way that truly motivates your listeners toward change. For example, in a presentation on childhood obesity, the fact that overweight children have a 70% risk of becoming overweight adults might be a powerful motivator.[21]

The use of a behavioral learning objective can help you identify the key elements of your presentation. A well-written objective is a statement of audience behavioral expectations. As we discussed in Chapter 1, learning involves the three domains of knowledge (*cognitive*, dealing with facts; *psychomotor*, dealing with performable skills; and *affective*, dealing with attitudes). Regardless of the domain of learning, behavioral objectives involve four components that can be remembered as ABCD (audience, behavior, conditions, and degree). These components are illustrated in **Figure 12-6**.

The recognized leader in the development of behavioral objectives was an educational psychologist by the name of Benjamin Bloom. He created a taxonomy for writing objectives which includes a spectrum of increasing levels of difficulty and appropriate verbs to go with each of these. A detailed description of Bloom's important work is beyond the scope of this text, however useful information can be obtained online.[22]

A set of well defined behavioral objectives is instrumental in facilitating effective preparation. By clearly outlining your presentation and developing one or two objectives for each major point, you will have gone a long way toward assuring a clear, organized presentation that is easy to prepare and deliver in a transformative manner.

AUDIENCE: Who is responsible for the behavior?

"The *student* will..."
"The *patient* will..."
"The *learner* will..."

BEHAVIOR: What observable action (verb) will the learner perform or demonstrate?

Cognitive domain: "The student will *perform a manual muscle test on the elbow.*"

Psychomotor domain: "The patient will *ambulate.*"

Affective domain: "The learner will *demonstrate* respect for patient confidentiality."

CONDITIONS: Under which circumstances is the audience expected to perform the behavior?

"*Following instructor demonstration*, the student will perform a manual muscle test on the elbow."

"The patient will ambulate 100 feet *indoors on level surfaces with a front-wheeled walker.*"

"*Following a lecture on HIPAA-related protected information,* the student will demonstrate respect for patient confidentiality."

DEGREE: The accuracy, extent, duration, or frequency with which the behavior will be performed.

"Following instructor demonstration, the student will perform a manual muscle test of the elbow that is within one grade *of the instructor's reading.*"

"The patient will ambulate 100 feet indoors on level surfaces with a front-wheeled walker and *standby supervision.*"

"*Following a lecture on HIPAA-related protected information,* the student will demonstrate respect for patient confidentiality *in accordance with HIPAA policy.*"

Figure 12–6. Elements of behavioral learning objectives. (Adapted from Bloom, 1984)[22]

Talking Points/Field Notes

Defining Behavioral Objectives

Having now defined your presentation topic, list the major points you want to convey to your audience. Next, construct one or two behavioral objectives related to each of these points. Be sure to include the audience, behavior, conditions, and degree of these.

Transformative Teachers ENGAGE Their Audiences

Transformative teachers do not merely talk *to* their audiences but also *with* them. This involves the ability to empathically connect with learners in a way that invites dialogue and the exchange of ideas. As we have discussed before, empathic connection begins with unconditional positive regard and a sincere concern with the welfare of another. In the context of transformative teaching, this involves doing all we can to provide meaningful information that will, in some way, promote positive change in our learners. Engaging our audience first entails stimulating interest in our information and then inviting them to become active participants in their learning process.

Being sold on our message and having it be well prepared are important ways of strengthening the potential for audience engagement. However, the next step is to create an interactive learning environment and then to provide opportunities for audience participation in the context of our message. Consider the following example:

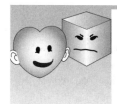

Champ and Blockhead Give a Talk

Champ and Blockhead are physical therapy students on their first internship. As part of the requirements for this experience, they must prepare and deliver a 30-minute presentation to the staff on a topic of their choice. As presentation day approaches, Champ and Blockhead are discussing their teaching strategies and putting the finishing touches on their talks.

"I was really psyched to be able to talk about the principles of exercise prescription," says Champ, as he looks over his computer-based slides. "I lost 25 pounds last year by doing an aerobic exercise program that followed the principles I'm going to talk about. I'm also going to have them do a couple of activities to assess their fitness, and I'll ask them about activities they might enjoy."

"I really had a rough time coming up with a topic," said Blockhead. "I really don't like public speaking, so I want to talk about something really straightforward and easy so I don't look like an idiot. So I'm going to present on total knee replacement exercise protocols and have as many anatomy slides as possible to fill up the time."

On the day of the presentation, Blockhead is nervous. In the minutes before his presentation, he has been caught up in a cascade of negative self-talk (which went along the lines of "this is going to be awful, you are going to be miserable the whole time"). He stands in front of the PT staff with a joyless expression, his hands clasped tightly in front of him. He looks down at his notes and as he begins to talk and suddenly wishes that he had rehearsed his talk the night before. "Uh, I'm going to talk about total knee replacement protocols," he begins. Then he turns out the lights in the room, obscuring his audience's view. He turns on his computer and when his slides fail to appear, he spends a few frantic moments trying to figure out the problem. Once he retrieves his slides, Blockhead begins moving them quickly as he reads off the screen with his back to his audience (who sit quietly as Blockhead does this). When his talk is over, he says "that's it" and turns off his computer before anyone in the audience has time to ask a question. When Blockhead turns on the lights and looks at his watch, he realizes that he has spoken for only 15 of the allotted 30 minutes.

When it is Champ's turn, he too is nervous, but he has been practicing deep breathing and visualizing himself giving a relaxed and enjoyable presentation. These strategies have helped him channel his anxiety more toward a state of energized anticipation. Thus Champ now stands in front of his audience with his arms relaxed at his sides. Having rehearsed his talk several times the night before, Champ has a good idea of what he wants to say and how he will come across to his audience. He smiles at everyone, making eye contact all around the room. "I don't know a single physical therapist who doesn't want to be as healthy as possible," he begins. "Although we are always encouraging our patients to exercise, how many of us are actually doing this ourselves?" When only two hands go up in

Continued

the room, he laughs and smiles again. "I get it. Exercising can be hard to fit into a busy day; but after I'm done sharing some new research about how important it is, I hope that, as a group, we can try to make that happen." Champ then sets the "ground rules" for his presentation. "I want us to enjoy this presentation, so I will be having you do a few short fitness activities. I also want you to stop me and ask questions and to share your thoughts and ideas whenever you wish." Finally, after sharing his objectives, he outlines an idea for a friendly fitness competition for the staff as a way to enable them to apply the presentation concepts. Champ's talk is fun and enjoyable for everyone, with plenty of discussion and exchange of ideas. Despite the energy generated by his presentation, Champ ends the presentation on time.

Questions

1. Consider the different approaches used by Champ and Blockhead in selecting their presentations. How would these affect their being sold on their message and being able to engage their audiences?
2. Champ and Blockhead are both nervous before their talks and each uses the preceding minutes in different ways. Comment on how these different approaches would affect their outlook and ability to deliver an effective talk.
3. What impact might the different postures and body language of Champ and Blockhead have on their audience's first impression? How might Champ and Blockhead's nonverbal communication affect audience engagement during their presentations?
4. Consider the impact of Champ's opening statements. How might these affect audience engagement and presentation?
5. In giving a presentation such as the one described, how important is rehearsal? In which specific ways can this enhance the effectiveness of the presentation?
6. What message might be conveyed by a presenter who has not checked his audiovisual equipment prior to his talk? How could Blockhead have prevented the unnecessary delay with his slides?

As this example illustrates, the process of engaging our audiences is a multifaceted approach that begins with topic selection and preparation. Rehearsing a talk (preferably in front of a mirror or a video camera for later review) is essential for identifying patterns of verbal and nonverbal communication that either enhance or detract from an engaging delivery. When one wishes to convey relaxed confidence, the best posture is simply to stand with both arms relaxed at one's sides. In contrast, hands in pockets can convey affected nonchalance, and arms tightly clenched in front (in what Koegel calls the "T. rex" position) conveys tension.[8]

Setting the "ground rules" for audience interaction at the beginning of a presentation can be extremely helpful. In the example above, Blockhead's nervous posture and lack of eye contact conveyed the message that he saw his talk as a painful experience to get through quickly. This unfortunate attitude was reinforced by the way he jumped into his presentation without inviting his audience to participate. Blockhead created further audience distance by turning out the lights, reading his presentation, and essentially hiding behind his slides. Furthermore, by not having his slides ready to go on his computer, he conveyed a lack of preparation and consideration for his audience.

In contrast, Champ engaged his audience immediately by making eye contact throughout the room. Eye contact is an important behavior for establishing a connection with the audience. Furthermore, maintaining this connection throughout a presentation enables you to assess both audience interest and understanding of your content.

The adult attention span is 20 minutes for retention-based learning.[23] Thus, in order to maintain audience attention and interest, it is recommended that the pace of a presentation change at least every 20 minutes and that audience participation be included at least every 8 minutes.[24]

There are countless methods of engaging audiences to interact with their presenter and the material involved.[25]

The following are some examples of active approaches to engaging audiences.

1. Think-pair-share: Pose a question to the audience and have them reflect on their own personal answer (1 minute). Then have them pair with a partner and share their reflections (2 to 3 minutes). Having pairs share their ideas can defuse audience anxiety about speaking up in front of the entire group

2. IQ (insight/question): After speaking for a period of time, have audience members write down one *insight* (something they have learned, a new way of looking at the subject at hand, a new application for the material), and one *question* (pertaining to the material or their insight). Then have audience members share their IQs in groups of three or four. The IQs can then be shared as part of larger class discussion. This technique is very helpful in assessing audience understanding of the material.

3. Anonymous cards: Hand out index cards to each audience member. Pose a question to the group and have the audience members write their responses on the cards anonymously. Collect the cards, shuffle them, and return them to the audience. When called upon, they can share the comments on their cards. This is a great way to share challenging or sensitive information.

4. Fishbowl discussion: A small group of audience members (up to about 10 people) sit in a circle. These persons have the floor. The rest of the audience sits outside of the circle and act as observers. A question is posed to the inner circle and a discussion begins. If a member of the observer group wishes to participate in the discussion, he or she must tap the shoulder of one of the inner-circle members to make an exchange. The number of persons in the inner circle is kept constant. This technique is excellent for brainstorming and generating creative ideas.

FISH BOWL SET UP

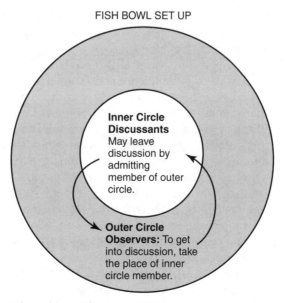

Adapted from Silberman, 1990[25]

Public speaking has been reported in several studies to be the top fear of many Americans.[26] Fear of public speaking has been associated with lack of career advancement and is thus an issue of considerable importance for those affected. For many individuals, fear of public speaking diminishes with thorough preparation and rehearsal. In addition, as experience in public speaking accumulates, many persons also find that they are less anxious and actually find themselves enjoying their teaching interactions.

For those who still find themselves experiencing strong negative reactions to teaching situations regardless of preparation or experience, there are several approaches that can be helpful.

Slow diaphragmatic breathing (one variation of which involves deep inhalation through the nostrils, holding for the count of six, then exhaling through the mouth to the count of eight) has been shown to be effective in reducing test anxiety in medical students.[26] As we have discussed previously, mindfulness-based stress reduction (MBSR) techniques can be of tremendous help in instilling a calm, centered presence amid anxiety-provoking situations. Finally, one intriguing study explored the efficacy of a brief intervention known as the Lefkoe method (TLM). Forty subjects with high levels of public speaking anxiety reported a statistically significant reduction in fear and anxiety (as measured by the SUDS scale) with a concurrent increase (also statistically significant) in confidence, subjective sense of relaxation, and teaching satisfaction after treatment with TLM.[27] TLM is a systematic method of eliminating the underlying beliefs that contribute to the fear of public speaking. Treatment can be accomplished either by use of a self-paced instructional video or through a guided telephone session with a TLM trainer. Both methods have been shown to be equally effective.[28]

When confronting "stage fright" related to public speaking, it may be helpful to realize that a little anxiety can actually be beneficial in terms of creating energy and a feeling of "firing on all cylinders." Even experienced, award-winning teachers feel the stirrings of tension before presenting. These emotions are a testimonial to their continued commitment to being the best they can be at their craft. After 22 years of teaching, I am still a little nervous before most of my talks. In addition, I will always remember the words of my father, an award-winning professor of psychiatry who taught at a major university medical school for over 30 years: "When I quit feeling a little anxious, I will likely be dead."

Transformative Teachers Are AUTHENTIC, Open, and Genuine

As we have discussed previously, authenticity is a measure of communicating in a way that conveys our most genuine self. In interacting with our closest, most trusted friends or family members, this genuine self is easily conveyed. Even when one is presenting in front of a large group, there is no reason to withhold these best aspects of oneself; in fact, these elements can endear us to our audience and facilitate our effectiveness. For example, I have a colleague with a zany, spontaneous sense of humor. Over the years, she has learned to use this inborn talent to lessen students' anxiety and provide memorable (and often hilarious) examples to illustrate application of the material. In contrast, if I were to attempt the same humor in my presentations, it would likely appear artificial and forced. Instead, when appropriate, I like to embellish my presentations through storytelling, which is a passion I have had since a very early age (when some of my more outrageous yarns got me into hot water at school).

Each of us has elements of self that flow naturally in our communication. Our presentations will be more enjoyable and effective if we remain true to these elements regardless of our audience. Certainly we might make adjustments depending on the context (e.g., if our sense of humor tends towards the ribald, we might do well to tone this down in a professional talk), but there is no reason to abandon this attribute altogether.

As is true in all interpersonal interactions, an open and relaxed posture (enhanced by a warm smile and eye contact) is the best way to convey confidence and approachability to our best self, regardless of our various personal attributes.

Talking Points/Field Notes

Bringing My Best Self to My Presentations

Directions

1. Earlier in the text, you were asked to identify attributes of your best self. You can revisit these or, if you prefer, you can generate this list again. Aim for a list of between three and five attributes.

2. After completing your list, review the active techniques for engaging learners and select two or three of these approaches. You can even make up your own. Keep in mind that an element of effective preparation is to first determine the activities you will use, then to consider the specific ways in which you will do so.

3. Consider how you can bring your most authentic self to your selected approaches. For example, if you are energetic and talkative, you might enjoy an IQ, where you can comment on your audience's insights and respond to their questions. If you are more reflective in nature, a think-pair-share enables you to consider your audiences' ideas in response to the questions you ask.

Discuss your answers to the above questions in a small group and record your observations in your field notes. The following suggestions can guide your discussion:

1. Share both your list of attributes and your active techniques.

2. Discuss your rationale for selecting your active techniques.

3. In which ways will you be able to apply your best personal attributes to the active techniques that you selected?

4. Consider the specific parts of your presentation into which you will insert these active techniques (e.g., after lecturing for a period of time as a means of assessing audience understanding).

5. How will you assess the effectiveness of your active learning techniques?

Transformative Teachers Are KNOWLEDGEABLE (But Not Know-It-Alls)

In most cases, you will be asked to present on a specific topic because of a recognized expertise. Accordingly, many physical therapists enjoy sharing their knowledge by presenting at continuing education courses and professional meetings. Such events involve both national and international audiences. For example, the World Confederation of Physical Therapy (WCPT) meets every 4 years and provides a vibrant international forum for professional education.[29]

Regardless of the setting or context of a presentation, audiences expect information to be up to date and inclusive of the newest evidence.

Given the considerable increase in our professional body of knowledge, it is important to maintain a "cutting edge" in representing oneself as an expert in a given topic. Thankfully, it is now easier than ever to stay on top of our content. Professional databases such as PEDro (the Physiotherapy Evidence Database)[30] provide access to a wide array of international journals from which current and emerging knowledge can be gleaned. Members of APTA also have access to numerous medical literature databases through Hooked on Evidence[31] and Open Door.[5]

Whenever possible, it is helpful to provide your audience with a bibliography. In addition, when you are presenting research evidence, it is important to include appropriate citations so that audience members can access the supporting literature. Although assembling these resources can be tedious, these efforts go a long way toward establishing both your credibility and your reputation as a committed teacher.

Despite the most thorough preparation, every speaker will invariably be asked a question to which he or she does not know the answer. Although it is tempting to bluff a response, most audiences will quickly catch on and your credibility will be diminished. It is more authentic (and assertive) to simply admit in a straightforward, unapologetic manner that you don't know. Your audience will greatly appreciate your honesty and humility. If you feel that the audience might benefit from further exploration of the question, you have several options. One is to redirect the question to everyone in the group and discuss any insights that arise. Often the answer will begin to emerge during this process. Even if it does not, this approach can still generate an interesting and worthwhile discussion. If you will be presenting to the same audience again in a short while, you can offer to find the answer and return with it to your next meeting (just be sure to follow through!).

In rare instances, an audience member may appear to ask questions in a challenging or intimidating manner. If left unchecked, this person may begin to dominate the discussion and distract you (and the rest of the audience). When this happens, you might consider acknowledging the value of this person's questions and then inviting him or her to continue the discussion with you after the presentation.

Transformative Teachers Are FAMILIAR With the Needs of Their Audience

One of the most important ingredients of transformative teaching interactions is an appropriate intersection between the needs of the audience and the knowledge of the presenter. Most content can be modified to adapt to differences in audience age and background. For example, physical therapists often talk about the value of exercise and personal fitness to groups of school-age children, modifying the same content (through their language, examples, and level of detail) for delivery to adult patients and other team members.

Another important contextual element in effective preparation is familiarizing yourself about the teaching environment you will share with your audience. For example, if the presentation will occur during a meal, activities that require physical participation (e.g., practicing a treatment technique) would not be the best choice. A list of audience considerations is presented in **Figure 12-7**.

In order to address these considerations in your preparation, it is important to identify them well in advance. When you are initially invited to give a presentation, you can inquire immediately. You can also ask your host about what he or she is hoping to learn from your presentation. If you are being asked to provide ideas for immediate application (as would be the case in a continuing education course), you might inquire about issues of particular interest to address in your talk. These preliminary inquiries will enhance the effectiveness of your presentation and help you to connect with your audience. Furthermore, they will assure your host that you are committed to giving an effective presentation.

Transformative Teachers Are ORGANIZED

In many ways, the elements of SPEAK FORTH address the concept of organization on a comprehensive scale. Thus far you have been asked to consider your objectives, teaching methods, and audience needs.

As you have explored each of these factors, you have essentially built a "screenplay" for your talk, complete with a "synopsis" (your topic and objectives), "stage props" (your teaching methods and audiovisuals), and setting (your audience's background and environment). The final element of organization involves developing a logical script for your presentation, which takes the form of an outline (or lesson plan).

EXPLORING EACH OF THESE CONSIDERATIONS WELL BEFORE YOUR PRESENTATION
CAN HELP YOU MEET AUDIENCE NEEDS

CONSIDERATION	IMPLICATION FOR PRESENTATION
Audience background	• Level of education (elementary students vs. PT clinicians) • Prior knowledge of presentation subject • Homogeneity (Do they all have the same level of knowledge?)
Audience size	• Format (lecture vs. demonstration) • Activities (may be difficult to supervise practice of skills) • Use of microphone (consider use if more than 50)
Seating and room set-up	• If chairs are fixed (auditorium style), activities requiring movement might be challenging. • Tables are helpful for small groups and activities. • Will everyone be able to see AVs? • Are you at liberty to change the seating? (Ask before you do this!) • What AV's are available? Do you need to bring your own computer or slide projector? If you are showing a video or DVD, is the necessary equipment available?
Setting	• Outdoor locations may preclude use of slides, videos, etc. • If audience is eating, they will likely prefer just to listen. Save activities for afterward.
Purpose of presentation	• Education? Entertainment? Inspiration? This will impact content and style of delivery.
Intended outcome	• What does audience hope to do as a consequence of attending your presentation? • How will you assure that they will be able to meet this need?

Figure 12–7. Considerations for assessing audience needs.

Effective outlines may vary in their level of detail. They may include skeleton versions with bulleted headings for major points and brief phrases of supporting information for each. This approach is often preferred by experienced speakers who are knowledgeable about their content, as it allows (and in fact, requires) a spontaneous, conversational delivery. On the downside, the lack of detail may also lead to tangents and digressions that frustrate the audience.

More detailed outlines can be written out almost word for word, just as with the lines in a script. For speakers who are presenting new content or who are inexperienced with presentations, this is a helpful approach for organizing thoughts in a logical and understandable fashion. Then, through the process of rehearsal, the main ideas of the script can be memorized sufficiently to also allow a level of spontaneity during the actual presentation. As you might know from experience, nothing generates audience boredom faster than a speaker who is glued to the podium reading her notes.

Writing out your lectures can be useful in other ways. First, it can build confidence and a sense of control. For example, as a new faculty member, this approach provided me with a mental life jacket in the greatly feared event that my lecture would evaporate from my brain. Second, writing out your talk provides you with the opportunity to rehearse. Although I still write out my talks, I do so mostly for this reason. I also add reminders and cues such as "slow down here" or "tell dog story." These additional cues ensure that I don't forget a helpful enhancement of my content. Although many of my colleagues might consider this exercise to be a neurotically tedious ritual, this approach has served me well over the years.

Whatever level of detail you choose, outlines can be written out, condensed into index cards, or shared with the audience as part of a digital slide presentation. Slide programs such as PowerPoint[32] provide space for speaker notes to be added below each slide and printed out for use during the presentation.

Effective organization also requires sequencing content in a logical manner. Perhaps you have heard the saying that an effective presentation is made up of three elements: the introduction (telling the audience what you are going to tell them), the main body (delivering the message), and closure (summarizing the message and assessing learning). **Figure 12-8** illustrates these three organizational elements.

Handouts have many advantages if used effectively. Of primary importance is their organization, clarity, and relevance to your presentation. If your audience will be taking notes, your handout may include an outline of your talk along with areas for note taking. Computer programs such as PowerPoint allow you to generate handouts that include each of your slides along with designated writing areas. Handouts can also be generated by scanning material into PDF files, which can be uploaded to a computer, modified, and printed. You will just have to be aware of copyright restrictions related to duplication of peer-reviewed journal articles and other online materials.

Even though computer slide programs afford a level of sophistication to your handouts, you will still need to pay attention to careful slide development. There are numerous resources for the effective use of PowerPoint, including online tutorials.[33,34]

ELEMENT	SPEAKER TASKS	AUDIENCE TASKS
INTRODUCTION	**Introduce self.** Connect with audience. Introduce topic and its relevance. Generate interest. Share objectives. Share planned activities.	**Impression formation** Focusing attention "Buying in" (Will this be worth my time?)
MAIN BODY	**Provide information in logical sequence which corresponds to objectives.** **For each objective:** Introduce main point. Introduce unfamiliar terminology. Provide supporting information. Reinforce with evidence/examples, demonstrations or audiovisuals. Involve audience when possible. Provide activity/change in teaching format at least every 60 minutes to maintain attention and interest. Reinforce learning with questions or activity.	 Attending, processing, participating
CLOSURE	**Summarize major points.** Provide take home message. Assess learning. Answer questions. Instill a sense of accomplishment. Provide suggestions for future learning. Create anticipation for next presentation (if applicable).	**Assessing value** Assessing learning
THROUGHOUT PRESENTATION	**Maintain eye contact.** Survey audience for interest and attention (adapt activities and teaching strategies as needed). Reinforce learning.	

Figure 12–8. Organizational elements of a presentation.

Talking Points/Field Notes

Organizing Your Presentation

Using the objectives you previously developed for your presentation, list these in a way that effectively builds audience understanding. This list will now be the skeleton for your presentation's "screenplay." From this skeleton of major objectives, list the major supporting points that you will include in your presentation, along with teaching methods, approximate amount of time, and specific learning activities. The APTA requires this information for all educational proposals submitted for their two national conferences, the Combined Sections Meeting (CSM) and the Annual Conference and Exposition. **Figure 12-9** illustrates the application of these guidelines through an example of a conference proposal that was accepted for presentation at the 2008 APTA annual conference.

Completion of this form is required when submitting a proposal for an APTA national conference presentation. The following is an example of a successful (accepted) proposal

Session Title:
End-of-Life Care: Issues of Living and Dying in Clinical Practice

Description of Course (about 150 words):
End-of-life issues present significant clinical and personal challenges when they arise in any setting: acute care, rehabilitation, outpatient, home health, or hospice. Recognizing that a patient is living with a life-limiting condition is significant in the way we approach care. This course will provide practitioners with the specialized knowledge and unique clinical tools to ensure sensitive and appropriate care in a variety of settings. All aspects of the dying process from physical, psychosocial, and spiritual perspectives will be explored using the most comprehensive care models, with opportunities for individual and small group reflection. Organizational, cultural, and ethical issues will also be addressed. A panel of expert clinicians will review clinical cases, professional development, and opportunities for personal growth from the ultimate life experience.

Course Objectives (no more than five):

Upon completion of this course, attendees will be able to:

1. Identify signs and symptoms of terminal disease processes.
2. Problem-solve clinical issues of life-limiting conditions.
3. Describe common syndromes and barriers to adequate pain relief at the end of life.
4. Discuss both pharmacological and nonpharmacological approaches to symptom control.
5. Differentiate five clinical practice patterns in palliative and hospice care.

Material Gain: There is no financial support for this course.

Bibliographical References:

1. Briggs R. Models for physical therapy practice in palliative medicine. *Rehabilitation Oncology*. 2000;18(2):18–19.
2. Callahan M., Kelley P. *Final Gifts*. New York: Poseidon Press; 1992.
3. City of Hope and American Association of Colleges of Nursing End-Of-Life Consortium (ELNEC). *Advancing End of Life Nursing Care: Core Curriculum*. American Association of Colleges of Nursing; 2000.
4. Doyle D, Hanks G, Cherny N, Calman K. *Oxford Textbook of Palliative Medicine* (3rd ed.). New York: Oxford University Press; 2005.
5. Kubler-Ross E. *On Death and Dying*. New York: Macmillan; 1969.
    Ferrell BR, Coyle N (eds.). *Textbook of Palliative Nursing* (2nd ed.). New York: Oxford Press; 2006.
6. Gudas SA. Terminal illness. In *Psychology in the Physical and Manual Therapies*. New York: Churchill Livingstone; 2004; 333–350.
7. Levine S. *A Year to Live*. New York: Crown; 1997.
8. Longaker C. *Facing Death and Finding Hope*. New York: Doubleday; 1997.
9. National Institute of Medicine. *Approaching Death: Improving Care at the End of Life*. Washington, DC: National Academy Press; 1997.
10. Nuland S. *How We Die*. New York: Alfred A. Knopf; 1994.
11. Reis E. A special place: Physical therapy in hospice and palliative care. *PT Magazine*. 2007;15(3):42–47.

Category: Home health
Theme: Oncology
Presentation Type: Preconference course: 1 day
Course Outline/Timeline:
Note: This level of detail is required in order to exact amount of instructional time to determine continuing education units. Breaks are not included as instructional time.)

15 min: Introduction
15 min: Being with Dying
30 min: How We Die – Physiology of Life's End
30 min: Clinical Issues Solutions – Tips, Unique Interventions
15 min: Morning break
30 min: Practice Patterns in Palliative Care and Hospice
60 min: Pain and Symptom (Anxiety, Dyspnea) Management
45 min: Cultural Differences in Grief Work
60 min: Lunch Break
45 min: Ethical concerns
15 min: Final Gifts – Special Needs, Awareness and Communication of the Dying
45 min: Personal and Professional Grief Work
15 min: Afternoon Break
15 min: A Year to Live – How to Live This Year as if It Were Your Last
15 min: End-of-Life Issues in Pediatric Care
15 min: Practice Development
30 min: Case Studies Panel
15 min: Q and A, Closing Remarks

Figure 12–9. Guidelines of respectful presenters.

Talking Points/Field Notes—cont'd

Speakers/Institutions and Contact Information:

R. Briggs, Enloe HomeCare and Hospice, Chico, CA
K. Mueller, Program in Physical Therapy, Northern Arizona University, Flagstaff, AZ
Northland Hospice and Palliative Care, Flagstaff, AZ
A.L. Leiserowitz, Physical Therapy, Seattle Cancer Care Alliance, Seattle, WA

Speaker Bios:

Richard Briggs, PT, MA has had a clinical practice specializing in palliative care and hospice for the past 22 years. He has presented on this and related topics at the Annual APTA Conference (1999) and CSM (2006, 2007), the National Hospice and Palliative Care Organization (NHPCO) Clinical Conference (2002, 2004, 2005, 2007), California Hospice Foundation (2000), and lectures at California State University, Sacramento. His writing has been published in *Rehabilitation Oncology, Home Health Section Quarterly, NHPCO Insights,* and *Topics in Geriatric Rehabilitation*. He currently is chair of NHPCO Allied Therapist Section and the APTA Hospice and Palliative Care SIG.

Karen Mueller, PT, PhD of physical therapy at Northern Arizona University, where she has taught end-of-life content for the past 20 years. She has also been a hospice volunteer for 17 years and a hospice physical therapist since 2000. Karen is the author of *Seasons of Loss: A Guided Experiential Process for Understanding the Transitions of Illness and End of Life* (Slack Inc., 2006).

Andrea Leiserowitz, MPT, has specialized in oncology for the past 10 years. She received clinical training in oncology rehabilitation at the National Institutes of Health, worked as a staff PT at MD Anderson Cancer Center, and opened the inpatient Seattle Cancer Care Alliance oncology rehabilitation program at the University of Washington in 2000. In 2003, she developed and opened the outpatient physical therapy department at the Seattle Cancer Care Alliance where she currently evaluates and treats pediatric and adult oncology patients and is a certified lymphedema therapist. She is an adjunct clinical faculty member at the University of Puget Sound Doctoral PT Program, and owns a private PT practice in Seattle, Pacific Northwest Physical Rehabilitation.

Keywords:
Palliative and hospice care, psychosocial and spiritual awareness

Teaching Methods:
Case study, demonstration, lecture, panel discussion, question and answer, small group discussions

Evaluation Method: Question and answer

Participant Level: Intermediate

A/V Equipment: Cordless lavalier microphone, LCD projector, screen, VCR

Participant Limitations: None (course is not restricted to a certain number)

Unique Considerations: No other special requirements

Figure 12–9. cont'd

If you do not intend to use handouts to facilitate note taking, consider providing these after your presentation to avoid audience distraction.

Transformative Teachers Are RESPECTFUL of Their Audience

Respectful interaction between the presenter and the audience is critical for creating an authentic and empowering learning environment. A respectful learning environment engenders a sense of welcoming inclusion by which audience members feel free to contribute questions and comments. Presenters can foster this by limiting unwelcome distractions (such as ringing cell phones) by starting and ending on time and by the judicious use of humor, language, and teaching methods that create comfort for everyone. There are several other steps a presenter can take to assure a respectful learning environment. These are illustrated in **Box 12-2.**

Transformative Teachers Are TENACIOUS in Their Quest for Excellence

Like many well-developed skills, transformative teaching requires an ongoing commitment to excellence. This commitment can be demonstrated by ongoing self-assessment as well as the solicitation of audience feedback. Excellence can also be developed through involvement in educational programs directed at improving teaching skills.

BOX 12-2:   Guidelines for Respectful Presenters

The respectful presenter...

1. Arrives early to assure the optimal setup for the presentation
2. Greets audience members as they arrive
3. Thanks any presentation sponsors for the opportunity to speak
4. Starts and ends on time
5. Ascertains that everyone in the audience is able to hear
6. Avoids humor directed at audience members (you can laugh *with* them but not *at* them)
7. Dresses professionally (one guideline is to dress slightly more formally than your audience)
8. Limits sources of audience distraction (many presenters ask audience members to turn off cell phones, especially if the audience is large)
9. Has determined that the audiovisual technologies are working *before* the audience arrives
10. Avoids slang, offensive humor, or any material that might create audience discomfort
11. Repeats audience questions for everyone to hear before answering
12. Thanks the audience for their attention and contributions at the end of the presentation

---

One of the first programs for the improvement of teaching effectiveness in health education was known as the Teaching Improvement Project System (TIPS). It was developed at the University of Kentucky School of Medicine at Lexington in 1975 and included several topics related to effective teaching, including the development of objectives, structure (body and closure), questioning techniques, and effective use of audiovisual aids. One of the most valuable aspects of TIPS was the "microteaching session," where participants presented a brief lecture to a small group of peers. This lecture was videotaped for later participant viewing in a feedback session with a course faculty member. The effectiveness of the TIPS approach to teaching excellence was documented in two studies involving medical school students and faculty.[35,36] Specifically, the opportunity to objectively view oneself in a teaching interaction and to receive honest, supportive feedback resulted in a statistically significant improvement in teaching effectiveness (as determined by student evaluations) and instructor confidence. Most importantly, the improvements were sustained at a 2-year follow-up self-assessment. These studies support the value of deliberately working to improve one's teaching. TIPS workshops are currently presented through over 30 university-based training sites in the United States.[37]

In our profession, the clinical instructor credentialing course provides valuable information that can be used to enhance teaching effectiveness. Although the context of this course pertains to clinical student supervision, the skills are relevant for teaching in more formal contexts.[10] Furthermore, in the spirit of ongoing development of teaching excellence, APTA now offers an advanced clinical instructor education and credentialing program (CIECP). It provides further content in the effective application of the patient/client management model, evidence-based practice, and professionalism.[38] Finally, APTA offers experienced clinical instructors the opportunity to become trainers for both clinical instructor training courses.[39] Interested applicants must apply to the APTA Clinical Instructor Education Board (CIEB). Acceptance into this course is by invitation only. Trainers must teach a minimum number of courses over a 3-year period in order to retain this credential. As of October 2008, there were 168 credentialed CI trainers in the United States, Puerto Rico, and Canada.

Talking Points/Field Notes

Teaching Self-Evaluation: The Video Microteach

As part of your preparation for a transformative teaching experience, you will present all or part of the talk you have been preparing to an audience of peers. Your talk will be videotaped and you will then have the opportunity to view this for the purpose of self-assessment. If you wish, you may work with a partner, where each of you view each other's videotape and share feedback. To guide your self-assessment, use the checklist in **Table 12-1.**

Instructor note: The value of the microteach will be greatly enhanced by having the course instructor or other faculty member view the videotaped teaching segment with students and providing feedback.

Table 12–1. Teaching Self-Assessment Checklist

Use the following rating scale to assess your performance on each of the following:

A = Always   F = Frequently   I = Infrequently   N = Never   NA = Not Applicable

Introduction	A F I N NA
Relaxed and open posture	_____
Eye contact with audience	_____
Statement of presentation topic	_____
Shares objectives for presentation	_____
Shares importance of topic	_____
Gains audience attention and interest	_____
Organization	A F I N NA
Content reflects objectives	_____
Content builds in logical fashion	_____
Content at appropriate level	_____
New content is reinforced for learning	_____
Delivery	A F I N NA
Conveys enthusiasm for topic	_____
Can be heard by all audience members	_____
Speaks clearly	_____
Minimal use of "filler" (um, uh, etc.)	_____
Speed is appropriate for understanding	_____
Conveys confidence, professionalism	_____
Dressed appropriately for context of presentation	_____
Appears knowledgeable about topic	_____
Maintains eye contact with audience throughout	_____

Talking Points/Field Notes—cont'd

Table 12–1.	**Teaching Self-Assessment Checklist—cont'd**
Audio Visual	**A F I N NA**
Audiovisuals work properly	_____
Does not read slides	_____
Faces audience when referencing slides	_____
Slides are legible and clear	_____
Handouts add to presentation effectiveness	_____
Demonstrations can be seen by all	_____
Audience Engagement	**A F I N NA**
Involves audience when appropriate	_____
Creates inclusive learning environment	_____
Addresses questions appropriately	_____

Teaching Self-Assessment Checklist Adapted from Teaching Improvement Project Systems (TIPS). Faculty workshop, Northern Arizona University, March 1990.

1. Depending on time constraints, you will offer all or part of the presentation that you have building throughout this chapter. Whatever approach you choose, be certain that your presentation is well prepared so that your performance can reflect an optimal teaching experience.

2. Your presentation will be videotaped for your later review. It is suggested that you review the tape at least twice so that you can fully evaluate all elements of your performance. As you review your videotape, use the checklist from Table 12-1 to guide your observations. Note: Most persons find it awkward to view themselves on videotape, and the tendency when doing so is to be highly critical. The point here is to objectively examine your teaching so you can assess areas for future growth.

3. If you select a partner for this exercise, each of you will view each other's videotape and use the checklist to exchange objective, helpful feedback. Questions 4 and 5 below can be incorporated into your discussion.

4. Once you have completed your assessment, consider your areas of *performance strength*. How can you continue to develop these attributes for even more effective presentations in the future?

5. Which areas would you consider your *performance challenges?* How might you continue to develop these attributes for even more effective presentations in the future?

6. How would you describe this teaching experience? Which elements were the most enjoyable? Which areas will improve with practice?

Transformative Teachers Approach Their Work With HUMILITY

The ability to engage in transformative teaching is, first and foremost, a privilege. The elements of SPEAK FORTH will not be fully evident with an attitude of arrogance or complacency. Thus, whenever we share information, it is helpful to keep the core values of our profession in mind (accountability, altruism, caring and compassion, integrity, excellence, professional duty, and social responsibility). By intentionally modeling these values in any element of our communication, we can "get out of our own way" and teach with the conviction, "I am here only to be truly helpful."[40]

Speaking Forth in Practice: The Importance of Mentorship

As we discussed at the beginning of this chapter, teaching involves "demonstration" and "inculcation" or indoctrination of attitudes and behaviors. The most powerful use of such teaching is to shape the professional development of a promising colleague (called a protégé) in the form of *mentorship*.

The word *mentor* originates from Homer's *Odyssey*. In this story, the goddess Athena assumes the identity of a wise old man named Mentor, who guides and protects Telemachus, the young son of Odysseus, as he goes off to war.

The word *protégé* derives from the French word meaning "protected."[41] Accordingly, effective mentors guide the career development of their protégés through the appropriate delegation of opportunities and responsibilities. In most cases, there comes a time when the protégé succeeds in his own right, sometimes even eclipsing the accomplishments of the mentor. In the *Odyssey*. Mentor guides Telemachus so effectively that he becomes a hero by freeing his father from captivity during the Trojan War.

The Qualities of Effective Mentors

The qualities of effective mentors have been examined at great length in medicine and the health professions. On an organizational level, effective mentors cast a wide net in terms of their scope of influence.

In a study of physicians, the presence of outstanding role models in the workplace was associated with improved job satisfaction.[42] In contrast, poor physician satisfaction was linked to adverse effects on patient care.

In a study of exemplary medical school faculty, extensive interviews were conducted with 24 clinically excellent department of medicine physicians (defined as exemplifying excellence in their daily work) at eight different academic institutions.[43] Eight domains of clinical excellence emerged. Interestingly, these faculty viewed "reputation" as the most important indicator of clinical excellence, which suggests that years of consistently outstanding professional behavior are required before one is recognized as a mentor by peers. Such longevity also speaks of genuine passion and commitment to one's work. Not surprisingly, the remaining seven domains of excellence included communication and interpersonal skills, professionalism and humanism, diagnostic acumen, skillful negotiation in the health-care system, knowledge, a scholarly approach to medicine, and a passion for clinical medicine.

The elements of exemplary practice have also been described in the PT profession.[44] These include (1) a knowledge base that grows through experience with patients, reflection, and ongoing learning; (2) grounding the clinical reasoning process in the context of the patient partnership in order to effect meaningful change; (3) linking movement assessment to functional outcomes; and (4) the consistent demonstration of caring and commitment to patients. In the context of our profession, these qualities pertain to the judicious and compassionate use of an expert knowledge to enhance movement, function, and quality of life. Accordingly, the slogan "*The science of healing, the art of caring*" is prominently displayed on the APTA website's home page.[45]

Regardless of the setting or professional context, both mentor and protégé must contribute to a successful and productive relationship. **Figure 12-10** illustrates key attributes for each role.

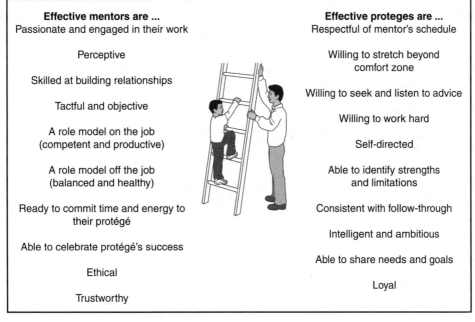

Effective mentors are ...
Passionate and engaged in their work

Perceptive

Skilled at building relationships

Tactful and objective

A role model on the job
(competent and productive)

A role model off the job
(balanced and healthy)

Ready to commit time and energy to
their protégé

Able to celebrate protégé's success

Ethical

Trustworthy

Effective proteges are ...
Respectful of mentor's schedule

Willing to stretch beyond
comfort zone

Willing to seek and listen to advice

Willing to work hard

Self-directed

Able to identify strengths
and limitations

Consistent with follow-through

Intelligent and ambitious

Able to share needs and goals

Loyal

Figure 12–10. Attributes of successful mentors and protégés.

Talking Points/Field Notes

My Skills as Mentor and Protégé

As you progress through your career, you will hopefully seek and develop many opportunities to serve as both mentor and protégé. Many successful individuals engage in both relationships simultaneously, which enables them to continue their own professional development while supporting that of a younger colleague. This exercise is thus designed to help you identify the attributes you would bring to either role. It is never too early to engage in this process from either perspective. For example, as a physical therapy student, you have already gained valuable skills that might help aspiring younger colleagues to achieve admission to a PT program.

PART I

Examine the list of mentor attributes in Figure 12-10 and discuss the following questions in a small group. You can also record your observations in your field notes.

1. Which qualities do you think are the most important for being a successful mentor?

2. Successful mentors choose their protégés carefully. First of all, it is important to feel an emotional connection, and many mentors state that they "see themselves" in their protégés. Thus, consider the attributes which would be important for you in selecting a person to mentor.

3. What are your particular strengths as mentor?

4. Which areas of mentor attributes might you want to strengthen?

5. In which specific ways would being a mentor help you in your own personal and professional development? (Perhaps you can speak from experience!)

Continued

Talking Points/Field Notes—cont'd

Part II

Examine the list of protégé attributes in Figure 12-10 and discuss the following questions in a small group. You can also record your observations in your field notes.

1. What qualities do you think are the most important in being a successful protégé?

2. Successful protégés seek mentors based on their admiration of certain personal and professional characteristics. What sort of attributes would you look for in approaching a potential mentor?

3. What are your particular strengths as a protégé?

4. In which specific areas might you seek the guidance of a mentor?

5. Which protégé attributes might you want to strengthen?

Developing a Culture of Mentorship

In contrast to the often impersonal processes that pair supervisors and subordinates with little consideration of their compatibility, mentorship is based upon a personally driven, consciously chosen relationship. Thus it requires deliberate effort to foster a "culture of mentorship" where novice clinicians learn from experienced colleagues in the context of a caring relationship.

For example, in 2008, the Association of PeriOperative Registered Nurses (AORN) established a position statement on mentoring that identifies the qualities of both effective mentors and protégés. In a recent article describing this initiative, the AORN president quipped, "Not only must we overcome the battle of 'eating our young,' we must understand the unique perspective that new generations bring to our profession."[38]

APTA also has two positions related to mentorship.[46] The first, entitled, "Mentoring for American Physical Therapy Association (APTA) Involvement," was approved by the APTA House of Delegates in 1996. This statement speaks to the responsibility of each member to "foster the involvement of other members in the Association" and "for those in leadership roles in the Association to mentor their fellow members."

The second position statement is entitled "Mentoring of Professionalism in Academic And Clinical Education" and was adopted by APTA in 2003 at the request of the student assembly. This statement reads "It is the responsibility of all academic and clinical faculty, clinical instructors, and professional mentors to actively promote to physical therapist students the importance of professionalism as a critical component of a doctoring profession."

In order to follow through with these directives, APTA has established an online "Members Mentoring Mentors" program.[47] This is a volunteer process where members can post areas of expertise in which they can mentor others. Members who are seeking mentorship can also use the site to identify and contact colleagues who can assist them in their own development. Physical therapy student members of the APTA are encouraged to participate in the process.

More recently, the APTA has extended the culture of mentorship to include opportunities for students to assist others students. This program is entitled Student Mentoring: Achieving and Reaching Together (SMART).[48]

In addition to these APTA-based initiatives, several PT academic programs have established mentoring programs where more experienced students mentor incoming ones. These programs have proven to be highly successful for everyone involved.[49]

Talking Points/Field Notes

Developing a Culture of Mentorship in My Academic Program

In the exercise, you are asked to consider specific ways to develop either an informal or formal mentorship program in your academic setting and/or surrounding professional community. This can take many forms, including one-on-one partnerships between students at different points in the program. For example, some programs have a "big brother/big sister" approach, and others have a "buddy" system between practicing clinicians and students. Discuss the following questions in a small group and reflect on your insights in your field notes.

1. What would be two specific ways in which you develop a mentor–protégé program within your academic program and the surrounding professional community?

2. What would be the specific purpose of each program?

3. How might mentors and protégés be identified and paired?

4. Which kinds of activities might be involved in each program?

5. How long might each program last? (A semester? a month?)

6. How might each program be evaluated?

7. What benefits could arise from these programs?

Transformative Teaching to Promote Behavioral Change

In the context of the therapeutic alliance, we build a trusting, care-based relationship that allows us to promote favorable patient outcomes. This first step is described in considerable detail in Chapter 10.

As stated previously, our patients won't care how much we know until they know how much we care. Once we have gained their trust and confidence, we can then partner with them to develop and reinforce their health-related self-efficacy. For many patients, this may mean the adoption of long-term behaviors such as participation in a regular exercise program. As you likely know if you have ever made such a change in your own life, the development of beneficial health habits requires motivation, planning, and commitment. For many patients, the process of behavioral change for better health may also involve adjustments in social activities, such as avoidance of environments typically associated with the undesired behavior. Discouragement can also arise when the initial rate of progress slows despite consistent engagement in appropriate behaviors. One example is the weight-loss plateau that often occurs in the face of long-term activity and nutritional adjustments.

Thus, in engaging in transformative teaching with our patients, we must recognize the many stages and related challenges of long-term behavioral change in order to target our interventions appropriately.

The Transtheoretical Model of Behavior Change

The transtheoretical model of behavioral change (TTM) was developed in 1979 by psychologist James Prochaska.[50] The TTM is a five-stage model that explains the cognitive and psychological processes involved in the attainment of long-term behavioral change. Furthermore, the model can help explain and even predict the likelihood of success in either adoption of positive behaviors such as exercise[51] as well as the extinction of negative ones such as smoking. The TTM involves five specific levels of specific patient attitudes and behaviors. Successful progression through these stages can be enhanced by specific types of interventions within each. Thus, by adapting interventions to facilitate success and prevent relapse, clinicians can optimize and reinforce their patients' health-care self-efficacy. The following discussion applies the five stages of TTM to a patient case scenario. In addition, we will consider the TTM in terms of an exploration of your own experiences with behavioral change.

Clinical Scenario

A Patient in Need of a Change in Health Behavior

Max Bennett is a 48-year-old advertising executive with a stressful career that involves extensive travel. Two weeks ago, he experienced a brief episode of blindness in the right halves of each eye and difficulty speaking. Although the episode resolved after 10 minutes, Max went to the emergency department, where subsequent follow-up revealed that he had sustained a transient ischemic attack (a dire warning sign of possible impending stroke).

Max was warned that his being sedentary, 40 pounds overweight, and a one-pack a day cigarette smoker were contributing to his risk of heart disease and stroke. Max was thus referred to an interdisciplinary cardiovascular fitness center for comprehensive lifestyle management. As the physical therapist in this setting, your role will be to assist Max in developing an aerobic exercise program. Max will also be working with a nutritionist to develop a weight-management program and a psychologist to address smoking cessation and stress reduction.

Talking Points/Field Notes

Precursors to Behavior Change in Your Own Life

In the context of our exploration of TTM, it will be helpful to apply the related stages to a successful behavior change in your own life (consider this to be a change that you were able to sustain for at least 6 months). Discuss the following questions and reflect on your observations in your field notes.

1. How did you first become aware of the need to make this change? Did this awareness arise from your own perceptions or was it pointed out to you by another person?

2. How was the undesirable behavior impacting your life? How did you minimize this impact?

3. What were the positive gains of the undesirable behavior?

4. What were the social, environmental, and behavioral "triggers" for the undesirable behavior? How did you manage these?

TTM Stage 1: Precontemplation ("That'll Be the Day!")

For persons in the precontemplation stage, the idea of successfully engaging in a specific health-promoting behavior is the furthest thing from their minds. If Max were in this stage with respect to exercise, he would likely say "There's no way I am going to fit exercise into my crazy schedule, so don't even ask!"

Max may have several reasons for this attitude. First, he might not understand the relationship between exercise and cardiovascular health. He may not be aware of the benefits of exercise in terms of assisting weight loss, reducing stress, and reinforcing a nonsmoking lifestyle. Max may also be discouraged by his inability to make exercise a regular part of his life, having tried and failed several times. One or more of these factors might lead Max toward an avoidant approach to exercise, so that he will not be willing to learn about the importance of this behavior in the context of his overall health.

Patients in the precontemplation stage are often labeled "noncompliant" and dismissed from a potentially supportive health-care environment ("We can't help you unless you're willing to change, so call us when you're ready"). This approach may result in further discouragement and reinforcement of such resistance to change. Most unfortunately of all, should the patient begin to reconsider his or her position, they may no longer be in a position to acquire the necessary support.

Transformative teaching in the precontemplation stage involves exploring the possibility of *readiness* for change. Factors which can improve readiness are feelings of *confidence* that change might be successful as well as a sense that making the change is *important*.[52] Thus questions for Max at this stage might proceed as follows:

Physical Therapy Questions for Max at the Precontemplation Stage

1. How ready are you to talk about starting an exercise program?

2. What concerns do you have about engaging in a regular exercise program?

3. How might you know when you are ready to explore the option of exercising?

4. What have been your experiences with exercise thus far? What did you learn from these experiences?

5. If you were unsuccessful with exercise in the past, what might you do differently now? How confident are you that you could make these changes?

6. What do you think might be the benefits of a regular exercise program?

7. What do you think are the biggest challenges to a regular exercise program?

8. How important do you think exercise is for overall health?

9. Do you have any friends or family members who exercise? What have you learned from them?

10. How can I support you right now?

The answers to each of these questions can provide useful information which can be used in the context of transformative teaching. Studies on the prevailing mindset of precontemplators suggest that there are several differences which distinguish this group. Accordingly, precontemplators can be reluctant, resigned, resisting, rebellious, or rationalizing.[53]

Regardless of the patient's mindset, the most important precursor for successful behavior change is that the patient bring a positive expectation for success.[53] Barriers to a positive expectation may be that patients do not view the change as important, that they are not confident of their ability to change, or that they do not have the resources (time, money, convenience, knowledge) to be successful. Thus the previous questions can help you discern which barriers might have to be addressed in your patient discussion.

For example, patients who do not clearly understand the benefits of behavioral change will obviously benefit from *consciousness raising*,[53] which involves assimilating information that will increase their awareness of the importance and value of the change. Patients at this stage also need assurance that their health-care team supports them despite their current inability to commit to behavioral change. Finally, patients need to know that you will be available for support when they are ready to move to the next level. In the case of Max, your discussion may reveal that he is overwhelmed by what he views as the simultaneous recommendations for so many behavioral changes all at once. This leads to a productive discussion in which Max is asked to prioritize the areas he would most like to address. It is decided that he needs to reduce his stress first and foremost. Thus, he begins with mindfulness meditation training. He agrees to a follow-up appointment with you in 6 weeks.

Talking Points/Field Notes

My Own Precontemplation

1. How would you describe a "precontemplation" experience in your own life?
2. How did you react to suggestions that you change your behavior?
3. What were your reasons for not being interested?
4. How might you have responded to the "PT Questions for the Precontemplation Stage" listed above?
5. From your own experience, how can you best help patients in the precontemplation stage?

TTM Stage 2: Contemplation

Persons in the contemplation stage are aware that they are facing a health issue that is creating problems for them. They realize that a change in behavior would be helpful and they now begin to consider the option of taking action in the "foreseeable future" (which is typically defined in the TTM literature as 6 months).[54]

These individuals are capable of identifying the pros and cons of the behavioral change but are often stuck more in the "cons." Accordingly, this stage has been described as one of "behavioral procrastination." Thus, when Max visits for his follow-up appointment to assess his readiness to begin an exercise program, he states "I know that exercise would help me be calmer and lose weight, and I have been thinking that I probably should do something about this." At this point, Max vacillates between feeling optimistic about his potential for change and pessimistic that he can address the barriers preventing it.

Despite the intellectual recognition that change is important, many contemplators are stuck in the compulsive patterns which drive the unhealthy behavior. Thus, discussions about readiness, importance, and confidence are still important at this stage; one helpful approach is to identify progress in each of these domains. If Max can appreciate that he is moving toward change, he may feel encouraged to consider further exploration. To quantify these changes, a rating scale of 1 to 10 can be used, as described below.[54]

Physical Therapy Questions for Max at the Contemplation Stage

1. If 0 was "completely not ready" and 10 was "completely ready," where would you rate yourself on your readiness to begin an exercise program?
2. What are your reasons for rating yourself as you did?

3. What might it take for you to feel more ready?

4. What is getting in your way of feeling more ready?

5. If 0 was "completely lacking in confidence" and 10 was "completely confident," where would you rate yourself on your confidence that you could be successful in maintaining an exercise program?

6. What might it take for you to feel more confident?

7. What is getting in your way of your feeling more confident?

8. If 0 was "completely unimportant" and 10 was "completely important," where would you rate yourself on the importance you attach to engaging in an exercise program?

9. What might it take for you to feel that exercise is important?

10. What do you think are the major pros and cons of exercising at this point?

11. How might you minimize the cons?

12. How might you strengthen the pros?

13. How might I help you become more ready, more confident, and more convinced of the importance of exercising?

At the contemplation stage, consciousness raising continues to be helpful and even more productive as the patient becomes more aware of the issues that may be limiting his willingness to engage in the behavioral change. Support and encouragement for patients at this stage remains critical.

Sometimes this support may involve networking with persons who have been successful in making behavioral changes in their own lives. Thus, patient-to-patient buddy systems can provide additional encouragement as well as practical assistance in moving toward change.

In your follow-up with Max, he states that his extensive travel schedule makes it "impossible" to exercise on a regular basis. At this point, you ask him if he would like to meet Sharon, another patient who also travels extensively while maintaining a regular exercise program. Max agrees and has an enjoyable discussion with her. At the end of their session, Max tells you, "I have a lot of thinking to do, so I will call you for another appointment in 2 weeks."

Talking Points/Field Notes

My Own Contemplation

1. How would you describe a "contemplation" experience in your own life?

2. How did you assess the pros and cons of making the behavior change?

3. What do you think were the biggest reasons for not taking action?

4. What were useful things that others said or did to help you feel more ready for change?

5. How might you have responded to the "PT Questions for the Contemplation Stage" listed above?

6. From your own experience, how can you best help patients in the contemplation stage?

TTM Stage 3: Preparation

Persons at this stage have now decided that they will take action in the immediate future (defined as within 1 month).[54] At this point, they have usually taken definitive action to move them toward the activity. When Max calls for his next appointment, he informs you that he has purchased exercise gear and that he has identified hotels with on-site gyms.

At this point, interventions can become more *action-oriented*. Of equal importance is to provide praise and encouragement for patient progress while also offering goals to encourage success. Thus, when Max calls for his appointment, you provide this support and also encourage him to bring his gear. In order to begin slowly and give Max his first taste of success, you decide to have him walk on the treadmill for 15 minutes at his normal speed. Max is relieved to discover that he is able to do this with no discomfort, which leads to your recommendations for a walking program. You instruct Max in the use of a pedometer and structure an exercise program that will slowly build towards 11,000 steps a day. You encourage him to wear his pedometer at all times, even when he is traveling. You suggest that for the next week, he measure and chart his daily walking in order to get a baseline. Finally, to support your recommendation, you provide evidence that identifies this level as a minimum needed for weight control in men between the ages of 40 to 50.[55]

When Max returns from his week of baseline monitoring, he informs you that he walks an average of 5,000 steps a day. Basing your recommendations on evidence, you tell him to add 20% to the average number steps every week until he is walking over 11,000 steps a day.[56]

This steady but gradual progression will be helpful in continuing to increase Max's confidence without making significant (and potentially overwhelming) changes at this early stage.

Although these recommendations are definite leads into the action stage, they are not yet at a sufficient level to be clinically significant for health improvement. Therefore you will have to use an evidence-based approach to determine the appropriate level of activity for your patients in light of their health concerns.[55] For example, Max also shares that he has begun to cut back on his cigarette habit. While this is definitely encouraging, he will not achieve measurable health benefits until he stops completely.

Finally, as Max makes progress, regular encouragement will ensure his continued resolve. Accordingly, another important intervention strategy is to help Max resolve any obstacles that may arise. To that end, much to his delight, he discovers that he can continue his walking program even while he is in an airport. Because of this, he no longer feels that his travel schedule is a major limitation to his pursuit of regular exercise.

Talking Points/Field Notes

My Preparation

1. Describe the specific preparations you made in order to institute your desired behavior change.

2. How did these preparations affect your sense of confidence and readiness to move toward action?

3. In what ways did other persons help and support you at this point?

4. How can we best support our patients at this stage?

TTM Stage 4: Action

Persons in the action stage have now made specific and measurable lifestyle changes at a clinically relevant level. Accordingly, they may experience noticeable changes in their subjective state of well-being, physical function, and appearance. Often, these changes are noted by friends and family, and this reinforcement can be highly gratifying. To that end, it can be helpful to question your patients about the changes they notice as well as their impact.

At this stage, patients also have greater internal awareness of the environmental, social, and attitudinal factors that either support or distract them from their new behavior. If they are unable to manage these elements, they may relapse to an undesired behavior (smoking again) or abandon the new one (stop exercising).

In your next visit with Max, he shares that he is now aware of his tendency to go home exhausted at night and thus feeling too tired to exercise. Thus he learns that it is important for him to get his walking in before he goes home. Max has now discovered many ways to get walking into his workday. For example, he shares that by parking his car further away in his company lot, he can get a good number of his steps in before his day even starts. He now often has "walking meetings" with colleagues and has even considered having a walking contest with his friends from work. Finally, Max discovers that he enjoys walking even more while listening to books on tape.

Talking Points/Field Notes

My Action Phase

1. Describe your early actions in adopting your desired behavior change.

2. What were some of the most rewarding elements of this stage?

3. What sort of environmental, social, and behavioral factors did you learn to manage?

4. Which of these were the most challenging and why?

5. How can physical therapists best assist patients in the action stage?

Stage 5: Maintenance

At this stage, persons have successfully integrated the desired behavior change as a regular part of their lives for longer than 6 months.[57] They are now more easily able to manage their environment, social network, and behaviors to promote ongoing success.

Persons can be in the maintenance phase for a lifetime. Accordingly, some versions of TTM suggest a final stage, termination, in which the patient reframes his or her identity to include the behavior as a measure of self (I am a runner, I am a nonsmoker). This stage suggests that the specific behavioral change is no longer an issue.[57]

Nevertheless, relapse can occur at any point, even after several years. This is likely to occur in the presence of significant life stressors or changes. For example, should Max injure himself or become seriously ill, he might be unable to resume his walking program. Should he experience a significant life stress (such as losing his job), he might become depressed and thus unable to summon the energy required to continue his exercise. In these situations, additional support may be needed to help maintain the behavior or to prevent the relapse from becoming permanent. Patient follow-up at regular intervals can also be useful in providing ongoing encouragement or to address changes that could contribute to relapse.

Other reasons for relapse are more insidious. Boredom or lack of continued noticeable gains (plateaus) are common. The impact of these can be minimized by ongoing support and encouragement so that patients don't feel that they are alone.

Support for ongoing health-care change is an important aspect of PT management in wellness and prevention programs and should be a part of our regular practice. Just as most of us visit our physicians for yearly health checkups, we should also visit our physical therapists for fitness support.

In the case of Max, after a month of supervised walking in your PT clinic, his insurance would no longer provide coverage. However, Max agreed to monthly follow-ups for a year after his TIA, during which time Max also joined a community hiking club, which kept him walking in a socially enjoyable way.

Talking Points/Field Notes

My Maintenance

1. Describe a health behavior that you have maintained for at least 6 months. How were you (or have you) able to continue your success?

2. How did you address any relapses that occurred? What strategies were the most helpful?

3. What are the most important things you do to assure continued involvement in the behavior?

4. What role do physical therapists have in supporting patients in their maintenance of health behavior change?

Implications for Physical Therapy

Although teaching for behavioral change may not be as formal as some of the other situations described in this chapter, the potential for transforming patient lives is enormous. Knowing the stages of TTM and the appropriate intervention strategies are important tools for optimizing our effectiveness with all patients. Without such skills, we can truly limit the scope of our therapeutic impact. Furthermore, as health care moves toward a greater appreciation of wellness and health promotion, effective application of the TTM model can provide new opportunities for clinical practice, research, and education.

Chapter Summary

1. Teaching is a central element of PT practice. Transformative teaching is an important tool for professional development and career advancement.

2. Transformative teaching involves SPEAKING FORTH. This includes:
   a. Being SOLD on your message
   b. Being PREPARED
   c. ENGAGING your audience
   d. Being AUTHENTIC
   e. Being KNOWLEDGEABLE
   f. Being FAMILIAR with your audience's needs

    g. Being ORGANIZED

    h. Being RESPECTFUL of your audience

    i. Being TENACIOUS in your quest for excellence

    j. Approaching your teaching with HUMILITY

3. Mentorship involves transformative teaching by example.

4. In the context of patient care, transformative teaching involves promoting desirable behavioral change.

5. A useful model of behavioral change is known as the transtheoretical model of change (TTM). By understanding the five component stages of TTM, interventions can be targeted to address the prevailing concerns, needs, and attitudes of our patients.

Take-Home Menu

1. Transformative teaching movies. Watch one of the following films for uplifting examples of transformative teaching.

    a. *The Miracle Worker* (1962). Patty Duke and Anne Bancroft play Helen Keller and her teacher Annie Sullivan in a powerful depiction of mentorship.

    b. *The Dead Poets' Society* (1989). Robin Williams plays a passionate teacher of classic literature in an ivy league boys' school. This film popularized the saying *carpe diem* ("seize the day").

    c. *Mr. Holland's Opus* (1996). Richard Dreyfuss plays an ambitious musician who must "settle" for teaching music as a day job. Instead of the boredom he expected, he discovers his passion for teaching as well as the power of transformation.

    d. *The Emperor's Club* (2002), starring Kevin Kline. A riveting film about education and ethics in action set in a private boys' school.

    e. *Mona Lisa Smile* (2003), starring Julia Roberts. A history teacher in a private girls' school exchanges lessons about life and love with her students.

2. Speakers' Bureau. Many organizations have a speakers' bureau through which members offer their educational services on a variety of topics. See if your state APTA chapter has such a group and volunteer to add a talk on the PT student perspective for elementary or high school students. If your chapter does not have this, offer to provide such a talk at a community school career day.

3. Submit a school project for presentation at an APTA meeting. The APTA welcomes platform or poster submissions from students. If your program requires a clinical or research project, consider submitting it for presentation. At the minimum, this will provide you with an opportunity to use the APTA proposal format to organize your presentation. At best, you might get to present to a national audience!

4. Attend the APTA student conclave at some point during your PT education. This will provide a marvelous opportunity for mentorship and inspiration for effective teaching.

References

1. Accurate and Reliable Dictionary: A Free English-English Online Dictionary: http://ardictionary.com/Teach/1175. Accessed August 11, 2008.

2. American Physical Therapy Association, Sections on Neurology and Pediatrics. III Step Conference: Linking Movement Science and Intervention. Salt Lake City, UT, July 15-21, 2005.

3. American Physical Therapy Association. *Hooked on Evidence:* http://www.hookedonevidence.com/. Accessed August 20, 2008.

4. American Physical Therapy Association. *Guide to Physical Therapist Practice,* 2nd rev ed. Alexandria, VA: American Physical Therapy Association; 2003.

5. American Physical Therapy Association. *Open Door: APTA's Portal to Evidence Based Practice* (to APTA members only): http://www.apta.org. Accessed August 12, 2008.

6. American Physical Therapy Association. PT CPI: Version 2006 Update: http://www.apta.org/AM/Template.cfm?Section=Home&CONTENTID=50666&TEMPLATE=/CM/ContentDisplay.cfm. Accessed August 19, 2008.

7. American Physical Therapy Association. *Physical Therapy: Journal of the American Physical Therapy Association:* http://www.ptjournal.org/. Accessed August 20, 2008.

8. Koegel T. *The Exceptional Presenter: A Proven Formula to Open Up and Own the Room.* Austin, TX: Greenleaf Book Group; 2007.

9. Emery MJ. Effectiveness of the clinical instructor: Students' perspective. *Phys Ther.* 1984;64(7):1079-1083.

10. American Physical Therapy Association. Clinical Instructor Credentialing Course: http://www.apta.org/AM/Template.cfm?Section=Clinical&TEMPLATE=/CM/ContentDisplay.cfm&CONTENTID=30905. Accessed October 22, 2008.

11. Kelly SP. The exemplary clinical instructor: A qualitative case study. *J Phys Ther Educ.* 2007;21(1):63-69.

12. Harden RM, Crosby M. AMEE Guide No. 20: The good teacher is more than a lecturer: The twelve roles of the teacher. *Med Teacher.* 2000;22(4):334-347.

13. American Physical Therapy Association Media Room. American Board of Physical Therapy Specialties recognizes board certified specialists: http://www.apta.org/AM/Template.cfm?Section=Media&CONTENTID=51618&TEMPLATE=/CM/ContentDisplay.cfm. Accessed September 11, 2008.

14. Telephone conversation with Kristine Stoneley, Assistant Director, APTA Department of Academic/Clinical Education. September 4, 2008.

15. Schmidt RA. Motor learning principles for physical therapy. In *Contemporary Management of Motor Control Problems: Proceedings of the II-STEP Conference.* Alexandria, VA: Foundation for Physical Therapy; 1991.

16. Carnegie Mellon. July 25: In Memoriam: Randy Pausch, innovative computer scientist at Carnegie Mellon, launched education initiatives, gained worldwide acclaim for last lecture: http://www.cmu.edu/news/archive/2008/July/july25_pausch.shtml. Accessed September 11, 2008.

17. American Medical Student Association. The Profession: http://209.85.173.104/search?q=cache:994UqLNoqYJ:www.amsa.org/meded/PROFESSion.doc+professor+speak+forth&hl=en&ct=clnk&cd=1&gl=us. Accessed September 13, 2008.

18. American Medical Association. *Declaration of Professional Responsibility.* December 4, 2001: http://www.ama-assn.org/ama/pub/category/7491.html. Accessed September 13, 2008.

19. Singh M, Balasubramanian SK, Chakraborty G. A comparative analysis of three communication formats: advertising, infomercial, and direct experience. *J Advertising.* 2000;29(4):59-67.

20. Bell J. "The Last Lecture" and me: Randy Pausch's timeless words inspire virtuoso violinist Joshua Bell to change his life. September 14, 2008. USA Weekend.Com: http://www.usaweekend.com/08_issues/080914/080914joshua-bell.html. Accessed September 21, 2008.

21. U.S. Department of Health and Human Services: Surgeon General's Office: Overweight Children and Adolescents: http://www.surgeongeneral.gov/topics/obesity/calltoaction/fact_adolescents.htm. Accessed September 21, 2008.

22. Bloom BS. *Taxonomy of Educational Objectives.* Boston, MA: Allyn and Bacon; 1984.

23. Major categories in the taxonomy of behavioral objectives: http://krummefamily.org/guides/bloom.html. Accessed September 25, 2008.

24. Pike RW. *Creative Training Techniques Handbook, Tips, Tactics, and How-To's for Delivering Effective Training,* 3rd ed. Amherst, MA: HRD Press; 2003.

25. Silberman M. *Active Training: A Handbook of Techniques, Designs, Case Examples and Tips.* San Francisco: Jossey-Bass; 1990.

26. Cunningham V, Lefkoe M, Sechrest L. Eliminating fears: An intervention that permanently eliminates the fear of public speaking. *Clin Psychol Psychother.* 2006;13:183-193.

27. Paul G, Elam B, Verhulst SJ. A longitudinal study of students' perceptions using deep breathing meditation to reduce testing stresses. *Teach Learn Med.* 2007;19(3):287-292.

28. The Lefkoe Institute: http://www.lefkoeinstitute/com

29. World Confederation of Physical Therapy. http://www.wcpt.org/congress/index.php. Accessed October 8, 2008.

30. PEDro Physiotherapy Evidence Data Base: http://www.pedro.fhs.usyd.edu.au/supporters.html. Accessed October 2, 2008.

31. American Physical Therapy Association. Hooked on evidence: http://www.hookedonevidence.org/search.cfm?CFID=36985782&CFTOKEN=6569204. Accessed October 2, 2008.

32. Microsoft Corporation. One Microsoft Way, Redmond, WA 98052.

33. Cyrus J. *Presentation Principles.* Author Stream: http://www.authorstream.com/Presentation/jcyrus-87907-presentation-principles-slide-presentations-education-ppt-powerpoint/. Accessed October 17, 2008.

34. Baruch College, City University of New York, Digital Media Library. Gareis E, Belland J, Varveris S, Parascandola M. *Effective Use of Powerpoint: Online Media Tutorial.* 2006: http://www.baruch.cuny.edu/dml/engine.php?action=viewAsset&mediaIndex=432. Accessed October 17, 2008.

35. Pandachuck KH, Harley D, Cook D. Effectiveness of a brief workshop designed to improve teaching performance at the University of Alabama. *Acad Med.* 2004;79(8):798-804.

36. Dennick R. Long term retention of teaching skills after attending the teaching improvement project: A longitudinal, self-evaluation study. *Med Teach.* 2003;25(3):314-318.

37. University of Texas Medical Branch. UTMB Teaching improvement project system: http://sahs.utmb.edu/cls/tips/. Accessed November 1, 2008.

38. American Physical Therapy Association. Advanced Clinical Instructor Education Program: http://www.apta.org/AM/Template.cfm?Section=Advanced_CIECP1&TEMPLATE=/CM/ContentDisplay.cfm&CONTENTID=47838. Accessed October 22, 2008.

39. American Physical Therapy Association. Process for becoming a credentialed clinical trainer: http://www.apta.org/AM/Template.cfm?Section=Professionalism1&TEMPLATE=/CM/ContentDisplay.cfm&CONTENTID=41469. Accessed October 22, 2008.

40. Foundation for Inner Peace. *A Course in Miracles: Workbook for Students.* Tiburon, CA: Foundation for Inner Peace; 1975.

41. Banschbach SK. The rewards of being both a mentor and a protégé. *AORN J.* 2008;2(88):175-176.

42. Menaker R, Bahn RS. How perceived physician leadership behavior affects physician satisfaction. *Mayo Clin Proc.* 2008;83(9):983-988.

43. Christmas C, Kravet SJ, Durso SC, Wright SM. Clinical excellence in academia: Perspectives from masterful academic clinicians. *Mayo Clin Proc.* 2008;83(9):989-994.

44. Shepard K, Hack LM, Gwyer J, Jensen G. Describing expert practice in physical therapy. *Qual Health Res.* 1999;6(9):746-758.

45. American Physical Therapy Association website home page: http://www.apta.org//AM/Template.cfm?Section=Home. Accessed October 26, 2008.

46. American Physical Therapy Association. Membership and Leadership: http://www.apta.org/AM/Template.cfm?Section=Mentoring_2&TEMPLATE=/CM/CoentDisplay.cfm&CONTENTID=42422.

47. American Physical Therapy Association. Membership and leadership. Mentoring members: http://www.apta.org/AM/Template.cfm?Section=Mentoring_2&Template=/TaggedPage/TaggedPageDisplay.cfm&TPLID=52&ContentID=19791. Accessed October 26, 2008.

48. American Physical Therapy Association SMART: student mentoring: Achieving and reaching together: http://www.apta.org/AM/Template.cfm?Section=Home&TEMPLATE=/CM/ContentDisplay.cfm&CONTENTID=48327. Accessed October 27, 2008.

49. Ries R. Peering into the future: Student-to-student mentoring programs are helping to prepare the PTs and PTAs of tomorrow for the challenges ahead. *PT Magazine.* June 2008:34-42.

50. Prochaska JO. *Systems of Psychotherapy: A Transtheoretical Analysis.* Homewood, IL: Dorsey Press; 1979.

51. Wilbur J, Vassalo A, Chandler P, et al. Midlife women's adherence to home based walking during maintenance. *Nurs Res.* 2005;54(1):33-40.

52. Rollnick S, Mason P, Butler C. *Health Behavior Change: A Guide for Practitioners.* London: Churchill Livingstone; 2002.

53. DiClemente CC. Motivational interviewing and the stages of change. In Miller WR, Rollnick S, eds. *Motivational Interviewing.* New York: Guilford Press; 1991.

54. Cancer Prevention Research Center. Detailed overview of the transtheoretical model: http://www.uri.edu/research/cprc/TTM/detailedoverview.htm. Accessed October 31, 2008.

55. Science News. For weight control you will need to walk more than 10,000 steps a day. *ScienceDaily.* Jan. 13, 2008.: http://www.sciencedaily.com/releases/2008/01/080111231316.htm. Accessed October 31, 2008.

56. America's Walking. The 20% Boost Program: Fit walking into your life. The realistic way to build up to 10,000 steps a day: http://www.pbs.org/americaswalking/health/health20percentboost.html. Accessed October 31, 2008.

57. Prochaska JO, DiClemente CC, Norcross JC. In search of how people change: Applications to addictive behavior. *Am Psychol.* 1992;47:1102-1114.

Index

Page numbers followed by "b" indicate a box reference, page numbers followed by "f" indicate a figure reference, and page numbers followed by "t" indicate a table reference.